CANCER ETIOLOGY, DIAGNOSIS AND TREATMENTS

FRONTIERS IN LEUKEMIA PHARMACOTHERAPY

CANCER ETIOLOGY, DIAGNOSIS AND TREATMENTS

Additional books and e-books in this series can be found on Nova's website under the Series tab.

CANCER ETIOLOGY, DIAGNOSIS AND TREATMENTS

FRONTIERS IN LEUKEMIA PHARMACOTHERAPY

LUNAWATI L. BENNETT
PHD, PHARMD
EDITOR

Nova Medicine & Health
New York

Library of Congress Cataloging-in-Publication Data

ISBN: 978-1-53614-960-9
Library of Congress Control Number: 2019931635

Published by Nova Science Publishers, Inc. † New York

CONTENTS

PREFACE

"*Frontiers in Leukemia Pharmacotherapy*" was designed as an educational resource for all oncology professionals involved in the care of leukemia. Chapter 1 is an introduction about leukemia. Leukemia is cancer of blood and bone marrow which is categorized into acute and chronic leukemia. Acute leukemias are: acute lymphoblastic leukemia (ALL), which is the most common childhood malignancy due to mutational events occurring in the precursor lymphoblasts preventing maturation and normal hematopoiesis, and acute myeloid leukemia (AML), which is the second most common leukemia in adults due to formation of immature blast cells of myeloid lineage. Chronic leukemia are: chronic myeloid leukemia (CML), which is more common in adult due to constitutively active tyrosine kinase, and chronic lymphoblastic leukemia (CLL), which is also more common in adult characterized by anemia and thrombocytopenia. Chapters 2 and 3 explain the mechanisms and genetic abnormalities that occur in acute and chronic leukemia. The most common aberrant signaling pathways are BCRL/ABL, P13k/Akt/JAK, NOTCH, and FLT3. Chapter 4 describes the mechanism of action and adverse events for common anti-leukemia drugs. Chapter 5 outlines the role of tyrosine kinases inhibitors in leukemia.

Chapters 6 to 13 discuss the epidemiology, etiology, pathogenesis, disease classification, clinical presentation, pathologic features, diagnosis, prognosis, and treatment guidelines for myelodysplastic syndrome (MDS), AML, ALL, acute promyelocytic leukemia (APL), CML, CLL, pediatric ALL, and pediatric AML, respectively. MDS is a heterogeneous disease with varying rates of disease progression that affect mostly older patients, therefore the goal of therapy for this subset of leukemia is for symptom management and improved quality of life rather than curing the patient. APL is clinically and biologically distinct subtype of AML associated with unique challenges requiring specialized management.

Chapter 14 highlights the general metastasis pattern in leukemia, followed by chapter 15 discussion on redox homeostasis occurring in leukemia and the role of antioxidants.

Not all antioxidants are useful for the treatment of leukemia; in fact, some may cause detrimental effects. Chapter 16 outlines supportive care for patients on chemotherapy experiencing fatigue, pain, or other complications such as tumor lysis syndrome, while chapter 17 discusses end of life care for those with leukemia. Chapter 18 covers pharmacometrics using computational modeling to support drug development and optimize drug therapy in leukemic patients. Finally, chapter 19 highlights novel antileukemia agents undergoing development for the treatment of leukemia.

This is a comprehensive book written by doctor of philosophy (PhDs) faculty that are doing research in the field of cancer, doctor of pharmacy (PharmDs) clinicians with advanced specialty certification (i.e., Board Certified Oncology Pharmacist), and by PhD or PharmD working as pharmacometric experts. Reputable books, journals, monograms, clinical trial results are used as the sources for this book. This expert knowledge make this book to be a valuable resource for healthcare providers such as pharmacists, physicians, oncology nurses, physician assistants, oncology scientists/fellows, and patients who are interested in learning about leukemia treatment.

Happy reading,

Lunawati L. Bennett MS, PhD, PharmD, FACN
Editor

IMPORTANT NOTICE FOR THE READER

Notice of Disclaimer

Medicine is powerful, and it is an ever-changing science. With new research and clinical experience, our knowledge of drug therapy are broaden. The author, contributor, and the publisher of this book have checked with scientific sources that believed to be reliable in their efforts to provide accurate and complete information. However, in view of the possibility of human error and changes in medical science, the author and the publisher of this book disclaim all responsibility for any errors or omissions results obtained from the information in this book.

No Advice

This Book contains general information for educational purposes only about medical conditions and possible medication and/or treatments. The information does not constitute medical advice or an invitation to use the treatments discussed, and should not be treated as such if the reader has any medical problems. Self-medication is neither advisable nor recommended. Readers are encourage to confirm the information with other sources such as package insert of the drugs, literature, or information from the pharmacy. Moreover, the reader must always consult medical or healthcare professionals or practitioners to address any medical condition.

In: Frontiers in Leukemia Pharmacotherapy
Editor: Lunawati L. Bennett
ISBN: 978-1-53614-960-9

Chapter 1

Overview of Acute and Chronic Leukemia

Lunawati L. Bennett**, PhD, PharmD
Union University, College of Pharmacy, Jackson, Tennessee, US

Abstract

Leukemia is cancer of blood and bone marrow which is categorized into acute and chronic leukemia. Acute leukemia further divided into acute lymphoblastic leukemia (ALL) which is the most common childhood malignancy due to mutational events occurring in the precursor lymphoblasts preventing maturation and normal hematopoiesis, and acute myeloid leukemia (AML) which is the second most common leukemia in adults due to the formation of immature blast cells of myeloid lineage. Chronic leukemia is divided into chronic myeloid leukemia (CML) which is more common in adult due to the constitutively active tyrosine kinase, and chronic lymphocytic leukemia (CLL) which is more common in adult characterized by anemia and thrombocytopenia.

This chapter highlights leukemia classification based on the French-American-British (FAB) system and World Health organization (WHO) classification, RAI and Benet staging systems.

Keywords: acute lymphoblastic leukemia, acute myeloid leukemia, chronic lymphocytic leukemia, chronic myeloid leukemia, FAB, RAI, Benet

* Corresponding Author Email: llbennett@uu.edu.

Abbreviations

ALL	acute lymphoblastic/lymphocytic leukemia
AML	acute myeloid leukemia
CLL	chronic lymphocytic leukemia
CML	chronic myeloid leukemia
APL	acute promyelocytic leukemia
MDS	myelodysplastic syndrome
SEER	Surveillance, Epidemiology and End Results
CNS	central nervous system
WHO	World Health Organization
BCR ABL	breakpoint cluster region- Abelson murine leukemia
NCCN	National Comprehensive Cancer Network

Introduction

Generally defines as cancer of the blood and bone marrow cells, leukemia is categorized based on the primary type of the cells being affected. Leukemia is characterized by unregulated blood-forming cells causing formation of immature cells or blasts which "crowd out" or inhibit normal cellular maturation in bone marrow, resulting in anemia, neutropenia, and thrombocytopenia. Leukemic blasts may also infiltrate a variety of tissues such as the central nervous system (CNS), lymph nodes, skin, liver, spleen, kidney, and testes [1].

Leukemia is classified based on the cell of origin and cell maturation. Myeloid leukemia develops from the common myeloid progenitor lineage which affects granulocytes, platelets and red blood cells. Lymphocytic leukemia occurs from progenitor lineage of lymphocytes affecting B cell, T cells, and NK (natural killer) cells [2]. Leukemia is further divided into acute lymphoblastic/lymphocytic leukemia (ALL), acute myeloid leukemia (AML), chronic lymphocytic leukemia (CLL), and chronic myeloid leukemia (CML). There are other leukemia types such as hairy cell leukemia, acute promyelocytic leukemia (APL), myelodysplastic syndrome (MDS), and others. MDS is malignant, heterogeneous leukemia that historically referred to as an oligoblastic leukemia which overtime can be transform into AML [3].

Acute leukemia is characterized by the overgrowth and rapid accumulation of immature malignant blood cells which can be fatal within weeks to months if untreated early and correctly. Chronic leukemia is characterized by slower growth of mature cells and may take months to years to progress [2]. However, CML can progress faster to cause cancer that resembled AML [2].

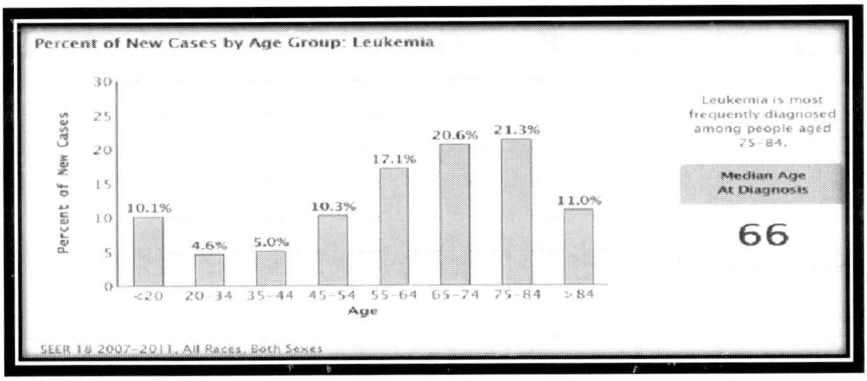

Figure 1. Percent of new cases of leukemia by age group [5].

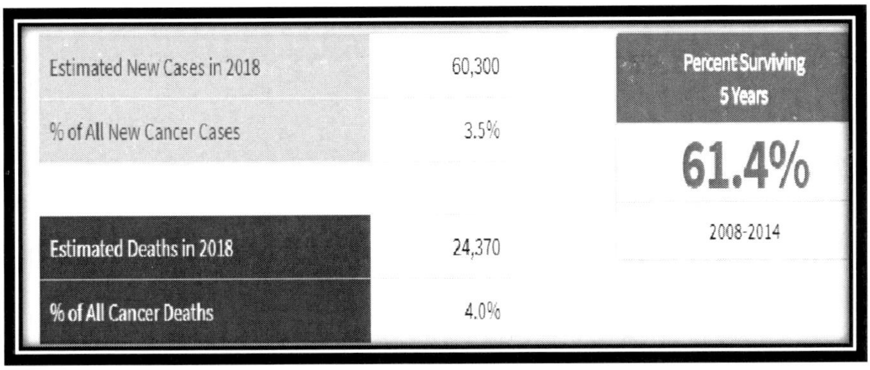

Figure 2. Estimated new cases and death due to leukemia [5].

It is estimated that in 2018, there are 5960 new cases of ALL, 19,520 of AML, 20,940 of CLL; and 8430 of CML, respectively in the United States [4]. An estimated death of 24,500 is expected of all leukemia, with 12,000 deaths are from acute leukemia (ALL and AML) and 4.5% death from CLL [5]. New cases of leukemia per year were estimated at 13.8 per 100,000 males and females. There are more than 455,000 people living in the US having leukemia [5]. Figure 1 and Figure 2 depicted percent of new cases by age group and 5 years percent of surviving. Hematologic malignancies account about 9% of all cancers and the fourth most frequently diagnosed cancer in men and women in the economically developed regions of the world [6].

ACUTE LEUKEMIA

Acute leukemia is more common in people younger than 20 years of age, with about 80% are ALL and 15-20% is AML. Three out of 4 pediatric patients with leukemia is usually diagnosed with ALL. Childhood ALL is about 30% more common in males than in females, peaks at 2 to 4 years of age and affects white more than African American children [6]. In developed countries, the incidence of ALL is the highest in children 2 to 5 years old. ALL can also occur in adult. Adult survival rate is about 40%, while pediatric survival is near 90% [5].

The incidence of AML is relatively low until the age of 35 and then rises almost exponentially [4]. The median age at diagnosis is estimated at 68 years and median age at death is 72. AML is projected to be the most deadly leukemia with estimated death of 10,670 in 2018. ALL and AML account for approximately one-third of all pediatric cancer. In the past several decades, progress has been made for the ALL treatment that the patients' 5-year survival rates have increased for up to 90% in children [7]. However, there are also up to 10-20% children with ALL have refractory to treatment or relapsed after treatment [8].

A multi factorial process involves in etiology of acute leukemia such as genetics, environments, social habits, exposure to toxins and viral and immunologic status. Genetic conditions such as having megakaryocytic thrombocytopenia, ataxia telangiectasia, Bloom syndrome, Diamon-Blackfan anemia, Down syndrome, Noonan syndrome, Shwachman syndrome, severe combined immunodeficiency syndrome, Wiskott-Aldrich syndrome have been identified to increase risk of developing acute leukemia. Children with Down syndrome have a tenfold to twentyfold increased risk of acute leukemia [9]. Maternal use of alcohol or drugs such as diet pills, amphetamine, and uterus exposure to antineoplastic such as alkylating agents, anthracyclines and epipodophyllotoxins, may associate with childhood AML [9].

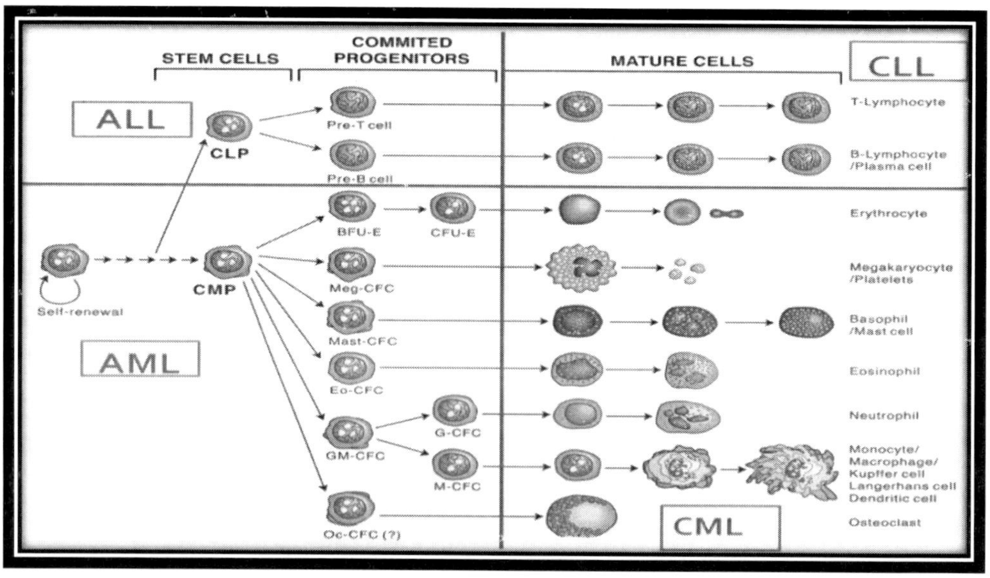

Abbreviation: ALL-acute lymphoblastic/lymphocytic leukemia; AML-acute myeloid leukemia; CLL-chronic lymphocytic leukemia; CML-chronic myeloid leukemia; CMP-chronic CLP BFU CFU CFC.

Figure 3. Classification of acute and chronic leukemia [10].

Prior to the 2008, the French American British (FAB) system was utilized frequently, but it has been replaced by the World Health organization (WHO) scheme. The WHO classification system incorporated factors such as chromosomal abnormalities, immunophenotyping, molecular and morphological features. Figure 3. shows classification of ALL, AML, CLL and CML [10]. Table 1 and 2 show FAB classification of ALL and AML, respectively [11]. Table 3 and 4 depicts WHO system of ALL and AML [11].

Table 1. FAB classification of ALL [2, 11]

FAB	Leukemia Cell	Description
L1	Pre-B or T cell	Small and homogenous, almost no cytoplasm, round to cleaved nucleoli, perinuclear chromatin Common in children. The most common type
L2	Pre-B or T cell	Large and heterogeneous, about 20% cytoplasm, nucleoli are more prominent More common in adults
L3	B cell	Large, mature cells (Burkitt's leukemia), basophilic, cytoplasm, cytoplasmic with vacuoles Uncommon and worst prognosis

Table 2. FAB classification of AML [2, 11]

Subtype	Bone marrow morphology	Immunophenotype
MO	Blasts > 30%	CD 13,33, 34, HLA-DR
M1	Blasts > 90%	CD 13, 4, 15, 33, 34, HLA-DR
M2	Blasts > 30%	CD 13, 14,33, 34 HLA-DR
M3	Blasts > 30%	CD 13, 15, 33
M4	Blasts > 30%, monocytes cells >20%,<80%	CD 13, 14, 15, 33, 34, HLA-DR
M4eo	M4 criteria, abnormal basophilic, eosinophil	CD 13, 14, 15, 33, 34, HLA-DR
M5A	Large blasts with >80% cells of monocytes lineage	CD 13, 14, 33, 34, HLA-DR
M5B	<80% of monocytes are blasts	CD 13,14,33 HLA-DR
M6	>30% blasts with > 50% erythroid cells	CD 13,33,41,71 HLA-DR, glycophorin A
M7	>30% blasts of megacyotic origin	CD 41, 61

Abbreviation: MO-undifferentiated AML; M1-AML with minimal maturation; M2-AML with significant maturation; M3-Acute Promyelocytic leukemia (APL); M4-Acute myelomonocytic leukemia; M4eo-Acute Myelomonocytic Leukemia with eosinophil; M5A- Acute monocytes Leukemia poorly differentiated; M5B-Acute monocytes leukemia well-differentiated; M6-Acute erythroleukemia; M7-Acute megakaryoblastic leukemia, CD= cluster of differentiation, HLA-DR= human leukocyte antigen.

Table 3. WHO classification of ALL [11]

Acute leukemia of ambiguous lineage	Acute undifferentiated leukemia
	Mixed phenotype acute leukemia (MPAL)
B cell lymphoblastic leukemia/lymphoma (B-ALL)	B-lymphoblastic leukemia/lymphoma
	B-lymphoblastic leukemia/lymphoma with t(9;22)
	B-lymphoblastic leukemia/lymphoma with TEL-AML1
	B-lymphoblastic leukemia/lymphoma with hyperdiploidy
	B-lymphoblastic leukemia/lymphoma with hypodiploidy
	B-lymphoblastic leukemia/lymphoma with t(5;14)
	B-lymphoblastic leukemia/lymphoma with t(1;19)
	B-lymphoblastic leukemia/lymphoma with recurrent genetic abnormalities
T cell lymphoblastic leukemia/lymphoma (T-ALL)	T cell lymphoblastic leukemia/lymphoma

Many of the signs and symptoms of acute leukemia are the result of low blood cells. Severe thrombocytopenia (<20,000 cells/mm^3) can cause bruising, petechia, and bleeding. Low red blood cells (RBC) (<7 g/dL) can result in fatigue, anemia, malaise and palpitation, while low white blood cells (WBC) can cause infection such as fever, chills, and rigor. Other clinical presentation includes seizures, headache, dyspnea on excretion, splenomegaly, hepatomegaly and lymphadenopathy, painless testicular due to enlargement and gum hypertrophy [12-14].

Besides complete blood count, uric acid, potassium, phosphate or calcium blood levels are also need to be tested. In addition, elevated prothrombin time, partial thromboplastin time, hypofibrinogemia are usually observed. Other laboratory testing includes bone marrow biopsy, chest radiograph, and lumbar puncture to determine if there any blasts in the central nervous system (CNS) are usually performed. Molecular testing for commonly mutated genes in leukemia such as FMS like tyrosine kinase 3 (FLT 3), nucleophosmin (NPM1), CCAAT enhancer binding protein alpha (CEBPA), BCR-ABL1 (breakpoint cluster region-Abelson proto oncogene), and others are performed to rule if patients have leukemia or other diseases [15-17].

Treatment for ALL is usually complex involving three distinct phases known as induction, consolidation and maintenance. Multi agent chemotherapy is usually used with vincristine, aminopterin, 6-mercaptopurine, and prednisone (VAMP). Other regimen is Hyper-CVAD consists of cyclophosphamide, doxorubicin, vincristine, dexamethasone, methotrexate and cytarabine. Tyrosine kinase inhibitors (TKIs) such as imatinib, dasatinib, or nilotinib have been used as well [18-22]. However, after achieving complete remission (CR), over 80% of adult with ALL ultimately relapsed. Several novel therapies have been indicated for relapse/refractory ALL such as blinatumomab, inotuzumab ozogomicin, nelarabine, and chimeric antigen receptor T cell therapy [23-26].

Philadelphia chromosome positive (Ph^+) ALL which is biologically distinct subtype of ALL due to chromosome t (9; 22) translocation [27-29]. Ph^+ is found in granulocyte and erythrocyte progenitors, macrophages, megakaryocytes, and lymphocytes. It is the consequences of breaks in chromosome 9 and 22 resulting in relocation ABL (Abelson proto-oncogene) from its normal site unto chromosome 9 of BCR (breakpoint cluster region). This hybrid BCR-ABL fusion gene is known as t (9; 22) (q34:q11) [27-29]. The hybrid fusion gene has a 210-kDa protein that is constitutively activated, which is different than normal 145-KDa ABL gene.

Table 4. WHO classification of AML [11]

AML with recurrent genetic abnormalities	
	AML with t(8;21)(q22;q21);RUNX1-RUNX1T1
	AML with inv(16)(p13.1q22) or t(16;16)(p13.1;q22);CBFB-MYH11
	APL with PML-RARA
	AML with t(9;11)(p21.3;q23.3);MLLT3-KMT2A
	AML with t(6;9)(p23;q34.1);DEK-NUP214
	AML with inv(3)(q21.3q26.2) or t(3;3)(q21.3;q26.2); GATA2, MECOM
	AML (megakaryoblastic) with t(1;22)(p13.3;q13.3);RBM15-MKL1
	AML with BCR-ABL1 (provisional entity)
	AML with mutated NPM1
	AML with bi-allelic mutations of CEBPA
	AML with mutated RUNX1 (provisional entity)
AML with myelodysplasia-related changes	
Therapy-related myeloid neoplasms	
AML, not otherwise specified	
	AML with minimal differentiation
	AML without maturation
	AML with maturation
	Acute myelomonocytic leukemia
	Acute monoblastic /monocytes leukemia
	Pure erythroid leukemia
	Acute megakaryoblastic leukemia
	Acute basophilic leukemia
	Acute panmyelosis with myelofibrosis
Myeloid sarcoma	
Myeloid proliferations related to Down syndrome	
	Transient abnormal myelopoiesis
	Myeloid leukemia associated with Down syndrome

Treatment of AML includes induction and consolidation phases. Common drug regimens used during induction in adults are: combination of cytarabine and idarubicin, cytarabine and daunorubicin, or high dose cytarabine (HiDAC) and daunorubicin [30-31]. Nearly 50% of older adults with AML never achieve CR following therapy due to refractory. Because of the poor prognosis in refractory AML, several intensive drug regimens exist including HiDAC, FLAGS (fludarabine, cytarabine, filgrastim), MEC (mitoxantrone, etoposide, cytarabine), and gemtuzumab ozogamicin [32-35].

Despite intensive treatment, 30% pediatric with AML relapsed and 5% to 10% patients die following treatment protocols. Undesirable adverse events such as cardiomyopathy due to anthracyclines illustrates that further intensification of chemotherapy seems no longer feasible [13]. Therefore, knowledge on the molecular and genetic background of acute leukemia is needed to detect novel patients-specific treatment targets with less severe adverse events.

CHRONIC LEUKEMIA

CML accounts for 15% cases of leukemia in the United States. CML has world-wide annual incidence of 1 in every 100,000 people [36]. The incidence of CML has not changed during the past few decades. The median age at diagnosis is 55 to 65 years. This disease is uncommon in children and adolescent, with only 2.7% of CML affect younger than 20 years [37]. CML is a disease due to malignant transformation of subpopulation of pluripotent hematopoietic stem cells leading to bone marrow hyperplasia, rapid accumulation of blast cells in the bone marrow, suppression of normal hematopoiesis, and Ph^+ chromosomal abnormality.

CML is a tri-phasic disease. It usually presents as chronic phase, accelerated phase, and blast crisis. Untreated CP phase can transform into acute phase resembling ALL or AML [37]. Table 5 depicts criteria for different phases of CML. First line treatment of CML is TKIs. Most patients respond favorably to TKIs. TKIs dramatically altered the landscape treatment of CML [38-41].

CLL is the most prevalent adult leukemia reported in 30% adult worldwide. This malignancy is detected in older patients (over 50 years) due to lymphocytosis for more than 3 months with clinical features of lymphadenopathy, organomegaly, fever and fatigue. About 25% of the patients are asymptomatic [42]. The most common chromosomal abnormalities are partial loss of one chromosome such as deletions on 6q, 11q, 17p and 13q, mutations in TP53, or gains of whole chromosomal such as trisomy 12 [43].

In order to anticipate survival rate of CLL patients, clinical staging system designed by Rai et al. and Binet et al. are usually used [44-46]. Rai staging system is used more often in the United States, while Binet system in Europe. The Rai system divides patient into 5 groups based on lymph, anemia, thrombocytopenia status and median survival of the patients. The Binet system classifies disease into 3 stages: low, intermediate and high risk. Staging systems are essential to understand disease, to predict the outcome and to decide the best therapeutic options for CLL patients [44-47].

Table 5. Criteria for different phases of CML [38-39]

Chronic Phase (CP)	Accelerated Phase (AP)	Blast Crisis (BC)
Clinical presentation: often asymptomatic, found incidentally during unrelated routine examination	*Clinical presentation*: increasing peripheral blood and bone marrow blasts and basophils, progressive splenomegaly	*Clinical presentation*: resembles acute leukemia that the leukemic clone dominates the bone marrow. Duration days to weeks before death
Sign and symptoms: fatigue, sweating, bone pain, weight loss, abdominal discomfort, spleen infection, gouty arthritis	*Sign and symptoms:* anemia, bone pain, fever, night sweat, weight loss	*Sign and symptoms*: fever, malaise
Laboratory findings: leukocytosis, less than 10% blasts in peripheral blood or bone marrow	*Laboratory findings*: 10-29% blasts in peripheral blood or bone marrow Platelet s less than 100,000 cells/mm3	*Laboratory findings:* more than 30% blasts in peripheral blood and bone marrow, large clusters of blast
Median survival without treatment: 47 months	12 – 24 months	3 – 6 months

Table 6. Rai classification system

Stage	Description	Median survival (months)	Risk status
0	Lymphocytosis, lymphocytes in blood >15,000/mcL and >40% lymphocytes in the bone marrow	150	Low
I	Stage 0 with enlarge node (s)	100	Intermediate
II	Stage 0-I with splenomegaly, hepatomegaly, or both	70	Intermediate
III	Stage 0 –II with hemoglobin < 11 g/dL or hematocrit < 33%	20	High
IV	Stage 0 –III with platelets < 100,000 mcL	20	High

From the 2008 National Cancer Institute (NCI) guidelines.

Table 7. The Binet classification system

Stage	Description *
A	Hemoglobin ≥ 10 g/dL and platelet ≥ 100,000/mm^3 and <3 involve nodal areas
B	Hemoglobin ≥ 10 g/dL and platelet ≥ 100,000/mm^3 and ≥ 3 involve nodal areas
C	Hemoglobin < 10 g/dL and platelet < 100,000/mm^3 and any number of involved nodal areas

*Areas of involvement considered lymphoid tissue groups (neck lymph nodes, groin lymph nodes, underarm lymph nodes, spleen, and liver) [46].

There was a study comparing both systems i.e., Rai and Binet in 133 CLL patients. The study concluded that both systems are comparable in terms of staging and predicting the outcomes. The Rai staging system appears to have an advantage over the Binet system by defining a subset of patients with excellent prognosis (stage 0) which is included within stage A of the Binet system [48].

Treatment for asymptomatic or early stage CLL usually observation rather than immediate treatment per NCNN guideline. If patients become symptomatic or if their absolute lymphocyte count doubled in the past 12 months, treatment therapy may be initiated [47]. The symptomatic treatment include combo of drugs such as FCR (Fludarabine, cyclophosphamide, rituximab), or combo of bendamustine and anti-CD20 monoclonal antibody obinutuzumab or ofatumumab, chlorambucil and rituximab or ofatumumab, and ibrutinib. Patients who experience relapsed or refractory to CLL treatment, defined as disease recurrence following a partial or CR that lasted at least six months, may include therapy like the initial therapy [48].

Conclusion

Leukemia is classified based on the cell of origin and cell maturation of blood and bone marrow. Acute leukemia is characterized by rapid accumulation of immature malignant blood cells and effect younger people, while chronic leukemia is more common in older people. AML is the most deadliest of the leukemia. Treatment options are differed between the four leukemia.

References

[1] Poon BB, Seung AH. Acute Leukemias. In: Dipiro JT, Talbert RL, Yee GE eds. *Pharmacotherapy: A Pathophysiologic Approach*, 9 ed. New York, NY: McGraw Hill; 2014; 2255-2276.

[2] Jabbour EJ, Faderl S, Kantarjian HM. Adult Acute Lymphobastic Leukemia. *Mayo Clin Proc*. 2005; 80(11):1517-1527.

[3] Vardiman JW, Harris NL, Brunning RD. The World Health Organization (WHO) classification of the myeloid neoplasms. *Blood* 2002;100:2292-2302.

[4] Siegel RL, Miller KD, Jemal A. *Cancer Statistics*, 2017. *CA Cancer J Clin* 2017;67:7-30.

[5] Noone AM, Howlader N, Krapcho M, Miller D, Brest A, Yu M, Ruhl J, Tatalovich Z, Mariotto A, Lewis DR, Chen HS, Feuer EJ, Cronin KA (eds). *SEER Cancer Statistics Review*, 1975-2015, National Cancer Institute. Bethesda, MD, 2018. https://seer.cancer.gov/statfacts/html/leukimias.html.

[6] Smith A, Howell D, Patmore R, et al. Incidence of hametological malignancy by sub-type: a report from the Hematological Malignancy Research Netwark. *Br. J Cancer* 2011; 105:1684-1692.

[7] Hunger S, Lu X, Devidas M et al. Improved survival for children and adolescents with acute lymphoblastic leukemia between 1990 and 2005: a report from the children's oncology group. *J Clin Oncol* 2012;30:1663-1669.

[8] Annesley CE, Brown P. Novel agents for the treatment of childhood acute leukemia. *Ther Adv Hematol* 2015;6(2) 61-79.

[9] Xavier AC, Taub JW. Acute leukemia in children with Down syndrome. *Haematologia* 2010; 95:1043-1050.

[10] Halford, Z. Lecture notes for oncology for Union University College of Pharmacy students. Unpublished work.

[11] Arber DA, Orazi A, Hasserjian R, et al. The 2016 revision to the World Health Organization classification of myeloid neoplasms and acute leukemia. *Blood* 2016;127(20):2391.

[12] Terwilliger T, Abdul-Hay M. Acute lymphoblastic leukemia: a comprehensive review and 2017 update. *Blood Cancer Journal* 2017; 7, e577; doi:10.1038/bcj.2017.53

[13] Kaspers GJ, Zimmermann M, Dworzk M et al. Improved outcome in pediatric relapsed acute myeloid leukemia: Results of a randomized trial on liposomal daunorubicin by the International BFM Study Group. *J Clin Oncol*. 2013; 31:599-607.

[14] De Rooij JDE, Zwaan CM, van den Heuvel-Eibrink M. Pediatric AML: from biology to clinical management. *J. Clin. Med* 2015; 4: 127-149.

[15] Moorman AV, Chilton L, Wilkinson J, et al. A population-based cytogenetic study of adults with acute lymphoblastic leukemia. *Blood* 2010;115:206-214.

[16] Roberts KG, GU Z, Payne-Turner D, et al. High frequency and poor outcome of Philadelphia chromosome-like acute lymphoblastic leukemia in adults. *J Clin Oncol* 2017;35:394-401.

[17] Mullighan CG, Su X, Zhang J, et al. Deletion of IKZF1 and prognosis in acute lymphoblastic leukemia. *N Eng J Med* 2009;360:470-480.

[18] Rowe JM, Buck G, Burnett AK, et al. Induction therapy for adults with acute lymphoblastic leukemia: results of more than 1500 patients from the international ALL trial: MRC UKALL XII/ECOG E2993. *Blood* 2005;106(12):3760-3767.

[19] Landau H, Lamanna N. Clinical manifestations and treatment of newly diagnosed acute lymphoblastic leukemia in adults. *Curr Hematol Malig Rep* 2006; 1: 171–79.

[20] Kantarjian HM, O'Brien S, Smith TL, et al. Results of treatment with hyper-CVAD, a dose-intensive regimen, in adult acute lymphocytic leukemia. *J Clin Oncol* 2000; 18:547-561.

[21] Evans WE, Hon YY, Bomgaars L, et al. Preponderance of thiopurine S-methyltransferase deficiency and heterozygosity among patients intolerant to mercaptopurine or azathipprine. *J Clin Oncol* 2001;19(8):2293-2301.

[22] Andersen JB, Szumlanski C, Weinshilboum RM, et al. Pharmacokinetics, dose adjustments, and 6-mercaptopurine/methotrexate drug interactions in two patients with thiopurine methyltransferase deficiency. *Acta Paediatr* 1998;87(1):108-111.

[23] Pulte ED, Vallejo J, Przepiorka D et al. FDA supplemental approval: blinatumomab for treatment of relapsed and refractory precursor b cell acute lymphoblastic leukemia. *Oncologist* 2018.doi: 10.1634/theoncologist.2018-0179.

[24] Al-Salama ZT. Inotuzumab ozogamicin: a review in relapsed/refractory B cell acute lymphoblastic leukemia. *Target oncol* 2018. doi: 10.1007/s11523-018-0584-z.

[25] Abaza Y, Kantarjian MH, faderl S et al. Hyper-CVAD plus nelarabine in newly diagnosed adult T cell acute lymphoblastic leukemia and T-lymphoblastic lymphoma. *Am J Hematol* 2018. 93(1):91-99. doi: 10.1002/ajh.24947.

[26] Maude SL, Frey N, Shaw PA et al. Chimeric antigen receptor T cells for sustained remissions in leukemia. *N Engl J med* 2014; 16;371(16):1507-17. doi: 10.1056/NEJMoa1407222.

[27] Fausel CA, Kiel PJ. Chronic Leukemias. In: DiPiro JT, Talbert RL, Yee GE, eds. *Pharmacotherapy: A Pathophysiologic Approach*, 9th ed. New York, NY: McGraw Hill; 2014: 2277-93.

[28] Chu E, Sartorelli AC. Cancer chemotherapy. In: Katzung BG, Trevor, AJ, Eds. *Basic & Clinical Pharmacology*. 13th ed. New York, NY: McGraw Hill 2015; pp. 918-40.

[29] Arora A, Scholar EM. Role of tyrosine kinase inhibitors in cancer therapy. *J Pharmacol Exp Ther* 2005; 315(3): 971-79.

[30] Löwenberg B, Pabst T, Vellenga E, et al. Cytarabine dose for acute myeloid leukemia. *N Engl J Med* 2011;364(11):1027.

[31] Li W, Gon x, Sun M, et al. High-dose cytarabine in acute myeloid leukemia treatment: a systemic review and meta-analysis. *PLoS One* 2014;9:e110153.

[32] Teuffel O, Leibundgut K, Lehrnbecher T, et al. Anthracyclines during induction therapy in acute myeloid leukemia: a systematic review and meta-analysis. *Br J Haematol* 2013;161:192-203.

[33] Ohtake S, Miyawaki S, Fujita H, et al. Randomized study of induction therapy comparing standard-dose idarubicin with high-dose daunorubicin in adult patients with previously untreated acute myeloid leukemia: the JALSG AML201 Study. *Blood* 2011;117(8):2358.

[34] Fernandez HF, Sun Z, Yao X, et al. Anthracycline dose intensification in acute myeloid leukemia. *N Engl J Med* 2009;361(13):1249.

[35] Burnett AK, Russell NH, Hills RK, et al. A randomized comparison of daunorubicin 90 mg/m2 vs 60 mg/m2 in AML induction: results from the UK NCRI AML17 trial in 1206 patients. *Blood* 2015;125(25):3878-3885.

[36] Alikian M, Gale RP, Apperley JF, et al. Molecular techniques for the personalized management of patients with chronic myeloid leukemia. *Biomol Detect Quantif* 2017;11:4-20. Doi: 10.1016/j.bdq.2017.01.001.

[37] Kantarjian H, Cortes J. Chronic myeloid leukemia. In *Abeloff's Clinical Oncology*, edited by John E. Niederhuber, James O Armitage, James H Doroshow, Michael B Kastan and Joel E Tepper, 1944-1957. Fifth edition. Philadelphia: Elsevier Saunders 2014.

[38] Cortes JE, Talpaz M, O'Brien S et al. Staging of chronic myeloid leukemia in the imatinib era. *Cancer* 2006; 106:1306-1315.

[39] Sokal JE, Cox EB, Baccarani M, et al. Prognostic discrimination in "good-risk' chronic granulocytic leukemia. *Blood* 1984; 63:789-799.

[40] *The NCCN Clinical Practice Guidelines in Oncology™ Chronic Myeloid Leukemia* (Version 4.2018). National Comprehensive Cancer Network, Inc. Available at: www.NCCN.org. Accessed June 10, 2018.

[41] Huang X, Cortes J, Kantarjian H. Estimations of the increasing prevalence and plateau prevalence of chronic myeloid leukemia in the era of tyrosine kinase inhibitor therapy. *Cancer*. 2012;118(12): 3123–3127.

[42] Dohner H, Stilgenbauer S, Benner A et al. Genomic aberrations and survival in chronic lymphoblastic leukemia. *N Engl J med* 2003; 343(26): 1910-1916.

[43] Baliakas P, Iskas M, Gardiner A et al. Chromosomal translocations and karyotype complexity in chronic leukemia: a systemic reappraisal of classic cytogenetic data. *Am J Hematol* 2014;89(3):249-255.

[44] Rahimi H, Sadeghian MH, Keramati MR et al. Cytogenetic abnormalities with interphase FISH method and clinical manifestation in chronic lymphocytic leukemia patients in north-east of Iran. *Int J Hematol Oncol Stem Cell Res* 2017;11(3):217-224.

[45] Rai KR, Sawitsky A, Cronkite EP et al. Clinical staging of chronic lymphocytic leukemia. *Blood* 1975; 46(2):219-234.

[46] Binet J, Leporrier M, Dighiero G et al. A clinical staging system for chronic lymphocytic leukemia.Prognostic significance. *Cancer* 1977;40(2):855-864.

[47] Fischer K, Cramer P, Busch R, eya la. Long-term remission after FCR chemoimmunotherapy in previously untreated patients with CLL: updated results of the CLL8 trial. *Blood* 2016;127(2):208-215.

[48] Zengin N, Kars A, Kansu E, et al. Comparison of Rai and Binet classification in chronic lymphocytic leukemia. *Hematology* 1997; 2:125-129. Doi: 10.1080/10245332.1997.11746327.

In: Frontiers in Leukemia Pharmacotherapy
Editor: Lunawati L. Bennett
ISBN: 978-1-53614-960-9

Chapter 2

MOLECULAR AND GENETIC BASES OF ACUTE LEUKEMIA

Lunawati L. Bennett*[1], PhD, PharmD and Qingyu S. Zhou, PhD[2]
[1]Union University, College of Pharmacy, Jackson, Tennessee, US
[2]University of South Florida, College of Pharmacy, Tampa, Florida, US

ABSTRACT

The pathogenesis of acute leukemia has now been identified better with the technology that can identify chromosomal abnormalities such as translocation of gene, point mutations, gene duplication in acute lymphocytic leukemia (ALL) and acute myeloid leukemia (AML). Alterations in the pathways of receptor tyrosine kinases (RTKs), FLT3, c-KIT, P13k/AKT/mTOR, RAS/RAF/MEK/ERK have been identified in AML, while mutations in NOTCH pathway and precursor of B-cell or T-cell receptor are known to relate to ALL pathogenesis.

This chapter highlights the review of common abnormal chromosomes and their cell signaling pathways, molecular and genetic aberrant of AML type I and type II, genes and cell signaling abnormalities in ALL, and diagnostic approach to unravel the biology of leukemia using methods such as reverse transcriptase polymerase chain reaction (RT-PCR), and next generation sequencing (NGS).

Keywords: Philadelphia chromosome, acute leukemia mutation, tyrosine kinase receptor, ALL, AML, lymphoid B cells, lymphoid T cells, NGS, RAS, JAK/STAT, FLT3, BCR-ABL, p13/Akt/mTOR

* Corresponding Author Email: llbennett@uu.edu.

Abbreviations

HSPC	hematopoietic stem and progenitor cells
AML	acute myeloid leukemia
ALL	acute lymphocytic leukemia
BCP-ALL	B cell precursor ALL
TCP-ALL	T cell precursor ALL
BCR	B cell antigen receptor
ERK	extracellular signal regulator kinase
NGS	Next Generation Sequencing
JAK	janus Kinase
ITD	internal tandem duplication
FLT3	FMS-like tyrosine kinase 3
BCR-ABL	breakpoint cluster region-Abelson murine leukemia
Ph^+	Philadelphia positive chromosome
TKIs	tyrosine kinase inhibitors
RTKs	receptor tyrosine kinases
PML	promyelocytic leukemia
RARα	retinoic acid receptor alpha
HD	histone deacetylase
NCoR	nuclear co-repressor
CBF	core binding factor
RUNX	runt-related transcription factor
NPMI	nuclear phosphoprotein with multiple function
EGFR	epithelial growth factor receptor
PDGFR	platelet derived growth factor receptor
GTP	guanosine-triphosphate-binding protein
MLL	mixed-lineage leukemia
RAS	rat sarcoma
RalGDS	RAS-like guanine nucleotide dissociation stimulator
MAPK	mitogen-activated protein kinase
TP53	tumor protein 53
NOTCH	neurogenic locus notch homolog protein 1
mTOR	mammalian target of rapamycin
PTEN	phosphatase and tensin deleted on Chromose 10
GPCRs	G-protein coupled receptors
TET2	ten-eleven translocation 2
DNMT3A	deoxyribonucleotide methyltransferase
IDH	isocitrate dehydrogenase
JARID1A	jumonji AT-rich interaction domain 1A

NSD1	nuclear receptor binding set domain
DOT1L	disruptor of telomeric silencing 1 like
CRLF-2	cytokine receptor-like factor 2
STAT	signal transducer and activator transcription
IL	interleukin
SCF	stem cell factor
MAML	mastermind like
MRD	minimal/measurable residual disease
FISH	fluorescence *in situ* hybridization

INTRODUCTION

Acute leukemia divided into acute myeloid leukemia (AML) and acute lymphoblastic leukemia (ALL). ALL disorders is originated from hematopoietic B-cell or T-cells precursor. Lymphoid cells are derived from pluripotent hematopoietic stem cells present in the bone marrow through stepwise maturation controlled by the hierarchical activation of transcription factors and selection through functional signal transduction [1]. Genetic alterations such as deletions, amplifications, mutations, and structural rearrangements are key transcription factors that disrupts lymphoid development and results in the arrest maturation of B-lineages and T-lineages of lymphoid cells [1].

ALL is considered a genetic disease that harbors a variety of chromosomal abnormalities, including chromosomal translocations which create novel fusion genes or dysregulation of gene expression such as t(12;21), t(1;19), t(9;22), t(4;11)), numerical chromosome copy number aberrations hyperdiploidy (>50 chromosomes) and hypodiploidy (<44 chromosomes), and gene-specific mutations [2]. Although chromosomal aberrations are the hallmark of ALL, they are insufficient to induce leukemia. In-cooperating lesions are required to develop cell cycle arrest, tumor suppression and chromatin modification following the initial event that confers self-renewal coupled with mutation which eventually leading to the establishment of leukemic clones [3].

AML is more prevalent in the adults as the result of the transformation of primitive hematopoietic stem and progenitor cells (HSPCs) causing formation of immature myeloid progenitors [4]. The molecular features of AML often connected to dysregulated signaling pathways, acquired somatic molecular alterations, chromosome abnormalities, and changes in microRNA expression and transcriptional regulatory networks. Treatment and prognosis for these two leukemia differ significantly due to the genetic and molecular heterogeneity between the two groups.

REVIEW OF COMMON MUTATED GENES

The identification of recurrent chromosomal abnormalities in acute leukemia including translocation of gene, point mutations, and gene duplications has provided important insights into the pathogenesis of the disease [5]. Several altered genes are more prominent in chronic or acute leukemia than other cancers.

BCR-ABL fusion kinase gene was the first alteration gene identified in chronic myelogenous leukemia (CML) and ALL. The breakage on chromosome 22 involves a gene referred to as "BCR" (breakpoint cluster region). Another breakage is identified on chromosome 9, this breakage is known as ABL (Abelson, name after the scientist who described this gene). The ABL gene translocates to chromosome 22 and fuses with the remaining part of the BCR gene (t 9, 22). This fusion between BCR and ABL leads to an abnormal fused gene, called "BCR-ABL" also known as Philadelphia chromosome (Ph^+). Drugs such as imatinib, dasatinib, nilotinib known as tyrosine kinase inhibitors (TKIs) have been shown to have efficacy and prolonged patients' lives for 3 years or more [6]. Prior to the availability of TKIs, Ph+ ALL patients had a very poor prognosis [5]. Figure 1. depicts the formation of BCR-ABL gene.

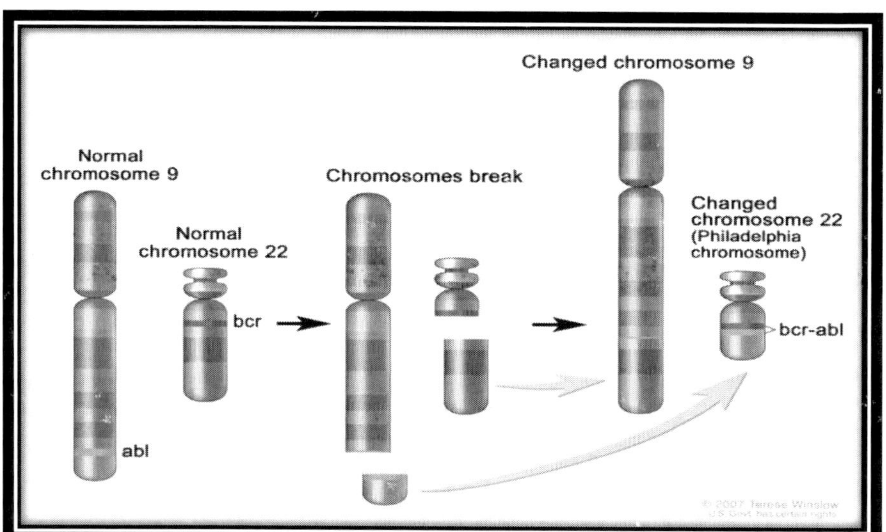

Figure 1. Philadelphia chromosome. A piece of chromosome 9 and a piece of chromosome 22 break off and trade places. The BCR-ABLgene is formed on chromosome 22 where the piece of chromosome 9 attaches. The changed chromosome 22 is called the Philadelphia chromosome. Down load from www.cancer.gov [7].

Recently, another BCR-ABL1 like fusion gene known as "Philadelphia chromosome -like" which have similar biological characteristics, except without BCR-ABL fusion, was identified. In ALL, this is called BCR-ABL1-like ALL [8-10]. This fusion can alter many other kinases such as BLNK, DGKH, FGFR1, IL2RB, LYN, NTRK3, PDGFRA, PTK2B, TYK2, and RAS signaling pathways [8-10]. This subtypes account for 15% of

B-ALL. Patients with BCR-ABL1-like ALL experience high relapse rates and are difficult to cure with conventional chemotherapy. This is due to rearrangements of CRLF-2 (cytokine receptor-like factor 2) with JAK1 and JAK2 point mutations [8, 11].

FLT3 (FMS-like tyrosine kinase 3) is a surface receptor tyrosine kinase (RTK) expressed on human $CD34^+$ hematopoietic stem. It is an early progenitor cells that play important role in cell proliferation and differentiation [12]. FLT3 receptor consists of an extracellular ligand-binding domain, a trans membrane domain, a juxtamembrane domain and two tyrosine kinase (TK) domains. Auto phosphorylation of the tyrosine residues on the receptor cause phosphorylation and activation of the RAS, SRC/JAK (janus kinase), P13K, ETS3 pathway which predict poor prognosis [13]. FLT3 is expressed on the majority of leukemic blasts causing decreased overall survival and increased relapse in patients with FLT3 mutations [14]. The mutations occur either as internal tandem duplication (ITD) in or near the juxta membrane domain, or as point mutations that result in single amino acids substitution within the activation loop of the TK domain. FLT3 mutation has been found in 30% to 35% of AML patients. Other TK receptor family include PDGFR (platelet derived growth factor receptors).

FLT3 inhibitors such as sorafenib and quizartinib inhibit only FLT3-ITD mutations, while midostaurin (PKC412, Rydapt®), crenolanib, and gilteritinib inhibit both FLT3-ITD and FLT3 TKD (tyrosine kinase domain). They had been investigated in several clinical trials and approved as orphan drugs by the Food and Drug Administration (FDA) [14]. Figure 2 shows FLT3 kinase signaling pathway and sites blocked by FLT3 inhibitors.

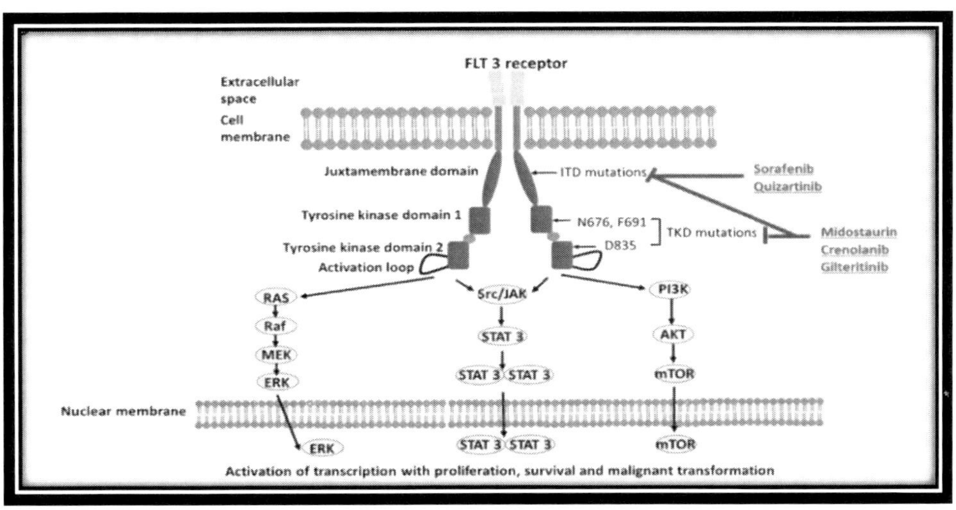

Figure 2. FLT3 kinase signaling pathway and sites blocked by FLT3 inhibitors. Sorafenib and quizartinib inhibit only FLT3-ITD mutations, while midostaurin, crenolanib, and gilteritinib inhibit both FLT3-ITD and FLT3TKD mutations [13].

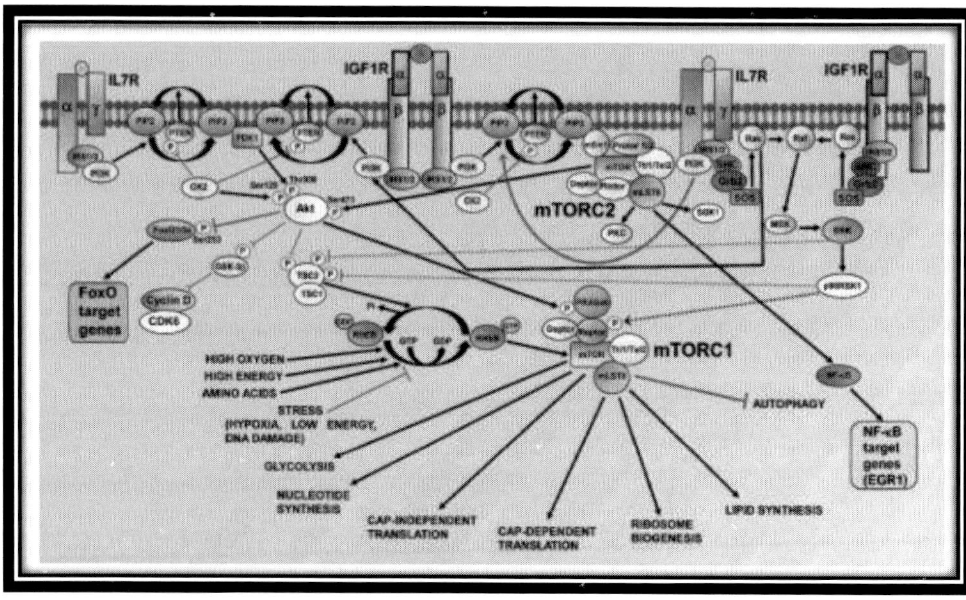

Figure 3. Regulation and functions mechanistic of mTOR1 and mTOR2. → Arrows indicate stimulatory events, while ⊣ lines indicate inhibitory events [16].

The constitutively active JAK(Janus kinase)/STAT (signal transducer and activator of transcription) signaling pathway results in uncontrolled proliferation of leukemic cells and has been associated with poor outcome [1]. Mutation in this pathways JAK1, JAK2, JAK3, interleukin 7 (IL7) have been observed in B-ALL and T-ALL [1]. Recently, JAK/STAT inhibitor ruxolitinib and mammalian target of rapamycin (mTOR) inhibitor were shown to have synergistic effect in the treatment of leukemia [15].

mTOR is a serine/threonine kinase that play important role in cell growth and proliferation. Constitutive activation of mTOR can cause cancer and occurs in the majority of AML and T-ALL [16]. mTOR inhibitors such as temsirolimus, sirolimus have been shown to arrest Go/G1 cell cycle and inhibit leukemic cells without affecting healthy $CD34^+$ bone marrow cells [17]. Figure 3. Showed regulation and function of mTOR.

The P13K/AKT/mTOR is involved in the regulation of cell growth, proliferation, motility, differentiation, inhibition of apoptosis, and modification of cells metabolism. These proteins also recruit RTKs and GPCRs (G protein-coupled receptors) [1]. Constitutive activation of this pathway impair apoptosis and cause inactivation of PTEN (Phosphatase and tensin deleted on Chromosome 10), the negative regulator of the P13K/AKT. Alteration in the P13K/AKT/mTOR pathway is predominant in T-ALL and AML which usually have poor prognosis and cause refractory to therapy [16, 18].

A translocation of genes that fuses the PML (promyelocytic leukemia) on chromosome 15 to the RARα (retinoic acid receptor alpha) on chromosome 17, result in formation of PML-RARα t (15;17) (q22;q11.2). This mutation recruits NCoR (nuclear co-repressor) and HD (histone deacetylase) which inhibits the expression of genes required for hematopoietic differentiation [5].

CBF (core binding factor) is a heterodimeric transcription made up of two subunits, CBFα (also known as RUNX-1) and CBFβ. These heterodimeric transcription factor regulates wider spectrum of genes. For example, fusion of RUNX1 on chromose 21 to MTG gene on chromose 8 t(8;21) has favorable prognosis in AML patients harboring this mutation [5]. C/EBPα (CCAAT/enhancer binding protein α) is a gene code for transcription factor which cause abnormal DNA binding of the transcription factor and loss of normal myeloid differentiation [5].

RUNX1(Runt-related transcription factor 1) and RUNX3 are genes responsible for encoding the DNA binding α-subunit of the RUNT domain that plays important role in the regulation of DNA transcription [19-20]. RUNX1 gene is located on chromose 21 (q21.22) plays important role in hematopoiesis during embryonic development [19]. RUNX3 gene which is located on chromosome 1 plays an important role in the regulation of other genes such as transforming growth factor-β and Notch 1 pathway, CBF1, ETS1, and ETS2 [21]. The RUNX1 and RUNX3 may serve as tumor promoter or tumor suppressor genes depending on the types of cancers [22-23].

NOTCH gene involves in signaling system found in multi cellular organism that regulate T-cell proliferation, cell differentiation, apoptosis, and development. NOTCH receptor genes encode a family of heterodimer trans membrane proteins (NOTCH1 to NOTCH4) [1]. NOTCH co-activates with Mastermind-like protein (MAML), FBXW7, MYC and NF-kβ. Mutation in NOTCH1and NOTCH2 genes have been identified in 50% of T-ALL patients [24]. Hairy and enhancer of split-1 (HES1) transcription factor downstream of NOTCH1 contribute to enhancing P13K/AKT/mTOR signaling in NOTCH1-dependent T-ALL [25].

IL7 plays a critical role in mTOR activation in T-ALL by causing activation of P13K/Akt/mTOR signaling pathway [26]. About 10% pediatric patient with T-ALL has been detected having IL7 mutation [26]. Together IGF1/IGF1R (insulin growth factor receptor) and IL7 not only activate P13K/AKT/mTOR but also involve in MEK/ERK (Mitogen-activated protein kinase kinase/ Extracellular signal-regulated kinase) pathways.

The Wnt signaling pathway is crucial for the normal development of HSPCs and B-cells. Wnt induces the formation of the Fzd (Frizzled)-LRP5/6 complex to activate the Wnt signaling pathway [1]. Without Wnt activation, β-catenin is phosphorylated by multiple protein destruction complex that degrade proteasome. Activation of Wnt to its receptors induces the destruction of β-catenin complex, which cause excess β-catenin to accumulate in the cytoplasm [1]. Some β-catenin is then able to enter the nucleus and activates gene expression of Wnt target genes such as LEF-1, c-MYC, and cyclin D1 [27]. NOTCH and Wnt plays important role to turn early T-lineage into T cells [1, 27].

Wnt pathway also involves in the inactivation of tumor suppressor genes such as FAT1 and FAT3 and activation of LEF1 gene which show poor prognosis in pediatric patients with T-ALL [28].

NPM1 (nuclear phosphoprotein with multiple function or nucleophosmin) is a heterozygous gene of the c-terminus of axon 12. NPMI mutations have been detected in 30% of AML. NPM1 mutation that does not relate to FLT3 usually have a better prognosis [5, 14].

AML patients who harbor MLL (mixed-lineage leukemia) abnormalities translocation of t(4;11) (q21;q23), t(9:11)(p22;q23), t (11;19)(q23;p13.3), t(10:11) (p12;q23) usually have inferior prognosis [5, 29]. MLL complexes with other genes such as SEC (super elongation complex), HOXA (homeobox A) cluster gene, and DOTL1 [30]. MLL-1 rearrangment are frequently found in leukemias of infant diagnose with ALL or AML [31].

RAS is a monomoric guanosine-diphosphate-binding protein(GTP) which is activated by various TKRs like the epithelial growth factor receptor (EGFR), PDGFR and the insulin receptors. RAS mutation preventing hydrolysis of RAS-GTP, keeping RAS in the "on" position. RAS genes include H-RAS (Harvey), K-RAS (Kisten), and N-RAS (neuroblastoma) [32]. Once activated, RAS also activate downstream pathways such as RAF family, MAPK (mitogen-activated protein kinase) and RalGDS (RAS-like guanine nucleotide dissociation stimulator) which participates in cell proliferation, survival, inflammation, and inhibition of apoptosis [5, 32-33]. RAS mutations has been identified in 15% to 30% of AML patients [5].

Tumor protein (TP53) plays important role in cell cycle arrest, apoptosis, DNA repair, and genomic stability. When DNA is damaged, TP53 is activated and induces cell cycle arrest that allow the cells to repair the damage. If the DNA is irreparable, TP53 can induce apoptosis. Under normal condition, TP53 levels are low. TP53 is a tumor suppressor gene located at 17q13. Mutation or deletion of this gene has been identified in 70% cases of AML [5]. Deletions of the CDKN2A/B, RB1 and T53 are also present in T-ALL and B-ALL which linked to poor prognosis and chemotherapy resistant [33]. Although TP53 mutation in ALL is rare in comparison to AML, mutation/deletion of TP53 are found to be significant in relapsed adult and children with ALL [34-35].

GENETIC ABERRANT IN AML

AML is thought to arise from two genetic abnormalities (mutations): type I and type II. Type I can induce proliferation or can inhibit apoptosis. Type I abnormalities result in increased uncontrolled proliferation and mutations of genes involved in signal transduction pathways such as BCR-ABL, FLT3, cKIT, N-RAS, K-RAS, PDGFR, FGFR, JAK2, JAK3, NF1, PTPN11 and inactivation of TP53 [36-38]. Type II abnormalities impair cells differentiation causing cells become immortalized, and induce genetic aberrations of hematopoietic transcription factors such as t(8;21)(q22;q22)/AML1-ETO, 11q23/MLL, NPMI, RUNX 1, RUNX3, PU1, MLL, PML-RARα, AMA1-ETO, and C/EBPα [38-40]. Figure 4. shows molecular mechanism involve in AML pathogenesis.

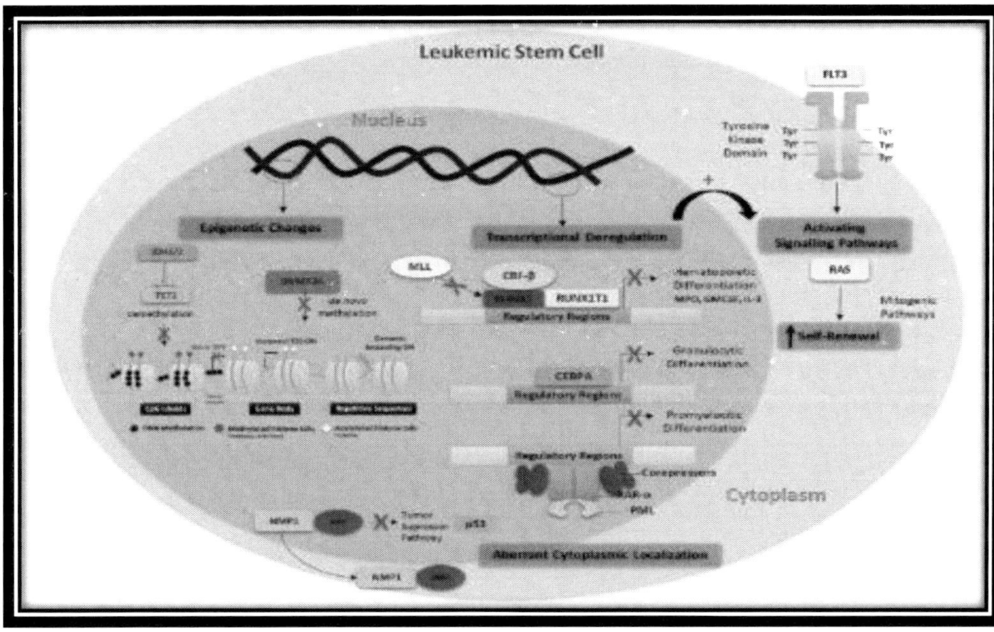

Figure 4. Molecular mechanisms involved in AML. Role of altered proteins shown in a leukemic stem cell. ***Nucleus***: epigenetic changes and transcriptional deregulation alter the gene expression profile. DNMT3A, IDH1/2 and TET2 mutants induce DNA methylation changes and histone code modification; therefore transcriptional repression in promoter regions (CpG Islands) and activation of incorrect transcriptional start sites (TSS) is observed. Hyper methylation of promoter regions results in silencing of TSS in target genes, while hypo methylation is associated with activation of proto-oncogenes and increase genomic instability. IDH11/2 and TET2 mutations are mutually exclusive. IDH1/2mutant forms inhibit only wild type TET2 function; CEBPA mutations and aberrant fusion genes like MLL, RUNX-1/RUNX1T1, and PML-RARα disrupts transcription of hematopoietic and myeloid differentiation specific genes by binding to regulatory regions. These events lead to activation of survival signaling pathways and stimulate self-renewal. Mutations in p53 affect tumor suppressor pathways enhancing abnormal proliferation. ***Cytoplasm***: FLT3 tyrosine kinase domain mutants induce activation of mitogenic signaling pathways and involve proliferation factors such as RAS to increase self-renewal. NMP1 mutant has aberrant cytoplasmic localization together with translocate interacting proteins (ARF) and blocks tumor suppressor pathway [36].

In children, type II cytogenetic abnormalities are common. The abnormalities of t(8;21)(q22;q22), inv (16)(p.13.1q22), t(15;17)(q22;q21), and 11q23/MLL together is referred to as CBF-AML [36, 41-42]. Some gene translocation t(91;22)(p13;q13), t(7;12)(q36;p13) and t(11;12)(p15:p13) are specific in children, but rarely found in adult [43-44]. C/EBPα plays role as type I or tyle II in inducing leukemiogenesis behaving as a tumor suppressors or tumor inducer of hematopoietic stem cells [38]. This alteration is thought due to mutations in C-terminal which disrupt DNA binding activity, while N-terminal mutations disrupt the full length of C/EBPα. Both mutations are found in 70% of AML patients. [38, 45]. More than 60 fusion genes have been identified in AML with the breakpoint of the MLL gene is highly conserved domain.

Combination of Type I and Type II mutations are more prevalent, such as that involve in RAS in combination with MLL-rearrangements, cKIT mutations in CBF-AML and FLT3-ITD in combination with PML/RARA and NUP98/NSDI [10, 12, 16]. Mutations in epigenetic regulators such as EZH2, ASXL1 and DNMT3A also involve in the development of AML [36, 40, 44-48]. Table 1 depicts genetic abberant involve in AML [48].

Specific frequently mutated RTK genes with poor prognosis such as FLT3, c-KIT, P13k/AKT/mTOR, and RAS/RAF/MEK/ARK pathways are explain in detailed below.

Table 1. Genetic abnormalities in AML. Extracted from Valerio [48]

Gene	Frequency	Effect
ASXL1	3%-5%	AML-MRC, MDS, Worse prognosis
BCOR	4% CN-AML	Possible worse prognosis
DNMT3A	20%	Possible worse prognosis
IDH1	6%-9% adult, 1% pediatric	Possible worse prognosis
IDH2	8%-12% adult 1%-2% pediatric	Contraversial. IDH2 R140 mutation with NPM1 associate with favorable prognosis in one study
MLL/KMT2A	4% -14%	MLL PTD shows worse prognosis in CN-AML
NRAS	8% adult 13% pediatric	No clear impact on prognosis
KRAS	2% adult 9% pediatric	No clear impact on prognosis
PHF6	2%-3%	Associated with adverse outcome
RUNX1	5%-18%	Poor prognosis. Transplant better outcome
TET2	7%-10% adult 1.5%-4% pediatric	Unclear, some shows adverse outcome in AML with isolated CEBPA or NPM1
TP53	2%-9% adult 1% pediatric	Unfavorable prognosis. Check Li-Fraumeni syndrome in young people
WT1	4%-11%	Poorer outcome, in CN-AML
CEBPA	10%	Better prognosis
KIT	2%-14%	Worse prognosis
FLT3	14%-25%	Worse prognosis
NPM1	30%	Favorable prognosis

Abbreviation: CN-AML: cytogenitically normal AML, MDS: myelodysplastic syndrome, MRC: myelodysplasia related changes, PTD: patial tandem duplication.

FLT3 MUTATIONS

Upon activation by the FLT3 ligand in HSPCs, FLT3 induces signaling downstream via the PI3K/Akt and the RAS/RAF pathways necessary for the proliferation and development of HSPC and B-cell progenitors involved in early hematopoiesis [24-25, 36] (Figure 4).

It has been reported that *FLT3*-ITD mutation upregulates the PI3K/AKT pathway via constitutive activation of AKT and inhibition of FOXO3a, which belongs to the forkhead transcription factors controlling apoptosis and cell cycle regulation [49-50]. Many studies in AML have demonstrated that the *FLT3*-ITD mutation is associated with inferior clinical outcomes in the long run [51-52]. Although patients with *FLT3*-ITD mutant AML have complete remission rates compare to those with wild-type FLT3 AML, the presence of *FLT3*-ITD mutations significantly increases the risk of relapse and decreases disease-free and overall survival [53-54]. However, patients with AML that harbors both *FLT3*-ITD mutation and a nucleophosphomin (*NPM1*) mutation have improved response rates and disease-free and overall survival as compared with those with *FLT3*-ITD mutant only AML [5, 14].

In contrast to FLT3-ITDs in the juxtamembrane domain, point mutations at position D835 within the activation loop of the TK domain of FLT3, referred to as FLT3-TKD mutations, are less common (~7%) and do not shows a clinical significance [55-56]. Although one study has found a correlation of FLT3-TKD mutations with leukocytosis at diagnosis and worse prognosis, the prognostic impact of FLT3-TKD remains less evident than the FLT3-ITD mutations. Nonetheless, it has been reported that FLT3-ITD-TKD dual mutants, which occurs in 1~2% AML patients, confer resistance to FLT3 TKIs and cytotoxic drugs by inducing hyper activation of STAT5, which subsequently upregulates the STAT5-target protein RAD51 and the apoptotic protein BCL-XL and result in cell-cycle arrest at the G2M checkpoint [57]. This finding suggests FLD-TKD mutations may represent an important mechanism of drug resistance in AML [58].

C-KIT MUTATIONS

The c-Kit proto-oncogene (CD117) encodes a trans membrane type III RTK, which interacts with its ligand, stem cell factor (SCF) to play an important role in regulating HSPCs functions [59-62]. Following the SCF binding and the initial auto phosphorylation of c-Kit, a molecular signaling switch in the c-Kit pathways occurs during differentiation in the hematopoietic system whereby immature HSPCs employ a PI3K-sensitive pathway to activate both ERK and AKT, which is then switched to the PI3K–independent MAP kinase pathway upon differentiation [63]. Among normal bone marrow cells, c-Kit expression has been found in about half of the $CD34^{+}$ precursors, including progenitors committed to the erythroid, granulomonocytic, and megakaryocytic cell lineage. It is also expressed in up to one third of the primitive $CD3^{-}CD4^{-}CD8^{-}$triple negative (TN) thymocyte precursor population, and in up to 4% of the mononuclear cell population, and in $CD56^{bright}$ natural killing cells [64-66]. High expression of c-Kit has been detected in 60-80% AML cases [67-68]. The constitutive activation of c-Kit found in AML blasts elicits the formation of large multi protein signaling complexes including PI3K/AKT, RAS-ERK, the SRC family kinases (SFK), phospholipase Cγ, and JAK/STAT pathways, leading to the excessive proliferation and aberrant differentiation of leukemic cells [69-71]. Mutations in *c-Kit* gene are exclusively associated with CBF-AML, which represents 5-8% of all AMLs. While CBF-AML has a relatively favorable prognosis, high incidence of relapse has been seen in patients with c-Kit mutant CBF-AML [5]. In CBF-AML, c-Kit mutations consist predominantly point mutations in exon 17, which encodes the activation loop in the kinase domain, and less frequently insertions and deletions in exon 8, which encodes the extracellular portion of the KIT receptor [72]. These mutations are observed in 20–25% of t (8; 21) and about 30% of inv (16) CBF-AML cases [73-74]. The c-Kit mutation Asp816 seen in 10.5% of t (8; 21) AML is associated with poor outcome due to its ability to constitutively activate the JAK/STAT pathway [1, 75].

PI3K/AKT/mTOR Signaling

The PI3K/AKT and the mTOR signaling pathways are two highly interconnected signaling pathways that play a pivotal role in mediating many aspects of cell survival and growth in both physiological and pathological conditions. In particular, the PI3K/Akt pathway is a key regulator of hematopoiesis, while the mTOR integrates signals initiated by upstream cellular stimuli to regulate ribosomal translation of mRNA into proteins necessary for cell cycle progression and cell growth through its downstream effector 4EBP1 and P70S6 kinase (S6K) [76-78]. The PI3K family consists of eight members that can be grouped into three classes [79-80]. Among the three classes of the PI3K family, the only class that has been implicated in regulation of hematopoiesis is Class I PI3K, which are heterodimers composed of a p110 catalytic and a p85 or p101 type regulatory/adaptor subunit [77, 81]. See Figure 3.

Upon the activation of RTKs and subsequent auto phosphorylation on tyrosine residues in their cytoplasmic tails, PI3K is recruited to the cell membrane by directly binding to phosphotyrosine consensus residues of RTKs through one of the two Src homology 2 (SH2) domains in the p85 subunit, leading to allosteric activation of the p110 catalytic subunit [82]. Following the activation of PI3K, the second messenger phosphatidylinositol-3, 4, 5-triphosphate (PI3, 4, 5-P_3) is produced from the substrate phosphatidylinositol-4, 4-bisphosphate (PI-4, 5-P_2), and then recruits a subset of signaling proteins with pleckstrin homology (PH) domains to the membrane, including protein serine/threonine kinase-3′-phosphoinositide-dependent kinase 1 (PDK1) and AKT [82-83]. AKT itself regulates several cell processes essential to cell survival and cell cycle progression.

AKT belongs to the AGC (PKA/PKG/PKC) superfamily of protein kinases and is related to AMP/GMP kinase and protein kinase C [85]. AKT contains an N-terminal pleckstrin homology (PH) domain, a central kinase CAT domain, and a C-terminal regulatory region [86]. Activation of AKT is mediated by phosphorylation at Thr308 by PDK1 and Ser473 by mTOR-raptor complex. AKT promotes cell survival by inactivating pro-apoptotic factors such as Bad and Procaspase-9, as well as phosphorylating FKHRL1, a member of the Forkhead family of transcription factors, which results in the retention of FKHRL1 in the cytoplasm and the inhibition of FKHRL1-dependent transcription, thereby suppressing the transcription of death genes, such as the *Fas* ligand gene [87-88]. AKT promotes cell growth primarily through the activation of the mTOR-raptor complex, which plays an evolutionarily conserved role in cell growth control [89-90]. Also, AKT activation can stimulate cell proliferation through multiple Akt downstream targets involved in cell cycle regulation, such as glycogen synthase kinase-3 (GSK3), insulin receptor substrate-1 (IRS-1), the cyclin-dependent kinase inhibitors $p21^{CIP1/WAF1}$ and $p27^{KIP1}$ [91-94].

The PI3K/AKT/mTOR pathway is constitutively activated in about 50–80% of AML cases [96-98]. Most of the clinical studies suggest that abnormal activation of PI3K/AKT/mTOR pathway is associated with poor prognosis in AML patients, whereas one study revealed that enhanced AKT phosphorylation positively correlates with the survival of AML patients [97-99]. The molecular mechanisms underlying the association between PI3K/AKT/mTOR activation and prognosis is still misunderstood. However, emerging evidence has revealed that constitutive activation of PI3K is involved in the spontaneous proliferation of primary AML cells and a reduced apoptotic response observed in AML blasts displaying enhanced PI3K/AKT activation [100-101]. Regardless of prognostic significance, it is clear that the PI3K/AKT pathway controls blast cell proliferation and the clonogenicity of leukemic progenitors, and thus may be an important therapeutic target of AML [96, 102-103].

RAS/RAF/MEK/ERK

The RAS/RAF/MEK/ERK cascade is an important signaling pathway involved in leukemogenesis, regulating diverse cellular functions including cell survival, proliferation, differentiation and invasion [5, 32-33, 104]. Typically, activation of the RAS/RAF/MEK/ERK pathway is initiated following ligand binding to RTKs at the plasma membrane, which activates the GTP-bound RAS with subsequent stimulation of RAF [32-33]. Upon activation, RAF transmits the signal by phosphorylating MEK1/2, which in turn activate their only known substrates, native ERK1/2, by phosphorylating both regulatory threonine and tyrosine residues of ERK1/2, leading to the regulation of gene transcription in the nucleus [105].

In patients with AML, N-RAS mutations are the most prominent RAS mutations and carried by 11% to 30% of patients [5, 32-33]. Although N-RAS mutations in AML were first reported three decades ago [100, 101], the role of N-RAS in oncogenic progression in AML is not well understood, nor are the prognostic implications of *NRAS* mutations in AML. Some studies have indicated that N-RAS mutations are associated with poor outcome or have the negative prognostic impact only in AML with favorable karyotype [107-109]. However, some have found no clear association of *RAS* mutations with the clinical outcome after AML therapy at all [109-112]. In contrast, results from a study of 2502 of patients with AML demonstrated that N-RAS mutations account for an improved prognosis in the subgroup with normal karyotype and non-mutated FLT3 status although the overall prognostic impact of N-RAS mutations was weak [113]. AML harboring wild-type RAS can have acquired activation of Ras pathway through constitutive gain-of-function alterations in upstream RTKs or mutations in RAS-regulated genes. Strong RAS activity was found in 22.2% and 25% of AML patients with and without a RAS mutation, respectively, suggesting that the state of RAS activity casts more light on clinical consequences of the RAS signaling pathways than the mutational analysis of RAS genes [110].

After activating RAS, growth factors and mitogens utilize the downstream RAF/MEK/ERK pathway to transmit signals from the cell surface to the nucleus to regulate the expression of target genes controlling cellular proliferation, differentiation, apoptosis and senescence. In AML, constitutive activation of the MEK/ERK pathway is attributable to aberrant activation of MEK, down regulation of phosphatase of activated cells (PAC1), and overexpression of ERK1/2 [104]. Alternatively, FLT3-ITD can eventually lead to constitutive MEK/ERK activation [114].

Genetic Aberrant in ALL

Acute lymphoblastic leukemia (ALL) represents a group of T- and B- precursor stage lymphoid cell malignancies and is characterized by clonal expansion of leukemic cells in the bone marrow, lymph nodes, thymus, or spleen [1-3]. In adults, 75% of the ALL cases develop from precursors of the B-cell lineage known as the precursor B-cell ALL (BCP-ALL) and about 25% of the cases from the precursor of T-cell (TCP-ALL).

As B cells of the immune system mature, each expresses a unique B cell antigen receptor (BCR) in the form of surface-bound immunoglobulin (Ig). In its monomeric form, the BCR consists of 2 parts: (1) the membrane immunoglobulin molecule that binds antigen, resulting in receptor aggregation, and (2) the Igα/Igβ heterodimer that functions as an antigen-binding subunit to transduce signaling to the interior of the B cell to regulate essential cellular functions. Structurally resembling the BCR, a pre-BCR comprises an immunoglobulin μ heavy chain pairing with a surrogate light chain (SLC) that is composed of *VPREB1* and λ5 (*IGLL1*) polypeptides and the signal-transducing heterodimer Igα/Igβ [115-116]. Both BCR and pre-BCR play a central role in regulating B-cell development through controlling cell-fate decisions at specific antigen-independent checkpoints.

In normal hematopoiesis, pre-BCR signaling controls differentiation of pre-B to immature B-cells by initiating and regulating diverse processes within the pre-B cell, including clonal selection, proliferation and subsequent maturation. Although the role of pre-BCR activity in BCP-ALL remains unclear, emerging evidence indicates that the role of pre-BCR signaling may differ depending on the stages of lymphoblast maturation and presence of oncogenic driver lesions. For example, in most BCR–ABL1$^+$ precursor B-cell acute lymphoblastic leukemia (BCR–ABL1$^+$ B-ALL), which is the most common molecular subtype of ALL in adults and comprise ~20% of cases, expression of functional pre-BCR is compromised in leukemic clones due to non-productive immunoglobulin heavy chain (*IGH*) gene rearrangement and/or dysregulation of other prominent effector proteins, such as IKAROS, SLP-65, and Bruton tyrosine kinase (BTK) [117-120]. On the other hand, malignant ALL blasts can hijack pre-BCR signaling to circumvent clonal extinction, resulting in B cell development arrested at the progenitor stage. Binding of antigen or ligand to pre-BCR initiates a cascade of tonic basal signaling transduced by the Igα/Igβ signaling chains, resulting in the phosphorylation of immune-receptor tyrosine-based activation motifs (ITAMs) by members of the SRC kinase family (including LYN, FYN, LCK and BLK) and subsequent recruitment of spleen tyrosine kinase (SYK). The primary substrate of SYK and ZAP70 in pre-B cells is the B cell linker protein BLNK (or SLP-65).

Phosphorylation of BLNK facilitates its association with BTK and phospholipase Cγ2 (PLCγ2), thereby promoting the activation of these two signaling molecules [119, 121]. Activation of PLCγ2 hydrolyzes inositol (4,5)-bisphosphate (PIP_2) into diacylglycerol (DAG) and inositol (1,4,5) triphosphate (IP_3), and the latter triggers the release of Ca^{2+} from ER stores and activation of CRAC channels, which is a critical event in the response of B cells to antigen stimulation [122-123]. In addition, PLCγ2 binds to activated RAS to promote the activation of extracellular signal-regulated kinase (ERK) [124-129]. For the continued survival of malignant B cells, pre-BCR signaling induces MAP kinase-mediated phosphorylation of B-cell lymphoma 6 (BCL6 protein) leading to BCL6 degradation by the ubiquitin–proteasome pathway [130]. Alterations in pre-BCR signaling via the SYK-BLNK axis can affect pre-B cell transformation. It has been shown that constitutive activation of SYK in mouse pre-B cells cause leukemic transformation, while BLNK-deficient pre-B cells express increased level of pre-BCR and exhibit uncontrolled growth [131-132]. BLNK can have both tumor promoting and tumor suppressing activity. The tumor suppressing activity of BLNK is independent of PLCγ2 but through the direct binding and inhibition of JAK3 [134-135].

It has been reported that silencing of BLNK in leukemic pre-B cells induces the production of IL-7, which promotes the proliferation and survival of pre-B cells in an autocrine manner that is dependent on JAK3–STAT5 signaling [134]. Moreover, suppression of IL-7 signaling results in upregulation of the transcription factors FOXO1 and PAX5, which co-activate many pre-B cell genes, including *BLNK, RAG1 and RAG2*. Induction of BLNK enables SYK mediated pre-BCR signaling and promotes immunoglobulin light-chain rearrangement [135]. In normal pre-B cells, BLNK expression can inhibits the activation of AKT, thereby promoting the nuclear translocation of FOXO1, which upregulates the gene that encodes the transcriptional repressor B cell lymphoma 6 (BCL-6) [135-138]. BCL-6 can induce cell-cycle exit via transcriptional repression of MYC [132]. In malignant pre-B cells, inactivation of BLNK by its somatic mutations releases its inhibition of both AKT and JAK3, and thus prevents the translocation of FOXO1 to the nucleus to activate BCL-6. Reduced BCL-6 expression relieves the suppression of cMYC-medicated cell cycle progression [139].

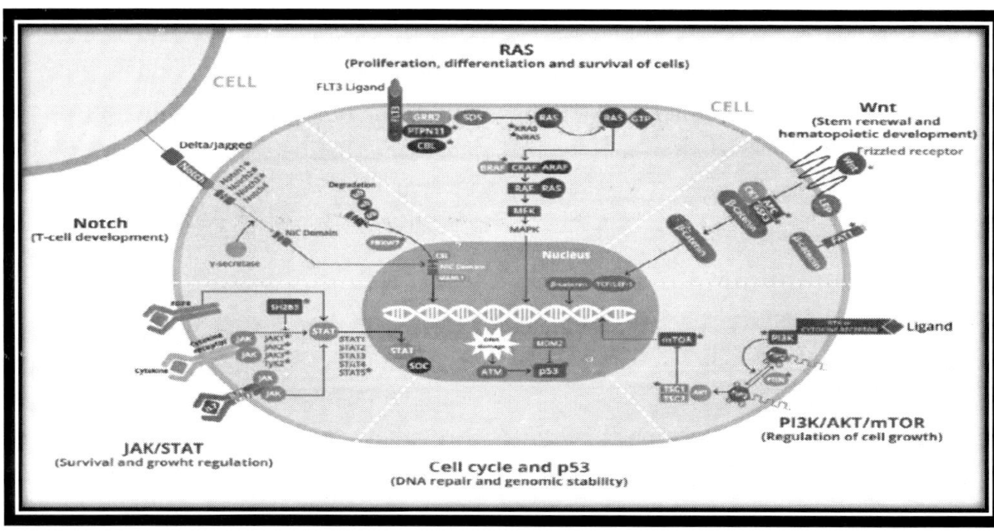

Figure 5. Cellular pathways affected by genes significantly mutated in ALL. Asterisks show the genes that are mutated in each cellular program and the biological effect of these mutations on the pathway (Green: activation mutation. Red: inactivating mutation [1].

Similar to BLNK, BTK also has both oncogenic and tumor suppressor functions. BTK exerts its tumor suppressor function independently of its kinase activity, but rather by acting as an adaptor protein in an SLP-65 independent pathway [140]. It has been demonstrated that deficiency of BTK increased the frequency of tumor formation in SLP-65- deficient mice and transgenic low-level expression of the E41K-Y223F mutant of

BTK, a constitutive active form of BTK, prevented tumor formation in BTK/SLP-65 double mutant mice, indicating that BTK can substitute for SLP-65 as a tumor suppressor [141]. Figure 5 depicts genes mutated in ALL. Table 2 summarizes pathway and genes aberrant using next generation sequencing (NGS) [1].

Table 2. Genes and pathways involve in ALL. Extracted from Montano et al. [1]

Pathway	Genes	Frequency
Cell cycle and p53 (DNA repair and genomic stability, tumor suppression)	ATM, CCND3,CDKN1B, RB1, CDKN2A, CDKN2B, STAG2, TP53	6% in B-ALL
JAK-STAT (survival and growth regulation)	CRLF2, IL2RB, IL7R, JAK1, JAK2, JAK3, PTPN2, SH2B3, STAT5A, STAT5B, TYK2	11% in B-ALL 30% in T-ALL
RAS (signal proliferation differentiation and survival of cells)	BRAF, CBL, CBLB, FLT3, KRAS, NF1, NRAS, PTPN11, RASGRP3	48% in B-ALL 15% in T-ALL
Lymphoid development and differentiation	Bcl11A, BTG1, CD200, EBF, EBF1, ETV6, IKZF1, IKZF2, IKZF3, LEF1, PAG1, PAX5, RAG1, RAG2, RUNX1, TCF3, TCF4, VPREB1, XBP1, BCL11B	18% in B-ALL
Transcriptional process	BCOR, CEBPA, c-MYC, DNM2, ERG, GATA3, LMO2, MEF2C, MGA, MYB, MYCN, RELN, TLX1, WT1	17% in T-ALL
NOTCH	DLL4, FBXW7, JAG1, JAG2, NOTCH1, NOTCH2, NOTCH3, HES1	60% in T-ALL
P13/AKT/mTOR	AKT1, AKT2, CSF3R, mTOR, PTEN, FGFR3, PIK3C2B, PIK3CA, PIK3CD, PIK3R1	85% in T-ALL
Wnt	FAT1, FAT3	13% in T-ALL
Epigenetic regulator and chromatin structure modifiers	WHSC1, TET2, SUZ12, SMARCA4, SETD2, PHF6, NCOR1, KMT2A, KMT2D, KDM2B, KDM5C, IDH1, IDH2, CREBBP, CTCF, GATA2, EP300, ARID1A, ARID2, ASXL1, ASXL2, EED, EZH2, HIST1H2AG, KDM6A, NR3C1, SETBP1, DNMT3	35% in T-ALL
Translational and RNA stability	CNOT1, CNOT3, DIS3, RPL10, RPL22, RPL5, ZCCHC7	23% in T-ALL
Splicing	DHX15, HNRNPA1, HNRNPR, PRPF40B, SF3B1, U2AF1, ZRSR2	16% in T-ALL
DNA repair	HERC1, MCH2, MCH6, ZFHX4	9% in T-ALL
ABL	ABL1, PDGFRG	14% in T-ALL
Other	BCR, IGH, LMO1, LYN, MEF2D, NT5C2, NTRK3, PICALM, TAI2, TCRA, TCRB, TCRD, TCRG, ZEB2, ZNF384	16% in B-ALL 53% in T-ALL

Specific genetic alteration in AML including STAT5 and NOTCH pathways explained more detailed below, follow by epigenetic regulation and chromatin modification highly prevalent in B-ALL and T-ALL are discussed below.

STAT5 SIGNALING IN BCP-ALL

It is well accepted that the development and homeostasis of lymphocytes are influenced by a number of regulatory cytokines including IL-2, IL-4, IL-7, IL-9, IL-15 and others [142-143]. Among those interleukins, IL-7 functions as an essential, non-redundant growth and anti-apoptosis factor for B- and T-cell (alpha/beta- and gamma/ delta-TCR + cells) precursors, and is essential for differentiation of gamma/delta-TCR+ cells [26, 143]. IL-7 binds to the γ_c-containing IL-7 receptor (IL-7R) to activate the constitutively associated JAK1 and JAK3 kinases. The activated JAK3 and JAK3 kinases phosphorylate themselves to create a docking site for Src Homology 2 (SH2) domain containing STAT proteins [144]. STAT5 is the predominant STAT protein activated by IL-7 and a key component of the JAK/STAT pathway regulating the transformation and function of B and T lymphocyte [145--146].

Activation of STAT5 in response to IL-7 stimulation promotes cell survival during the developmental transition from uncommitted common lymphoid progenitors (CLPs) to committed pro-B cells by activating the prosurvival *Mcl1* gene and ordering immunoglobulin gene recombination by suppressing the immunoglobulin κ light chain (IgK) gene rearrangements in pro-B cells [147]. Moreover, the STAT5-dependent regulation of the *Ccnd3* gene encoding for cyclin D3 is essential for proliferative cell expansion during the pro-B to pre-B cell transition [148]. Besides regulating genes that promote survival and proliferation, STAT5 also binds to a large subset of genes involved in the pre BCR pathway, including those for the upstream kinases SYK and BLK, the adaptors BLNK and CARMA1, and the downstream transcription factors IRF4, IRF8, IKAROS and AIOLOS, to ensure sufficient expansion of progenitor B cells and prevent premature B cell differentiation [149].

Although mutations in STAT5 gene have not been found in human BCP-ALL, it has been reported that STAT5 is constitutively activated in a subset of BCP-ALL harboring activating mutations in upstream signaling components of the JAK/STAT pathway, suggesting that STAT5 is functionally important in certain types of BCP-ALL [150]. For example, BCR-ALL with the t(9;22)(q34;q11) translocation, which encodes the constitutively active BCR–ABL1-TK, often have constitutive activation of STAT5, which is variably associated with a corresponding activation of JAK kinases suggesting the BCR–ABL1 kinase contributes to leukemogenesis via aberrant JAK/STAT signaling pathway [151-154].

NOTCH SIGNALING IN T-ALL

T-ALL is an aggressive lymphoid tumor resulting from the malignant transformation and subsequent clonal expansion of T-cell precursors expressing immature T-cell markers [24, 155-156]. *Over 60%* of *T-ALL cases* show aberrant activation of the notch homolog protein 1 (NOTCH1) rendering *NOTCH1* the most notable and prevalent oncogene in this disease [25, 157-158]. NOTCH receptors are multi-domain proteins expressed on the cell surface. The core elements of the NOTCH signaling system include the Delta and Serrate family of ligands (Delta-like 1, 3 and 4; and Jagged 1 and 2), four distinct NOTCH receptors (NOTCH1-4), and the RBPJ/CSL (CBF1/Su(H)/LAG-1) DNA binding protein [157].

In lymphocytes, NOTCH signaling is essential for specifying the T cell fate, and is directly involved in the regulation of T-cell precursor development with NOTCH1 functioning as the key receptor responsible for not only the T-cell lineage commitment but also the inhibition of alternative differentiation pathways [159]. NOTCH1 is most highly expressed in immature $CD4^-$ $CD8^-$ thymocytes while NOTCH ligands are expressed on thymic epithelial cells, and thus NOTCH signaling is initiated by ligand-receptor interactions that take place between adjacent thymocytes and thymic epithelial cells [160-163].

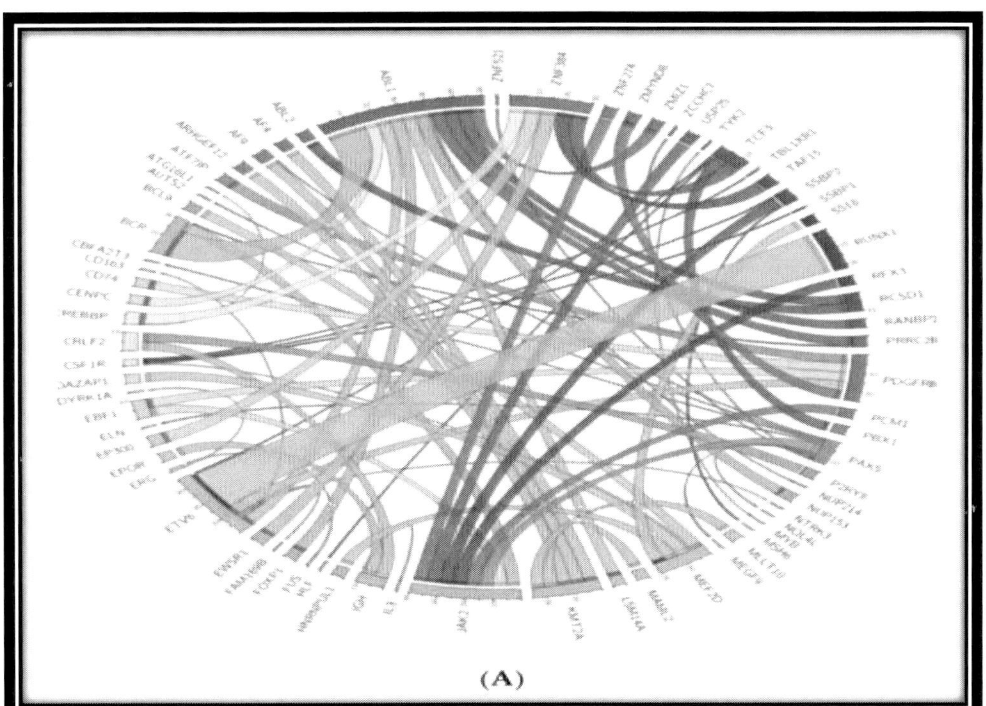

Figure 6A. New fusion genes identified by NGS approaches in B-ALL and their frequencies in B-cell ALL [1].

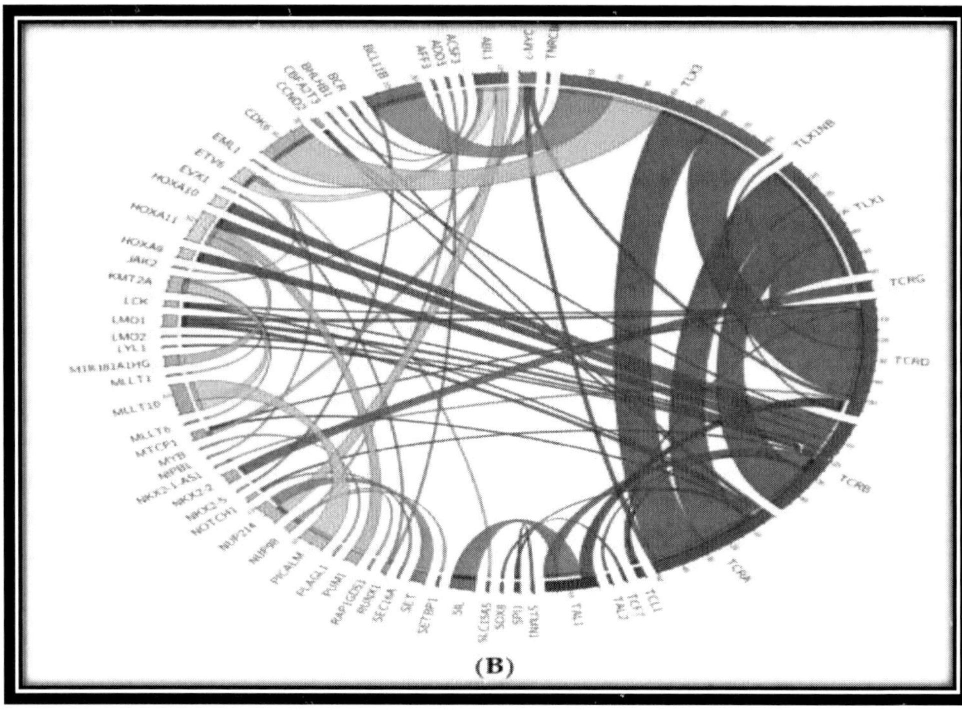

Figure 6B. New fusion genes identified by NGS approaches in T-ALL and their frequencies in T-cell ALL [1].

Interaction between NOTCH receptors and ligands of the Serrate and Delta families result in two successive cleavages, first in the extracellular domain mediated by ADAM metalloprotease, and second in the trans membrane domain by *presenilin-dependent γ-secretase*-like *protease,* which release the intracellular domain of NOTCH (ICN) and permit its translocation to the nucleus [164]. After ICN translocate to the nucleus, it binds the basic helix-loop-helix (bHLH) transcription factor CSL (for CBF1, Su (H), and LAG-1). CSL acts as a switch in that it binds co-repressors and inhibits transcription in its basal state, but induces transcriptional activation through displacing co-repressors and recruiting co-activators when interacting with ICN. Essential co-activators are proteins encoded by the Mastermind-like (MAML) gene family capable to form a multi protein complex with the ICN and CSL and recruit co-activators, such as p300 [24, 165].

Aberrantly enforced NOTCH1 signaling is a potent inducer of T-ALL in mouse models and is required to sustain the growth of a human t(7;9)-positive T-ALL cell line [166-169]. In most T-ALLs, NOTCH1 is not activated by chromosomal translocations, but result from activating mutations that disrupt the heterodimerization (HD) and PEST domains of the receptor [170]. Activating mutations in NOTCH1 co-occur frequently with the loss of cyclin-dependent kinase inhibitor 2A (CDKN2A) locus, which encodes tumor suppressor $p14^{ARF}$ and $p16^{INK4A}$, resulting in the dysregulated expression of a diverse group of T cell-specific transcription factors that can act as oncogenes, including MYC, MYB, T cell acute lymphocytic leukemia 1 (TAL1) and

TAL2, the T cell leukemia homeobox 1 (TLX1) and TLX2, NK2 homeobox 1 (NKX2-1) and NKX2-2, and homeobox A (HOXA)genes [171-180]. The two protein products of *CDKN2A*, $p14^{ARF}$ and $p16^{INK4A}$, are directly involved in cell cycle regulation. Given that $p14^{ARF}$ can down regulate mouse double minute 2 homolog (*MDM2),* thereby activating p53, NOTCH can suppress p53 by repressing the $p14^{ARF}$-MDM2-p53 surveillance network [181-182]. Although the relationship between NOTCH signaling and $p16^{INK4A}$ remains elusive, $p16^{INK4A}$ is known to inhibit cyclin-dependent kinases and G1 to S phase cell cycle progression and function as a master regulator of cell cycle entry via the Rb-E2F signaling axis [180-182].

Epigenetic Regulation and Chromatin Modification

Chromatin structure modification and epigenetic regulation which involve in DNA methylation and histone protein modification plays important role in cancer development. DNA hypo methylation can promote cancer development through chromosomal instability, reactivation of transposons, and loss of imprinting [183]. Epigenetic alterations are highly prevalent in B-ALL and T-ALL.

The term epigenetics was originally used to describe heritable changes in gene expression (phenotype) that were independent of DNA sequence alterations (genotype) [184]. Several histone modification and chromatin and gene regulation including enzymes that cause acetylation, methylation, hydroxyl methylation, phosphorylation and ubiquitination have been identified and known as "epigenetic writers," "epigenetic erasers," and "epigenetic readers" [185]. Epigenetic regulators that alter ALL include MLL1, CREBBP, WHSC1, and SETD2 [1].

In AML, epigenetic regulators involve in cancer are: IDH1 and IDH2 (isocitrate dehydrogenase), TET2 (ten-eleven translocation), DNMT3A (DNA methyltransferase), JARID1A (Jumonji AT-rich interaction domain 1A), NSD1 (nuclear receptor binding SET domain), DOT1L (disruptor of telomeric silencing 1 like), HDAC and many others [186]. DNMT3A is a DNA methyl transferase involves in epigenetic regulation of the genome through methylation. Mutations in DNMT3A occurring in 20% of AML due to substitution of the amino acid arginine. DNMT3A mutations often co-occur with FLT3-ITD, NPM1, IDH1 and IDH2 [48].

Oncogenic activating mutations in epigenetic modifiers such as IDH1, IDH2, EZH2 and DNMT3A and inactivating mutations in chromatin modifiers such as KDM6A, CREBBP, EP300 and SMARCB1 have been observed in ALL [187-188]. Mutations of histone acetyl transferase CREBBP, methyl transferase WHSC1, SETD1 and MLL1 have been identified in B-ALL [189]. Therefore, DNMT3A inhibitor such as azacitidine, HDAC inhibitors such as vorinostat, panobinostat, and DOTL1 inhibitors have potential therapeutic implication. They are currently on phase 1 or 2 clinical trials for the treatment of ALL or AML. For specific inhibitors of epigenetic regulators, see www.clinical trials.gov [190]. Figure 8 shows genes commonly aberrant in DNA methylation of AML, while Figure 9 depicts various possible drugs for therapeutic applications.

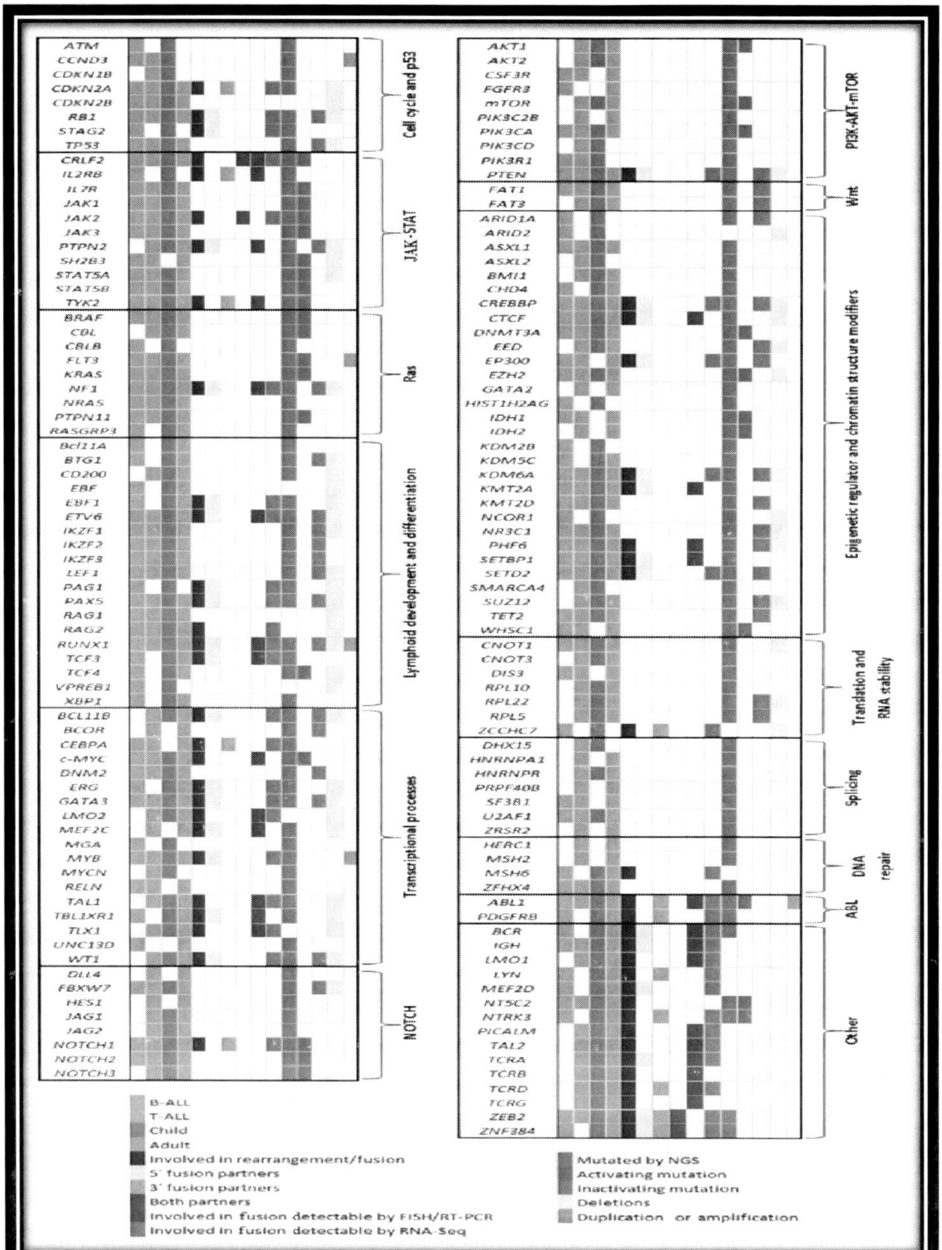

Figure 7. Summary of key genes altered in the different signaling pathways involve in ALL. This illustrates the genetic alterations (somatic mutations, rearrangement/fusion, deletions and duplications) presence in the main genes involves in the pathogenic pathways of ALL [1].

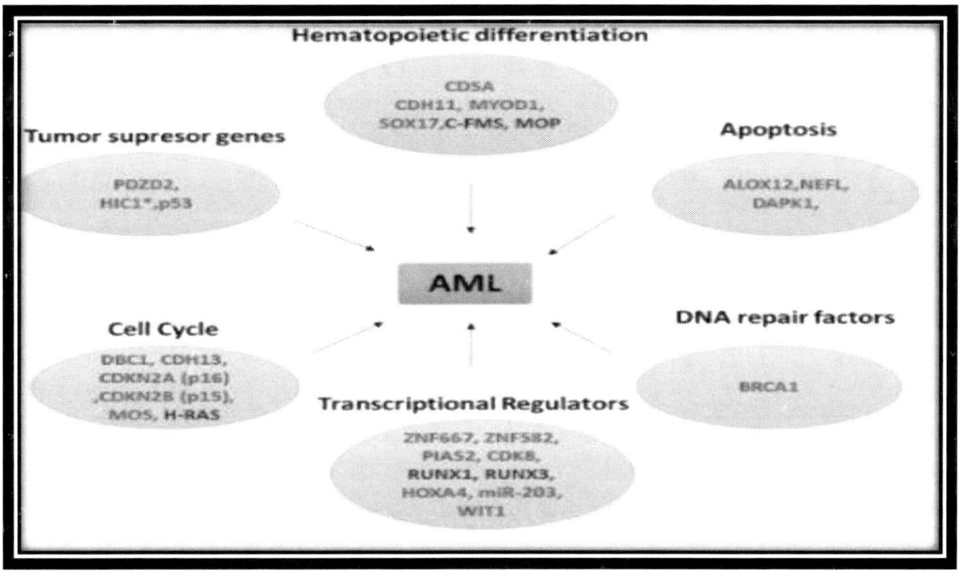

Figure 8. Genes with common aberrant DNA methylation in AML. RUNX1, RUNX3, HRAS, CFMS, MOP are hypo methylated genes with dysregulation increase of gene expression. Others are hyper methylated genes with silenced or down regulated gene expression [36].

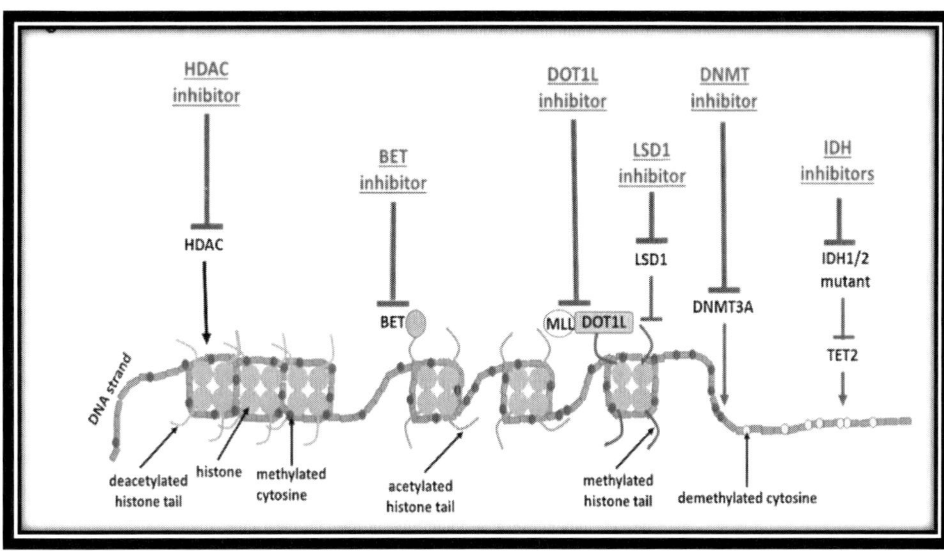

Figure 9. Epigenetic mechanisms of gene regulation through histone acetylation and histone and DNA methylation by various epigenetic modifiers. These epigenetic mechanisms can be blocked by inhibitors at various specified sites [13].

Diagnostic Approach and Analysis

In order to provide more insight into the heterogeneity and biology of acute leukemia and to monitor minimal/measurable residual disease (MRD), several methods to detect

DNA, RNA and proteins have been used in clinical research or clinical settings to integrate molecular information about specific genes, messenger RNA, and protein. These techniques include use of mass spectrometry, chromatography to detect microsphere antibody, Fluorescence *in situ* hybridization (FISH), reverse transcription quantitative polymerase chain reaction (RT-qPCR), gene expression profiling, flow cytometer, and alterations of gene using next generation sequencing (NGS). Consistent nomenclature of genes is also important when naming the specific genes.

Mass spectrometry (MS) is useful for large scale proteomic (protein) analysis. MS can uncover thousands of proteins or molecules without the need for prior probe selection. DNA or RNA detection; however, require prior steps such as RNA extraction, conversion of RNA to cDNA. However, MS techniques is not widely used in detection of leukemia [191]. Affinity proteomic using SEC (size exclusion chromatography) link to MAP (microsphere-based antibody proteins) arrays has been develop. The technique is known as SEC-MAP [192]. SEC-MAP enables the detection of hundreds of proteins in a single sample and provides information about the protein size [191]. MAP array is probed with fluorescent-labeled micro beads that carry specific antibody against specific antigen, while native cellular proteins are isolated from cellular compartments labeled with biotin. The antibody-protein binding is detected using phycoerythrin labeled streptavidin; follow by reading the color code of micro beads population with flow cytometer. The MAP arrays carry antibodies against proteins that are known for leukemia diagnosis such as BCR-ABL1, ETV6-RUNX1 and others, and cluster differentiation (CD) markers and against components of intracellular signaling pathways [193].

Fluorescence *in situ* hybridization (FISH) technique which is able to detect chromosomal abnormalities of leukemic cells was first introduced by Dohner et al. using specific DNA probes to detect single cell in interphase or metaphase. Abnormalities of normal cells can be detected by conventional cytogenetic combined with FISH, which play significant role in assessing risk of leukemia in children or adult [194-195].

RT-qPCR is the gold-standard and is used to monitor patients' responses to tyrosine kinase therapy. RT-qPCR was first used to detect minimal residual disease (MRD) after hematopoietic stem cell transplant in CML patients [196]. However, variability to quantify results from different laboratories need to be addressed first to get standardized and reliable results. The variable results from different laboratories are due to the differences in the RNA extraction, cDNA synthesis, and reverse transcription (RT), preparation of the reagents, platform controls, standard curve, and the possible loss of quantification sensitivity at lower transcript concentrations [197]. International Scale (IS) is used as a way to standardize baseline using 30 pre-treatment samples from the IRIS trial (Interferon and Cytarabine versus ST1571) [198]. The International Standardization Group worked in conjunction with World Health organization (WHO) to get validation. However, using the IS is a labor intensive method requiring confirmation of the local conversion factor on a regular basis, and when there is any change in RT-qPCR step

[196-197]. Several more robust calibrators and reference standards have been developed since. These are: armored RNA (ARQ) (Asuragen ™) technology and ERM-AD623™ that improve comparison of results between testing laboratories worldwide [197,199-200]. Other variation to PCR include LDI-PCR (long distance inverse) and AMP-E (anchored multiplex PCR-based enrichment [198]. When RT-PCR fully quantified correctly, this method provides high sensitive, easy, and fast way to diagnose leukemia.

Microarrays platform consist numerous regularly spaced DNA probes that are immobilized on a solid surface from patient sample labeled with a fluorescent dye [201]. The probe on the micro array may be cDNA or larger genomic fragments. With microarray technology, different approaches such as knowing the amount of RNA being transcript as GEP (Gene expression profiling) could predict the cytogenetic subtype of acute leukemia with accuracy [36, 201]. Mate par whole genome sequencing (MP-WGS) is a method to detect and to fine map specific structural rearrangements where the chromosome breaks [36]. Microarray also can detect genomic DNA level that allow exploration of hundreds to thousands of single nucleotide polymorphism (SNP). Current available microarrays includes Affymetrix™, Illumina™, and NimbleGen™ [202].

MFC (Multiparameter Flow Cytometer) uses panels of fluorochrome-labeled mAbs to identify aberrantly expressed antigens located on or within leukemic cells [203]. MCF with multiple laser is able to detect different fluorochromes by combining multiple mAbs to detect leukemic cells within white blood cells from 10^3 to 10^5 [204]. MFC can detect leukemia-associated immunophenotypes (LAIP) or different-from-normal (DfN) patterns [205]. Researchers continue to work on improving MFC methodology and technology

Next Generation Sequencing (NGS) is also known as massively parallel sequencing or high throughput sequencing technique. The NGS technology combines Sanger and pyro sequencing technique to sequence the synthesis of DNA or to chain terminate DNA but at a much higher throughput. NGS use fluidics technology to release nucleotide flows to synthesize nascent DNA strand enabling direct translation of DNA data to DNA sequence [1, 197]. NGS-DNA technology can sequence millions of small DNA fragments from evaluating a few genes to entire genes [206]. The NGS method can combine with different modern sequencing technologies allowing sequencing DNA and RNA quickly [197]. However, current NGS technique remains expensive and requires bioinformatics who know how to do data analysis. Several hindrances in using NGS includes template preparation, sequencing imaging, quantitative error and possible mistakes in comparing to reference data. Several available NGS technologies includes Illumina (Solexa™) sequencing, Roche 454™ sequencing and Ion Torrent™ (proton, PGM, or semiconductor) [197]. NGS has been proven to be a powerful tool to study the clonal evolution and to discover novel gene mutations [1, 207]. For more comprehensive review and platform comparison between the NGS sequencers, please refer to references #197, 208-210. An optional, but still in distance future is combining NGS with RT-qPCR and microarray analysis techniques. This technique will allow better understanding of gene expression signature and hematopoietic lineage chromosome rearrangement of acute leukemia.

MEASURABLE RESIDUAL DISEASE

Measurable residual disease or minimal residual disease (MRD) is defined as the presence of "post-therapy leukemic cells" below morphologic detection. The MRD is used as prognostic marker to detect risk of relapsed and survival rate of patients with AML [211]. More than 50% adult patients with AML relapsed after attaining complete remission (CR) with induction chemotherapy [212]. Traditionally, assessment of post-therapy remission is based upon cytomorphology. Relapsed AML conventionally defined as ≥ 5% blasts presence in the bone marrow not attributable to other causes [212]. The microscopic assessment using bone marrow or peripheral blood are sometimes unreliable due to the use of small number of cells (200-500) and due to the sample quality. The pathologist's expertise is also important in interpreting the data [205]. Flow cytometer and other molecular techniques for assessment of MRD are more sensitive than morphologic assessment [214]. Flow cytometry have been used to detect CD markers such as CD 13, CD 15, CD 33, CD 34, HLA-DR and others [79]. Other potential markers monitoring MRD includes NPM1, RUNX1, FLT3-ITD, IDH1/IDH2 [79]. Potential marker using RT-qPCR include CBFB/MYH11, NPM1, RUNX1, FLT3-ITD, IDH1/IDH2, t (10; 11)-KMT2A-MLLT10, t (9; 11)-KMT2A-MLLT3, and others [205].

MRD monitoring has become a routine clinical practice for the management of patients with ALL, acute promyelocytic leukemia (APL), and chronic myeloid leukemia (CML) [214]. The correlation between MRD status and relapsed risk has generated interest among clinicians to use MRD testing. Initiating or intensifying therapy after MRD may decrease risk of relapsed and improved overall survival of the patients [205].

CONCLUSION

Aberrant genetic in AML are different than ALL. In AML and ALL, genetic abnormalities such as FLT3, P13/AKT/MTOR, and RAS/RAF/MEK/ERK genes lead to poor prognosis. Epigenetic alterations and DNA methylation are prevalent in ALL and AML. There are similar gene mutations encountered in ALL and AML such as NOTCH or P13/AKT/MTOR. Due to the complex pathophysiologic of acute leukemia, approach using genetic, epigenetic, and proteomic to understand a more comprehensive picture of acute leukemia are needed. As molecular testing methods advancing, testing multiple genes will become more feasible and be done routinely.

REFERENCES

[1] Montano A, Forero-Castro M, Marchena-Mendoza D, et al. New challenges in targeting signaling pathways in acute lymphoblastic leukemia by NGS approaches: an update. *Cancer (Basel)*2018; 10(4):110. Doi:10.3390/cancers 10040110.

[2] Ma Y, Dobbins SE, Sherborne AL, et al. Developmental timing of mutations revealed by whole-genome sequencing of twins with acute lymphoblastic leukemia. *Proc Natl Acad Sci USA* 2013; *110*(18), 7429-7433, doi:10.1073/pnas.12210991
10.PMC3645544.

[3] Greaves MF, Wiemels J. Origins of chromosome translocations in childhood leukaemia. *Nat Rev Cancer.* 2003*: 3*(9), 639-649, doi:10.1038/nrc1164.

[4] Gilliland D, Tallman M. Focus on acute leukemias. *Cancer Cell* 2002;1:417-420.

[5] Applebaum, Frederick. "Acute Leukemias in Adults." In *Abeloff's Clinical Oncology*, ed. Niederhuber JE, Armitage JO, Doroshow JH, et al. 5th ed. Philadelphia: Elsevier Saunders 2014:1890-1906.

[6] Schltz K, Bowman W, Aledo A, et al. Improved early event-free survival with imatinib in Philadelphia chromosome-positive acute lymphoblastic leukemia: a children's oncology group study. *J Clin Oncol* 2009;27:5175-5181.

[7] https://www.cancer.gov/publications/dictionaries/cancer-terms/def/bcr-abl-fusion-gene.

[8] Tasian SK, Loh ML, Hunger SP. Philadelphia chromosome-like acute lymphoblastic leukemia. *Blood* 2017; DOI 10.1182/Blood-2017-06-743252.

[9] Mullighan CG, Su X, Zhang J et al. Children;s Oncology Group. Deletion of IKZF-1 and prognosis in acute lymphoblastic leukemia. *N Eng J Med* 2009; 360 (5):470-480.

[10] Den Boer ML, van Slegtenhorst M, De Menezes RX, et al. A subtype of childhood acute lymphoblastic leukemia with poor treatment outcome: a genome-wide classification study. *Lancet Oncol.* 2009; 10(2):125-134.

[11] Zhang Q, Shi C, Han L, et al. Inhibition of mTORC1/C2 signaling improves anti-leukemia efficacy of JAK/STAT blockade in CRLF2 rearranged and/or JAK driven Philadelphia chromosome-like acute B cell lymphoblastic leukemia. *Ontotarget* 2018;9(8):8027-2041. Doi:10.18632/oncotarget.24261.eCollection 2018.

[12] Small D, Levenstein M, Kim E, et al. STK-1, the human humolog of Flk-2/Flt-3, is selectively expressed in CD34+ human bone marrow cells and is involved in the proliferation of early progenitor/stem cells. *Proc Natl Acad Sci USA* 1994;91:459-463.

[13] Lim SH, Duvielecka PM, Raghunathan VM. Molecular targeting in acute myeloid leukemia. *J Transl Med 2017*; 15:183.

[14] Annesley CE, Brown P. Novel agents for the treatment of childhood acute leukemia. *Ther Adv Hematol* 2015;6(2) 61-79.

[15] Ishida S, Akiyama H, Umezawa Y, et al. Mechanisms for mTOR1 activation and synergistic induction of apoptosis by ruxolitinib and BH3 mimetics or authophagy inhibitors in JAK2-V617F expressing leukemic cells including newly established PVTL-2. *Oncotarget* 2018;9(42): 26834-26851. Doi:10.18632/oncotarget.25515.eCollection 2018.

[16] Evangelisti C, Charini F, McCubrey JA et al. Therapeutic targeting of mTOR in T-cell acute lymphoblastic leukemia: an update. *Int J of Mol Sci* 2018.

[17] Recher C, Dos Santos C, Demur C, et al. mTOR a new therapeutic target in acute myeloid leukemia. *Cell cycle* 2005;4:1540-1549.

[18] Simioni C, Ultimo S, Martelli AM, et al. Synergistic effects of selective inhibitors targeting the P13K/AKT/MTOR pathway or NUP214-ABL1 fusion protein in human acute lymphoblastic leukemia. *Oncotarget* 2016;7:79842-79853.

[19] Krygier A, Szmajda D, Zebrowska, M, et al. Expression levels of the runt-related transcription factor 1 and 3 genes in the development of acute myeloid leukemia. *Oncol Lett* 2018; 15(5):6733-6738.

[20] Ito, Y. Oncogenic potential of the RUNX gene family: “Overview.” *Oncogene* 2004; 23:4198-4208.

[21] Bangsow C, Rubins N, Glusman G, et al. The RUNX3 gene sequence, structure and regulated expression. *Gene* 2001; 279: 221-232.

[22] Fu L, Fu H, Tian L, et al. High expression of RUNX1 is associated with poorer outcomes in cytogenetically normal acute myeloid leukemia. *Oncotarget* 2016; 7:15828-15839.

[23] Cheng CK, Li L, Cheng SH, et al. Transcriptional repression of the RUNX3/AML gene by the t(8;21) and inv(16) fusion proteins in acute myeloid leukemia. *Blood* 2008; 112: 3391-3402.

[24] Neumann M, Vosberg S, Schlee C, et al. Mutational spectrum of adult T-ALL. *Oncotarget* 2015; 6:2754-2766.

[25] Palomero T; Sulis ML; Cortina M., et al. Mutational loss of PTEN induces resistance to NOTCH1 inhibition in T-cell leukemia. *Nat. Med.* 2007; 13: 1203–1210.

[26] Li Y, Buijs-Gladdines JG, Cante-Barrett K et al. IL-7 receptor mutations and steroid resistance in pediatric T cell acute lymphoblastic leukemia: A genome sequencing study. *PLoS Med.* 2016; 13, e1002200.

[27] Seke Etet PF, Vecchio L, Bogne KP, et al. Normal hematopoiesis and hematologic malignancies: Role of canonical Wnt signaling pathway and stromal microenvironment. *Biochim Biophys. Acta.* 2013; 1835:1-10. Doi: 10.1016/j.bbcan 2012.08.002.

[28] Gutierrez A, Sanda T, Ma W, et al. Inactivation of lef1 in T-cell acute lymphoblastic leukemia. *Blood* 2010;115:2845-2851. Doi:10.1182/blood-2009-07-234377.

[29] Campana, D and Pui, Ching-Hon. "Childhood Leukemia." In *Abeloff's Clinical Oncology*, ed. Niederhuber JE, Armitage JO, Doroshow JH, et al. 5th ed. Philadelphia: Elsevier Saunders 2014:1849-1872.

[30] Chen CW, Armstrong SA. Targeting DOT1L and HOX gene expression in MLL-rearranged leukemia and beyond. *Exp Hemal.* 2015;43 (8):673-684. Doi: 10.1016/j.exphem.2015.05.012.

[31] Deshpande AJ, Bradner J, Armstrong SA. Chromatin modifications as therapeutic targets in MLL-rearranged leukemia. *Trends Immunol.* 2012;33(11):563-570.

[32] Perentesis JP, Bhatia S, Boyle E, et al. Ras oncogene mutation s and outcome of therapy of childhood acute lymphoblastic leukemia. *Leukemia* 2004;18:685-692.

[33] Knight T, Irving JA. Ras/Raf/MER/ERK pathway activation in childhood acute lymphoblastic leukemia and its therapeutic targeting. *Front. Oncol* 2014;4:160. Doi:10.3389/fonc.2014.00160.

[34] Forero-castro M, Robledo C, Benito R, et al. Mutations in TP53and JAK2 are independent prognosic biomarkers in B-cell precuros acute lymphoblastic leukemia. *Br J Cancer.* 2017; 117:256-265. Doi: 10.1038/bjc.2017.152.

[35] Hof J, Krentz S, van Schewick C, et al. Mutations and deletions of the TP53 gene predict non-response to treatment and poor outcome in first relapse of childhood acute lymphoblastic leukemia. *J Clin Oncol.* 2011;29:3185-3193. Doi:10.1200/JCO.2011.34.8144.

[36] Prada-Arismendy J, Arroyave JC, Rothlisberger S. Molecular biomarkers in acute myeloid leukemia. *Blood Rev* 2017;31:63-76.

[37] De Rooij JDE, Zwaan CM, van den Heuvel-Eibrink MM. Pediatric AML: from biology to clinical management. *J. Clin. Med* 2015; 4: 127-149.

[38] Kitamura T, Inoue D, Okochi-Watanabe N, et al. The molecular basis of myeloid malignancies. *Proc. Japan Acad Ser B Phys Biol Sci* 2014; 90(10): 389-404.

[39] Hollink IH, van den Heuvel-Eibrink MM, Arentsen-Peters ST et al. Characterization of CEBPA mutations and promoter hypermethylation in pediatric acute myeloid leukemia. *Haematologica* 2011;96:384-392.

[40] Hollink IH, Arentsen-Peters ST et al. Integrative analysis of type I and type II aberrations underscores the genetic heterogeneity of pediatric acute myeloid leukemia. *Haematologica* 2011;96:1478-1487.

[41] Betts DR, Ammann RA, Hirt A, et al. The prognostic significance of cytogenetic aberrations in childhood acute myeloid leukemia. A study of the Swiss Paediatric Oncology Group (SPOG). *Eur J Haematol.* 2007;78;468-476.

[42] Von Neuhoff, Reinhardt D, Sander A et al. Prognostic impact of specific chromosomal aberrations in a large group of pediatric patients with acute myeloid

leukemia treated uniformly according to trial AML-BFM 98. *J Clin. Oncol.* 2010;28:2682-2689.

[43] Torres L, Lisboa S, Vieira J et al. Acute megakaryoblastic leukemia with a four-way variant translocation originating the RBM15-MKL1 fusion gene. *Blood Cancer* 2011;56:846-849.

[44] Hollink IH, van den Heuvel-Eibrink MM, Arentsen-Peters ST et al. NUP98/NSD1 characterizes a novel poor prognostic group in acute myeloid leukemia with a distinct HOX gene expression pattern. *Blood* 2011; 118:3645-3656.

[45] Pabst T, Mueller BU. Transcriptional dysregulation during myeloid transformation in AML. *Oncogene* 2007;26:6829-6837.

[46] Ley TJ, Ding L, Walter MJ. DNMT3A mutations in acute myeloid leukemia. *N Engl J Med.* 2010;363:2424-2433.

[47] Yan XJ, Xu J, Gu ZH, et al. Exome sequencing identifies somatic mutations of DNA methyltransferase gene DNMT3A in acute monocytic leukemia. *Nat Genet.* 2011; 43:309-315.

[48] Valerio DG, Katsman-Kuipers JE, Jansen JH. Mapping epigenetic regulator gene mutations in cytogetically normal pediatric acute myeloid leukemia. *Haematologica* 2014, 99. Doi:103324/haematol.2013.094565.

[49] Brandts CH, Sargin B, Rode M., et al. Constitutive activation of Akt by Flt3 internal tandem duplications is necessary for increased survival, proliferation, and myeloid transformation. *Cancer Res* 2005 65(21), 9643-9650, doi:10.1158/0008-5472.CAN-05-0422.

[50] Scheijen B, Ngo H, Kang H, et al. FLT3 receptors with internal tandem duplications promote cell viability and proliferation by signaling through Foxo proteins. *Oncogene.* 2004; 23(19), 3338-3349.doi:10.1038/sj.onc.1207456.

[51] Yoo SJ, Park CJ, Jang S, et al. Inferior prognostic outcome in acute promyelocytic leukemia with alterations of FLT3 gene. *Leuk Lymphoma*. 2006;47(9), 1788-1793, doi:10.1080/10428190600687927.

[52] Breccia M, Loglisci G, Loglisci MG, et al. FLT3-ITD confers poor prognosis in patients with acute promyelocytic leukemia treated with AIDA protocols: long-term follow-up analysis. *Haematologica*; 2013: 98(12), e161-163. doi:10.3324/haematol.2013.095380.PMC3856980

[53] Kiyoi H, Yanada M, Ozekia K. Clinical significance of FLT3 in leukemia. *Int J Hematol* 2005; 82(2), 85-92, doi:10.1532/IJH97.05066.

[54] Sheikhha, M H, Awan A, Tobal K, et al. Prognostic significance of FLT3 ITD and D835 mutations in AML patients. *Hematol J.* 2003; *4*(1), 41-46, doi:10.1038/sj.thj.6200224.

[55] Abu-Duhier FM, Goodeve AC, Wilson GA, Care RS, Peake IR, Reilly JT. Identification of novel FLT-3 Asp835 mutations in adult acute myeloid leukaemia. *British Journal of Haematology*. 2001;113(4):983-988.

[56] Yamamoto Y, Kiyoi H, Nakano Y, et al. Activating mutation of D835 within the activation loop of FLT3 in human hematologic malignancies. *Blood.* 2001;97(8):2434-2439.

[57] Bagrintseva K, Geisenhof S, Kern R, et al. FLT3-ITD-TKD dual mutants associated with AML confer resistance to FLT3 PTK inhibitors and cytotoxic agents by overexpression of Bcl-x(L). *Blood.* 2005;105(9):3679-3685.

[58] Smith CC, Wang Q, Chin CS, et al. Validation of ITD mutations in FLT3 as a therapeutic target in human acute myeloid leukaemia. *Nature.* 2012;485(7397):260-263.

[59] Sharma Y, Astle CM, Harrison DE. Heterozygous kit mutants with little or no apparent anemia exhibit large defects in overall hematopoietic stem cell function. *Experimental Hematology.* 2007;35(2):214-220.

[60] Thoren LA, Liuba K, Bryder D, et al. Kit regulates maintenance of quiescent hematopoietic stem cells. *J Immunol.* 2008;180(4):2045-2053.

[61] Waskow C, Madan V, Bartels S, Costa C, Blasig R, Rodewald HR. Hematopoietic stem cell transplantation without irradiation. *Nature Methods.* 2009;6(4):267-269.

[62] Wilson A, Laurenti E, Trumpp A. Balancing dormant and self-renewing hematopoietic stem cells. *Current Opin Genet Develop.* 2009;19(5):461-468.

[63] Wandzioch E, Edling CE, Palmer RH, Carlsson L, Hallberg B. Activation of the MAP kinase pathway by c-Kit is PI-3 kinase dependent in hematopoietic progenitor/stem cell lines. *Blood.* 2004;104(1):51-57.

[64] Escribano L, Ocqueteau M, Almeida J, Orfao A, San Miguel JF. Expression of the c-kit (CD117) molecule in normal and malignant hematopoiesis. *Leukemia & Lymphoma.* 1998;30(5-6):459-466.

[65] deCastro CM, Denning SM, Langdon S, et al. The c-kit proto-oncogene receptor is expressed on a subset of human CD3-CD4-CD8- (triple-negative) thymocytes. *Experimental Hematology.* 1994;22(10):1025-1033.

[66] Poli A, Michel T, Theresine M, Andres E, Hentges F, Zimmer J. CD56bright natural killer (NK) cells: an important NK cell subset. *Immunology.* 2009;126(4):458-465.

[67] Reuss-Borst MA, Buhring HJ, Schmidt H, Muller CA. AML: immunophenotypic heterogeneity and prognostic significance of c-kit expression. *Leukemia.* 1994;8(2):258-263.

[68] Cole SR, Aylett GW, Harvey NL, Cambareri AC, Ashman LK. Increased expression of c-Kit or its ligand Steel Factor is not a common feature of adult acute myeloid leukaemia. *Leukemia.* 1996;10(2):288-296.

[69] Ronnstrand L. Signal transduction via the stem cell factor receptor/c-Kit. Cellular and molecular life sciences*: CMLS.* 2004;61(19-20):2535-2548.

[70] Lennartsson J, Jelacic T, Linnekin D, Shivakrupa R. Normal and oncogenic forms of the receptor tyrosine kinase kit. *Stem Cells.* 2005;23(1):16-43.

[71] Kanakura Y, Ikeda H, Kitayama H, Sugahara H, Furitsu T. Expression, function and activation of the proto-oncogene c-kit product in human leukemia cells. *Leukemia & Lymphoma*. 1993;10(1-2):35-41.

[72] Park SH, Chi HS, Min SK, Park BG, Jang S, Park CJ. Prognostic impact of c-KIT mutations in core binding factor acute myeloid leukemia. *Leukemia Research.* 2011;35(10):1376-1383.

[73] Cairoli R, Beghini A, Grillo G, et al. Prognostic impact of c-KIT mutations in core binding factor leukemias: an Italian retrospective study. *Blood.* 2006;107(9):3463-3468.

[74] Malaise M, Steinbach D, Corbacioglu S. Clinical implications of c-Kit mutations in acute myelogenous leukemia. *Curr Hematol Malig Rep*. 2009;4(2):77-82.

[75] Ning ZQ, Li J, Arceci RJ. Signal transducer and activator of transcription 3 activation is required for Asp(816) mutant c-Kit-mediated cytokine-independent survival and proliferation in human leukemia cells. *Blood.* 2001;97(11):3559-3567.

[76] Datta SR, Brunet A, Greenberg ME. Cellular survival: a play in three Akts. *Genes & Development.* 1999;13(22):2905-2927.

[77] Polak R, Buitenhuis M. The PI3K/PKB signaling module as key regulator of hematopoiesis: implications for therapeutic strategies in leukemia. *Blood.* 2012;119(4):911-923.

[78] Shaw RJ, Cantley LC. Ras, PI(3)K and mTOR signalling controls tumour cell growth. *Nature.* 2006;441(7092):424-430.

[79] Harada K, Truong AB, Cai T, Khavari PA. The class II phosphoinositide 3-kinase C2beta is not essential for epidermal differentiation. *Molecular Cellular Biology.* 2005;25(24):11122-11130.

[80] Vanhaesebroeck B, Guillermet-Guibert J, Graupera M, Bilanges B. The emerging mechanisms of isoform-specific PI3K signalling. *Molecular Cell Biology.* 2010;11(5):329-341.

[81] Czupalla C, Culo M, Muller EC, et al. Identification and characterization of the autophosphorylation sites of phosphoinositide 3-kinase isoforms beta and gamma. *Journal of Biological Chemistry.* 2003;278(13):11536-11545.

[82] Vadas O, Burke JE, Zhang X, et al. Structural basis for activation and inhibition of class I phosphoinositide 3-kinases. *Science Signaling*. 2011;4(195):re2.

[83] Fruman DA, Meyers RE, Cantley LC. Phosphoinositide kinases. *Annu Rev Biochem.* 1998;67:481-507.

[84] Fresno Vara JA, Casado E, de Castro J et al. PI3K/Akt signalling pathway and cancer. *Cancer Treatment Reviews.* 2004;30(2):193-204.

[85] Bellacosa A, Testa JR, Moore R, Larue L. A portrait of AKT kinases: human cancer and animal models depict a family with strong individualities. *Cancer Biology & Therapy.* 2004;3(3):268-275.

[86] Kumar CC, Madison V. AKT crystal structure and AKT-specific inhibitors. *Oncogene.* 2005;24(50):7493-7501.

[87] Brunet A, Bonni A, Zigmond MJ, et al. Akt promotes cell survival by phosphorylating and inhibiting a Forkhead transcription factor. *Cell.* 1999;96(6):857-868.

[88] Testa JR, Bellacosa A. AKT plays a central role in tumorigenesis. *Proc Natl Acad Sci USA* 2001;98(20):10983-10985.

[89] Sabatini DM. mTOR and cancer: insights into a complex relationship. *Nature Reviews Cancer.* 2006;6(9):729-734.

[90] Wullschleger S, Loewith R, Hall MN. TOR signaling in growth and metabolism. *Cell.* 2006;124(3):471-484.

[91] Wang CD, Yuan CF, Bu YQ, et al. Fangchinoline inhibits cell proliferation via Akt/GSK-3beta/ cyclin D1 signaling and induces apoptosis in MDA-MB-231 breast cancer cells. *Asian Pacific Journal of Cancer Prevention.* 2014;15(2):769-773.

[92] Machado-Neto JA, Favaro P, Lazarini M, et al. Knockdown of insulin receptor substrate 1 reduces proliferation and downregulates Akt/mTOR and MAPK pathways in K562 cells. *Biochimica et Biophysica Acta.* 2011;1813(8):1404-1411.

[93] Rossig L, Jadidi AS, Urbich C, Badorff C, Zeiher AM, Dimmeler S. Akt-dependent phosphorylation of p21(Cip1) regulates PCNA binding and proliferation of endothelial cells. *Molecular and Cellular Biology.* 2001;21(16):5644-5657.

[94] Liang J, Slingerland JM. Multiple roles of the PI3K/PKB (Akt) pathway in cell cycle progression. *Cell Cycle.* 2003;2(4):339-345.

[95] Evangelisti C, Evangelisti C, Bressanin D, et al. Targeting phosphatidylinositol 3-kinase signaling in acute myelogenous leukemia. *Expert Opinion on Therapeutic Targets.* 2013;17(8):921-936.

[96] Xu Q, Simpson SE, Scialla TJ, Bagg A, Carroll M. Survival of acute myeloid leukemia cells requires PI3 kinase activation. *Blood.* 2003;102(3):972-980.

[97] Kornblau SM, Qiu YH, Bekele BN, et al. Studying the right cell in acute myelogenous leukemia: dynamic changes of apoptosis and signal transduction pathway protein expression in chemotherapy resistant ex-vivo selected "survivor cells." *Cell Cycle.* 2006;5(23):2769-2777.

[98] Min YH, Eom JI, Cheong JW, et al. Constitutive phosphorylation of Akt/PKB protein in acute myeloid leukemia: Its significance as a prognostic variable. *Leukemia.* 2003;17(5):995-997.

[99] Tamburini J, Elie C, Bardet V, et al. Constitutive phosphoinositide 3-kinase/Akt activation represents a favorable prognostic factor in de novo acute myelogenous leukemia patients. *Blood.* 2007;110(3):1025-1028.

[100] Kubota Y, Ohnishi H, Kitanaka A, Ishida T, Tanaka T. Constitutive activation of PI3K is involved in the spontaneous proliferation of primary acute myeloid

leukemia cells: direct evidence of PI3K activation. *Leukemia*. 2004;18(8):1438-1440.

[101] Rosen DB, Putta S, Covey T, et al. Distinct patterns of DNA damage response and apoptosis correlate with Jak/Stat and PI3kinase response profiles in human acute myelogenous leukemia. *PloS one*. 2010;5(8):e12405.

[102] Sujobert P, Bardet V, Cornillet-Lefebvre P, et al. Essential role for the p110delta isoform in phosphoinositide 3-kinase activation and cell proliferation in acute myeloid leukemia. *Blood*. 2005;106(3):1063-1066.

[103] Chapuis N, Tamburini J, Cornillet-Lefebvre P, et al. Autocrine IGF-1/IGF-1R signaling is responsible for constitutive PI3K/Akt activation in acute myeloid leukemia: therapeutic value of neutralizing anti-IGF-1R antibody. *Haematologica*. 2010;95(3):415-423.

[104] Kim SC, Hahn JS, Min YH, Yoo NC, Ko YW, Lee WJ. Constitutive activation of extracellular signal-regulated kinase in human acute leukemias: combined role of activation of MEK, hyperexpression of extracellular signal-regulated kinase, and downregulation of a phosphatase, PAC1. *Blood*. 1999;93(11):3893-3899.

[105] Wortzel I, Seger R. The ERK Cascade: Distinct Functions within Various Subcellular Organelles. *Genes Cancer*. 2011;2(3):195-209.

[106] Padua RA, West RR. Oncogene mutation and prognosis in the myelodysplastic syndromes. *British J of Haematology*. 2000;111(3):873-874.

[107] Paquette RL, Landaw EM, Pierre RV, et al. N-ras mutations are associated with poor prognosis and increased risk of leukemia in myelodysplastic syndrome. *Blood*. 1993;82(2):590-599.

[108] Kiyoi H, Naoe T, Nakano Y, et al. Prognostic implication of FLT3 and N-RAS gene mutations in acute myeloid leukemia. *Blood*. 1999;93(9):3074-3080.

[109] Neubauer A, Dodge RK, George SL, et al. Prognostic importance of mutations in the ras proto-oncogenes in de novo acute myeloid leukemia. *Blood*. 1994;83(6):1603-1611.

[110] Illmer T, Thiede C, Fredersdorf A, et al. Activation of the RAS pathway is predictive for a chemosensitive phenotype of acute myelogenous leukemia blasts. *Clinical Cancer Research* 2005;11(9):3217-3224.

[111] Bowen DT, Frew ME, Hills R, et al. RAS mutation in acute myeloid leukemia is associated with distinct cytogenetic subgroups but does not influence outcome in patients younger than 60 years. *Blood*. 2005;106(6):2113-2119.

[112] Radich JP, Kopecky KJ, Willman CL, et al. N-ras mutations in adult de novo acute myelogenous leukemia: prevalence and clinical significance. *Blood*. 1990;76(4):801-807.

[113] Bacher U, Haferlach T, Schoch C, Kern W, Schnittger S. Implications of NRAS mutations in AML: a study of 2502 patients. *Blood*. 2006;107(10):3847-3853.

[114] Hayakawa F, Towatari M, Kiyoi H, et al. Tandem-duplicated Flt3 constitutively activates STAT5 and MAP kinase and introduces autonomous cell growth in IL-3-dependent cell lines. *Oncogene.* 2000;19(5):624-631.

[115] Karasuyama H, Rolink A, Shinkai Y, Young F, Alt FW, Melchers F. The expression of Vpre-B/lambda 5 surrogate light chain in early bone marrow precursor B cells of normal and B cell-deficient mutant mice. *Cell.* 1994;77(1):133-143.

[116] Shimizu T, Mundt C, Licence S, Melchers F, Martensson IL. VpreB1/VpreB2/lambda 5 triple-deficient mice show impaired B cell development but functional allelic exclusion of the IgH locus. *J Immunol.* 2002;168(12):6286-6293.

[117] Moorman AV, Richards S, Harrison CJ. Involvement of the MLL gene in T-lineage acute lymphoblastic leukemia. *Blood.* 2002;100(6):2273-2274.

[118] Klein F, Feldhahn N, Herzog S, et al. BCR-ABL1 induces aberrant splicing of IKAROS and lineage infidelity in pre-B lymphoblastic leukemia cells. *Oncogene.* 2006;25(7):1118-1124.

[119] Feldhahn N, Rio P, Soh BN, et al. Deficiency of Bruton's tyrosine kinase in B cell precursor leukemia cells. *Proc Natl Acad Sci USA* 2005; 102(37): 13266-13271.

[120] Mullighan CG, Miller CB, Radtke I, et al. BCR-ABL1 lymphoblastic leukaemia is characterized by the deletion of Ikaros. *Nature.* 2008;453(7191):110-114.

[121] Chiu CW, Dalton M, Ishiai M, Kurosaki T, Chan AC. BLNK: molecular scaffolding through 'cis'-mediated organization of signaling proteins. *Embo Journal.* 2002;21(23):6461-6472.

[122] Berridge MJ. Inositol Trisphosphate and Calcium Signaling. *Nature.* 1993;361(6410):315-325.

[123] Vig M, Kinet JP. Calcium signaling in immune cells. *Nature Immunology.* 2009;10(1):21-27.

[124] Saijo K, Schmedt C, Su IH, et al. Essential role of Src-family protein tyrosine kinases in NF-kappaB activation during B cell development. *Nature Immunology.* 2003;4(3):274-279.

[125] Ubelhart R, Bach MP, Eschbach C, Wossning T, Reth M, Jumaa H. N-linked glycosylation selectively regulates autonomous precursor BCR function. *Nature Immunology.* 2010;11(8):759-765.

[126] Ohnishi K, Melchers F. The nonimmunoglobulin portion of lambda5 mediates cell-autonomous pre-B cell receptor signaling. *Nature Immunology.* 2003;4(9):849-856.

[127] Yasuda T, Sanjo H, Pages G, et al. Erk kinases link pre-B cell receptor signaling to transcriptional events required for early B cell expansion. *Immunity.* 2008;28(4):499-508.

[128] Herzog S, Hug E, Meixlsperger S, et al. SLP-65 regulates immunoglobulin light chain gene recombination through the PI(3)K-PKB-Foxo pathway. *Nature Immunology*. 2008;9(6):623-631.

[129] Eswaran J, Sinclair P, Heidenreich O, et al. The pre-B-cell receptor checkpoint in acute lymphoblastic leukaemia. *Leukemia*. 2015;29(8):1623-1631.

[130] Niu H, Ye BH, Dalla-Favera R. Antigen receptor signaling induces MAP kinase-mediated phosphorylation and degradation of the BCL-6 transcription factor. *Genes & Development*. 1998;12(13):1953-1961.

[131] Wossning T, Herzog S, Kohler F, et al. Deregulated Syk inhibits differentiation and induces growth factor-independent proliferation of pre-B cells. *Journal of Experimental Medicine*. 2006;203(13):2829-2840.

[132] Flemming A, Brummer T, Reth M, Jumaa H. The adaptor protein SLP-65 acts as a tumor suppressor that limits pre-B cell expansion. *Nature Immunology*. 2003;4(1):38-43.

[133] Halcomb KE, Contreras CM, Hinman RM, Coursey TG, Wright HL, Satterthwaite AB. Btk and phospholipase C gamma 2 can function independently during B cell development. *European Journal of Immunology*. 2007;37(4):1033-1042.

[134] Nakayama J, Yamamoto M, Hayashi K, et al. BLNK suppresses pre-B-cell leukemogenesis through inhibition of JAK3. *Blood*. 2009;113(7):1483-1492.

[135] Ochiai K, Maienschein-Cline M, Mandal M, et al. A self-reinforcing regulatory network triggered by limiting IL-7 activates pre-BCR signaling and differentiation. *Nature Immunology*. 2012;13(3):300-307.

[136] Amin RH, Schlissel MS. Foxo1 directly regulates the transcription of recombination-activating genes during B cell development. *Nature Immunology*. 2008;9(6):613-622.

[137] Dengler HS, Baracho GV, Omori SA, et al. Distinct functions for the transcription factor Foxo1 at various stages of B cell differentiation. *Nature Immunology*. 2008;9(12):1388-1398.

[138] Fernandez de Mattos S, Essafi A, Soeiro I, et al. FoxO3a and BCR-ABL regulate cyclin D2 transcription through a STAT5/BCL6-dependent mechanism. *Molecular and Cellular Biology*. 2004;24(22):10058-10071.

[139] Nahar R, Ramezani-Rad P, Mossner M, et al. Pre-B cell receptor-mediated activation of BCL6 induces pre-B cell quiescence through transcriptional repression of MYC. *Blood*. 2011;118(15):4174-4178.

[140] Middendorp S, Zijlstra AJ, Kersseboom R, Dingjan GM, Jumaa H, Hendriks RW. Tumor suppressor function of Bruton tyrosine kinase is independent of its catalytic activity. *Blood*. 2005;105(1):259-265.

[141] Kersseboom R, Middendorp S, Dingjan GM, et al. Bruton's tyrosine kinase cooperates with the B cell linker protein SLP-65 as a tumor suppressor in Pre-B cells. *Journal of Experimental Medicine*. 2003;198(1):91-98.

[142] Ryan DH, Nuccie BL, Ritterman I, Liesveld JL, Abboud CN. Cytokine regulation of early human lymphopoiesis. *J Immunol.* 1994;152(11):5250-5258.

[143] Appasamy PM. Biological and clinical implications of interleukin-7 and lymphopoiesis. *Cytokines Cell Mol Ther.* 1999;5(1):25-39.

[144] Harrison DA, McCoon PE, Binari R, Gilman M, Perrimon N. Drosophila unpaired encodes a secreted protein that activates the JAK signaling pathway. *Genes & Development.* 1998;12(20):3252-3263.

[145] Mullen M, Gonzalez-Perez RR. Leptin-Induced JAK/STAT Signaling and Cancer Growth. *Vaccines (Basel).* 2016;4(3).

[146] Heltemes-Harris LM, Farrar MA. The role of STAT5 in lymphocyte development and transformation. *Curr Opin Immunol.* 2012;24(2):146-152.

[147] Malin S, McManus S, Cobaleda C, et al. Role of STAT5 in controlling cell survival and immunoglobulin gene recombination during pro-B cell development. *Nature Immunology.* 2010;11(2):171-179.

[148] Cooper AB, Sawai CM, Sicinska E, et al. A unique function for cyclin D3 in early B cell development. *Nature Immunology.* 2006;7(5):489-497.

[149] Katerndahl CDS, Heltemes-Harris LM, Willette MJL, et al. Antagonism of B cell enhancer networks by STAT5 drives leukemia and poor patient survival. *Nature Immunology.* 2017;18(6):694-704.

[150] Hoelbl A, Schuster C, Kovacic B, et al. Stat5 is indispensable for the maintenance of bcr/abl-positive leukaemia. *EMBO Molecular Medicine.* 2010;2(3):98-110.

[151] Gleissner B, Gokbuget N, Bartram CR, et al. Leading prognostic relevance of the BCR-ABL translocation in adult acute B-lineage lymphoblastic leukemia: a prospective study of the German Multicenter Trial Group and confirmed polymerase chain reaction analysis. *Blood.* 2002;99(5):1536-1543.

[152] Chai SK, Nichols GL, Rothman P. Constitutive activation of JAKs and STATs in BCR-Abl-expressing cell lines and peripheral blood cells derived from leukemic patients. *J Immunol.* 1997;159(10):4720-4728.

[153] Xie S, Wang Y, Liu J, et al. Involvement of Jak2 tyrosine phosphorylation in Bcr-Abl transformation. *Oncogene.* 2001;20(43):6188-6195.

[154] Buettner R, Mora LB, Jove R. Activated STAT signaling in human tumors provides novel molecular targets for therapeutic intervention. *Clinical Cancer Research.* 2002;8(4):945-954.

[155] Hunger SP, Mullighan CG. Acute Lymphoblastic Leukemia in Children. *New England Journal of Medicine.* 2015;373(16):1541-1552.

[156] Litzow MR, Ferrando AA. How I treat T-cell acute lymphoblastic leukemia in adults. *Blood.* 2015;126(7):833-841.

[157] Aster JC, Pear WS, Blacklow SC. Notch signaling in leukemia. *Annu Rev Pathol.* 2008;3:587-613.

[158] Weng AP, Ferrando AA, Lee W, et al. Activating mutations of NOTCH1 in human T cell acute lymphoblastic leukemia. *Science.* 2004;306(5694):269-271.

[159] Goldberg JM, Silverman LB, Levy DE, et al. Childhood T-cell acute lymphoblastic leukemia: the Dana-Farber Cancer Institute acute lymphoblastic leukemia consortium experience. *Journal of Clinical Oncology*. 2003;21(19):3616-3622.

[160] Ellisen LW, Bird J, West DC, et al. TAN-1, the human homolog of the Drosophila notch gene, is broken by chromosomal translocations in T lymphoblastic neoplasms. *Cell.* 1991;66(4):649-661.

[161] Hasserjian RP, Aster JC, Davi F, Weinberg DS, Sklar J. Modulated expression of notch1 during thymocyte development. *Blood.* 1996;88(3):970-976.

[162] Anderson G, Pongracz J, Parnell S, Jenkinson EJ. Notch ligand-bearing thymic epithelial cells initiate and sustain Notch signaling in thymocytes independently of T cell receptor signaling. *European Journal of Immunology.* 2001;31(11):3349-3354.

[163] Allman D, Punt JA, Izon DJ, Aster JC, Pear WS. An invitation to T and more: notch signaling in lymphopoiesis. *Cell.* 2002;109 Suppl:S1-11.

[164] Mumm JS, Kopan R. Notch signaling: from the outside in. *Developmental Biology.* 2000;228(2):151-165.

[165] Wu L, Aster JC, Blacklow SC, Lake R, Artavanis-Tsakonas S, Griffin JD. MAML1, a human homologue of Drosophila mastermind, is a transcriptional co-activator for NOTCH receptors. *Nature Genetics*. 2000;26(4):484-489.

[166] Aster JC, Xu L, Karnell FG, Patriub V, Pui JC, Pear WS. Essential roles for ankyrin repeat and transactivation domains in induction of T-cell leukemia by notch1. *Molecular and Cellular Biology*. 2000;20(20):7505-7515.

[167] Feldman BJ, Hampton T, Cleary ML. A carboxy-terminal deletion mutant of Notch1 accelerates lymphoid oncogenesis in E2A-PBX1 transgenic mice. *Blood.* 2000;96(5):1906-1913.

[168] Hoemann CD, Beaulieu N, Girard L, Rebai N, Jolicoeur P. Two distinct Notch1 mutant alleles are involved in the induction of T-cell leukemia in c-myc transgenic mice. *Molecular and Cellular Biology*. 2000;20(11):3831-3842.

[169] Weng AP, Nam Y, Wolfe MS, et al. Growth suppression of pre-T acute lymphoblastic leukemia cells by inhibition of notch signaling. Molecular and *Cellular Biology*. 2003;23(2):655-664.

[170] Bhanushali AA, Babu S, Thangapandi VR, Pillai R, Chheda P, Das BR. Mutations in the HD and PEST domain of Notch-1 receptor in T-cell acute lymphoblastic leukemia: report of novel mutations from Indian population. *Oncol Res.* 2010;19(2):99-104.

[171] Van Vlierberghe P, Ambesi-Impiombato A, De Keersmaecker K, et al. Prognostic relevance of integrated genetic profiling in adult T-cell acute lymphoblastic leukemia. *Blood*. 2013;122(1):74-82.

[172] Erikson J, Finger L, Sun L, et al. Deregulation of c-myc by translocation of the alpha-locus of the T-cell receptor in T-cell leukemias. *Science.* 1986;232(4752):884-886.

[173] Weng AP, Millholland JM, Yashiro-Ohtani Y, et al. c-Myc is an important direct target of Notch1 in T-cell acute lymphoblastic leukemia/lymphoma. *Genes & Development.* 2006;20(15):2096-2109.

[174] Clappier E, Cuccuini W, Kalota A, et al. The C-MYB locus is involved in chromosomal translocation and genomic duplications in human T-cell acute leukemia (T-ALL), the translocation defining a new T-ALL subtype in very young children. *Blood.* 2007;110(4):1251-1261.

[175] Begley CG, Aplan PD, Denning SM, Haynes BF, Waldmann TA, Kirsch IR. The gene SCL is expressed during early hematopoiesis and encodes a differentiation-related DNA-binding motif. *Proc Natl Acad Sci USA* 2. 1989; 86(24):10128-10132.

[176] Xia Y, Brown L, Yang CY, et al. TAL2, a helix-loop-helix gene activated by the (7;9)(q34;q32) translocation in human T-cell leukemia. *Proc Natl Acad Sci USA* 1991;88(24):11416-11420.

[177] Hatano M, Roberts CW, Minden M, Crist WM, Korsmeyer SJ. Deregulation of a homeobox gene, HOX11, by the t(10;14) in T cell leukemia. *Science.* 1991;253(5015):79-82.

[178] Bernard OA, Busson-LeConiat M, Ballerini P, et al. A new recurrent and specific cryptic translocation, t(5;14)(q35;q32), is associated with expression of the Hox11L2 gene in T acute lymphoblastic leukemia. *Leukemia.* 2001;15(10):1495-1504.

[179] Homminga I, Zwaan CM, Manz CY, et al. *In vitro* efficacy of forodesine and nelarabine (ara-G) in pediatric leukemia. *Blood.* 2011;118(8):2184-2190.

[180] Soulier J, Clappier E, Cayuela JM, et al. HOXA genes are included in genetic and biologic networks defining human acute T-cell leukemia (T-ALL). *Blood.* 2005;106(1):274-286.

[181] Vousden KH, Lane DP. p53 in health and disease. *Nature reviews Molecular Cell Biology.* 2007;8(4):275-283.

[182] Eischen CM, Weber JD, Roussel MF, Sherr CJ, Cleveland JL. Disruption of the ARF-Mdm2-p53 tumor suppressor pathway in Myc-induced lymphomagenesis. *Genes & Development.* 1999;13(20):2658-2669.

[183] San-Jose Eneriz E, Agirre X, Rodriquez-Otero P, et al. Epigenetic regulation of cell signaling pathways in acute lymphoblastic leukemia. *Epigenomics* 2013;5:525-538.

[184] Waddington C. The epigenotype 1942. *Int J Epidemiol* 41:10-13.

[185] Dawson M, Kouzarides T, Huntly B. Targeting epigenetic readers in cancer. *N Engl J Med* 2012; 367:647-657.

[186] Gallipoli P, Giotopoulos G, Huntly BJP. Epigenetic regulators as promising therapeutic targets in acute myeloid leukemia. *The Adv Hematol.* 20115; 6(3):103-119.

[187] Yokota T, Kanakura Y. Genetic abnormalities associated with acute lymphoblastic leukemia. *Cancer Sci.*2016;107-721-725.

[188] Roy DM, Walsh LA, Chan TA. Driver mutations of cancer epigenomes. *Protein Cell* 2014;5:265-296. Doi;10.1007/s 13238-014-0031-6.

[189] Paulsson K, Liljebjorn H, Biloglav A, et al. The genomic landscape of high hyperdiploid childhood acute lymphoblastic leukemia. *Nat Genet* 2015;47:672-676.

[190] https://clinicaltrials.gov/.

[191] Kanderova V, Kuzilkova D, Stuchly J et al. High-resolution antibody array analysis of childhood acute leukemia cells. *Mol Cell Proteomics* 2016;15(4):1246-1261.

[192] Wu W, Slastad H, de laRosaCarrillo D et al. Antibody array analysis with label based detection and resolution of protein size. *Mol Cell Proteomics* 2009;8:245-257.

[193] Slasstad H, Wu W, Goullart L et al. Multiplexed immuno-precipitation with 1725 commercially available antibodies to cellular proteins. *Proteomics* 2011; 11: 4578–4582.

[194] Dohner H, Stilgenbauer S, Benner A et al. Genomic aberrations and survival in chronic lymphoblastic leukemia. *N Engl J Med* 2003; 343(26): 1910-1916.

[195] Goud TM, Al Salmani KK, Al harasi SM et al. Importance of FISH combined with Morphology, Immunophenotype and Cytogenetic Analysis of Childhood/ Adult Acute Lymphoblastic Leukemia in Omani Patients. *Asian Pac J Cancer Prev* 2015; 16 (16), 7343-7350. http://dx.doi.org/10.7314/APJCP.2015.16.16.7343.

[196] Cross NC, Feng L, Chase A, et al. Competitive polymerase chain reaction to estimate the number of BCR-ABL transcripts in chronic myeloid leukemia patients after bone marrow transplantations. *Blood.* 1993;82(6):1929-1936.

[197] Alikian M, Gale RP, Apperley JF, et al. Molecular techniques for the personalized management of patients with chronic myeloid leukemia. *Biomol Detect Quantif* 2017;11:4-20. Doi: 10.1016/j.bdq.2017.01.001.

[198] Hughes T, Deininger M, Hochhaus A et al. Monitoring CML patients responding to treatment with tyrosine kinase inhibitors: review and recommendations for harmonizing current methodology for detecting BCR-ABL transcripts and kinase domain mutations and for expressing results. *Blood* 2006; 108:28-37.

[199] Doleshal M, Magotra AA, Choudhury B et al. Evaluation and validation of total RNA extraction methods for microRNA expression analyses in formalin-fixed, paraffin-embedded tissues. *J Mol. Diagn* 2008;10:203-211.

[200] White H, Deprez L, Corbisier P et al. A certified plasmid reference material for the standardization of BCR-ABL1 mRNA quantification by real-time quantitative PCR. *Leukemia* 2014;29(2):369-376.

[201] Bacher U, Kohlman A, Haferlach T. Gene expression profiling for diagnosis and therapy in acute leukemia and other hematologic malignancies. *Cancer Treatment Reviews* 2010; 36:637-646.

[202] .Mullighan CG, Downing JT. Genome-wide profiling of genetic alterations in acute lymphoblastic leukemia: recent insights and future directions. *Leukemia* 2009;23;1209-1218.

[203] Tomlinson B, Lazarus HM. Enhancing acute myeloid leukemia therapy - monitoring response using residual disease testing as a guide to therapeutic decision-making. *Expert Rev Hematol*. 2017;10(6):563-574.

[204] D el Principe MI, Buccisano F, Maurillo L, et al. Minimal residual disease in acute myeloid leukemia of adults: determination, prognostic impact and clinical applications. *Mediterr J Hematol Infect Dis*. 2016;8(1):e2016052.

[205] Ravandi FWalter RB, Freeman SD. Evaluating measurable residual disease in acute myeloid leukemia. *Blood Adv* 2018; 2(11): 1356-1366. doi: 10.1182/ bloodadvances.2018016378.

[206] Behjati S, Tarpey PS. What is next generation sequencing? *Arch Dis Child Educ Pract Ed.* 2013;98(6):236-238.

[207] Balgobind BV, Zwaan CM, Reinhardt D, et al. High BRE expression in pediatric MLL-rearrnged AML is associated with favorable outcome. *Leukemia* 2010;24:2048-2055.

[208] Quail MA, Smith M, Coupland P et al. A tale of three next generation sequencing platforms: comparison of Ion Torrent, Pacific Biosciences and Illimina MnSeq sequencers. *BMC Genomics* 2012;13:341.

[209] Kircher M, Stenzel U, Kelso J. Improved base calling for the Illumina Genome Analyzer using machine learning strategies. *Genome Biol* 2009; 10(8):R83.

[210] Bragg LM, Stone G, Butler MK et al. Shining a light on dark sequencing: characterizing errors in Ion Torrent PGM data. *PloS Comput Biol* 2013;9(4):e1003031.

[211] Ossenkoppele G, Schuurhuis GJ. MRD in AML: time for redefinition of CR? *Blood.* 2013;121(12):2166-2168.

[212] Walter RB, Kantarjian HM, Huang X, et al. Effect of complete remission and responses less than complete remission on survival in acute myeloid leukemia: a combined Eastern Cooperative Oncology Group, Southwest Oncology Group, and M. D. Anderson Cancer Center Study. *J Clin Oncol*. 2010;28(10):1766-1771.

[213] Chen X, Xie H, Wood BL, et al. Relation of clinical response and minimal residual disease and their prognostic impact on outcome in acute myeloid leukemia. *J Clin Oncol*. 2015;33(11):1258-1264.

[214] van Dongen JJ, van der Velden VH, Brüggemann M, Orfao A. Minimal residual disease diagnostics in acute lymphoblastic leukemia: need for sensitive, fast, and standardized technologies. *Blood.* 2015;125(26):3996-4009.

In: Frontiers in Leukemia Pharmacotherapy
Editor: Lunawati L. Bennett
ISBN: 978-1-53614-960-9

Chapter 3

MOLECULAR AND GENETIC BASES OF CHRONIC LEUKEMIA

Qingyu Stephanie Zhou**, PhD
University of South Florida, College of Pharmacy, Tampa, Florida, US

ABSTRACT

Chronic lymphocytic leukemia (CLL) and chronic myelogenous leukemia (CML) are two different hematological neoplasms which are originate from immune cells. CLL is the *most common* form of leukemia in adults with no cure to date. It is a B-cell lymphoproliferative disorder characterized by the clonal expansion of mature, antigen-stimulated $CD5^+/CD23^+$ B cells in peripheral blood, bone marrow, and secondary lymphoid tissues. Those malignant B cells depend on constitutively activated *B-cell receptor signaling* for survival.

CML is a myeloproliferative disease characterized by the reciprocal translocation [t(9;22)(q34;q11) known as the Philadelphia chromosome (Ph)], which places sequences from the Abelson-leukemia-virus (*abl*) gene from chromosome 9 to the downstream of the Breakpoint Cluster Region (*bcr*) gene on chromosome 22. BCR-ABL oncoprotein are linked to multiple signaling pathways that promote CML cell survival and proliferation.

This chapter focus on the current knowledge of the common dysregulated signal transduction pathways and genetic abnormalities associated with the progression of CLL and CML. Understanding molecular mechanisms implicated in the pathogenesis and progression of CLL and CML is essential to the development of prognostic markers and effective treatment strategies targeting specific molecular events.

Keywords: chronic lymphocytic leukemia, chronic myelogenous leukemia, B-cell receptor, BCR-ABL

* Corresponding Author Email: qzhou1@health.usf.edu.

Abbreviations

ABL	Abelson leukemia virus
AID	activation-induced cytidine deaminase
AKT	protein kinase B
APC	adenomatous polyposis coli
BCR	Breakpoint Cluster Region protein
BCR	B-cell receptor
BLNK	B cell linker protein
BIM	BCL-2-interacting mediator of cell death
BTK	Bruton's tyrosine kinase
CLL	chronic lymphocytic leukemia
CML	chronic myelogenous leukemia
CSR	class switch recombination
DAG	diacylglycerol
DOK1	docking protein 1
EGFR	epidermal growth factor receptor
ERK	extracellular signal-regulated protein kinases
FGF	fibroblast growth factor
FOXO	Forkhead box O
GAB2	Grb2-associated binder
GC	germinal centers
GRB2	growth factor receptor-bound protein 2
GSK	*glycogen synthase kinase*
HCDR	heavy-chain complementarity determining region
HGF	hepatocyte growth factor
Hh	Hedgehog
IAP	inhibitor of apoptosis
Ig	immunoglobulin
IGF	insulin-like growth factor
IP3	inositol-1,4,5-trisphosphate
ITAM	immunoreceptor tyrosine-based activation motif
JAK	Janus kinase
c-Kit	stem cell factor receptor
MAPK	mitogen-activated protein kinase
MCL-1	myeloid cell leukemia sequence *1* protein
mTOR	mammalian target of rapamycin
PDGFR	platelet-derived growth factor receptor
PDK	protein kinase
PI(4,5)P2	phosphatidylinositol-4,5-bisphosphate

PH	pleckstrin homology domain
PKC	protein kinase C
PLC	phospholipase
PPII	polyproline type II
$P(3,4,5)P_3$	phosphatidylinostital-3,4,5-triphosphate
RAF	rapidly accelerated fibrosarcoma
RAS	*rat sarcoma viral* oncogene homolog
RSK	90 kDa ribosomal S6 kinase
SH	Src homology
SHIP1	SH2 domain-containing inositol-5-phosphatase 1
SLP-65	Src homology domain-containing leukocyte protein of 65 kDa SMOSmoothened
SOS	son-of-sevenless
STAT	*signal transducer and activator of transcription*
SYK	spleen tyrosine kinase
VEGFR	vascular endothelial growth factor receptor
ZAP-70	ζ chain–associated protein kinase of 70 kD

INTRODUCTION

Hematopoietic stem cells (HSCs) are mesodermal precursor cells able to self-renew and differentiate into all blood lineages [1]. The process by which self-renewing HSCs give rise to functionally specialized mature blood cells is called hematopoiesis. Under physiological conditions, hematopoiesis is strictly regulated by an intricate network of cytokines, growth factors, microRNA, and transcription factors that control the balance of cellular proliferation, differentiation, morphogenesis and functional maturation to ensure right quantity of different mature blood cell types being produced at the right time. Dysregulation of the molecular pathways involved in hematopoiesis can potentially lead to leukemogenesis, the induction, development and progression of leukemia. Leukemia is a hierarchically organized process similar to hematopoiesis, but originates from leukemic stem cells (LSCs) instead of HSCs. In many aspects, leukemia resembles normal hematopoiesis in that many intercellular and intracellular molecular mechanisms that regulate the normal hematopoiesis also control leukemogenesis.

Leukemogenesis is a multistep process involving the sequential acquisition and accumulation of genetic alterations in HSCs. In general, mutations required for leukemogenesis to occur can be categorized into Class I and Class II mutations [2]. Class I mutations are the activating mutations that confer a proliferative and/or survival advantage to the leukemic cells through constitutive activation of signal transduction pathways. Examples of Class I mutations include mutations leading to activation of the

RAS/RAF/MEK/ERK or PI3K/AKT/mTOR signaling cascades. In contrast to Class I mutations, Class II mutations comprise various loss-of-function mutations that affect transcription factors or components of the transcriptional activation complex, leading to impaired differentiation and apoptosis of hematopoietic cells and aberrant acquisition of self-renewal properties by hematopoietic progenitors. Examples of Class II mutations include the loss-of-function mutations in genes that regulate normal hematopoiesis, such as *AML1*, *CEBP*α and *GATA1*, and recurrent oncogenic fusion *BCR-ABL* at t [9, 22] translocation loci in chronic myeloid leukemia.

1. Chronic Lymphocytic Leukemia

Chronic lymphocytic leukemia (CLL), a B-cell lymphoproliferative disorder, represents the most common type of leukemia diagnosed in adults, accounting for 35% of all leukemia cases in the United States [Statistics adapted from the American Cancer Society's publication, Cancer Facts and Figures 2018]. CLL is characterized by the clonal expansion of mature, antigen-stimulated $CD5^+$/$CD23^+$ B cells in peripheral blood, bone marrow, and secondary lymphoid tissues [3]. During normal B cell development, B cells egress from the bone marrow at the transitional B cell stage and migrate through the periphery to complete their maturation by differentiating into the various B cell subsets, including follicular B cells, marginal zone B cells and germinal center B cells, depending on the distinct micro environmental influences of the spleen, lymph nodes and pleural cavity [4].

Mature B cells that recirculate through the blood and the follicular regions of lymphoid tissues and do not encounter their cognate antigen rely on the continued expression of functional B cell receptors that transduce tonic signals for their survival [5, 6]. In the case of activation and clonal expansion of mature B cells, antigen-induced B-cell receptor (BCR) signaling is required [7]. During adaptive immune, oligoclonal cluster of highly proliferating B lymphocytes within follicles of lymphoid tissues form an area called the germinal centers (GC), which is surrounded by a mantle of resting B lymphocytes. B lymphocytes that undergo intense clonal expansion in germinal centers differentiate into plasma cells secreting antibody and memory B cells expressing high-affinity BCRs [8].

BCRs undergo a process of affinity maturation that is driven by the expression of activation-induced cytidine deaminase (AID), which subsequently mediates the class switch recombination (CSR) of immunoglobulin (Ig) heavy chains to produce the secondary, or memory, repertoire of antibodies [9]. AID is also responsible for the introduction of point mutations in the V gene segments of Ig genes that can alter BCR specificity and affinity [10, 11]. The presence of mutations in the V gene segments of Ig genes is an important molecular indication of malignancies derived from germinal center B or memory B cells, such as B cell chronic lymphocytic leukemia (B-CLL).

1.1. Aberrant Activation of BCRs in Pathogenesis of B-CLL

The BCR is a multimeric *protein complex controlling* B cell homeostasis, differentiation and function [12]. BCR consists of Ig proteins that reside within an immunoreceptor tyrosine-based activation motif (ITAM) [13]. Mature B cells receive two types of signals from their BCRs, i.e., the antigen-dependent and the antigen-independent "tonic" signals [14]. Antigen-dependent BCR signaling is initiated by the activation of Src family tyrosine kinase such as Lyn that phosphorylates ITAM tyrosine residues on the cytoplasmic tails of Igα (also known as CD79A) and Igβ (also known as CD79B) [15]. The LYN-mediated monophosphorylation of ITAMs on Igα and Igβ subsequently activates spleen tyrosine kinase (SYK) through a docking protein 1 (DOK1) and/or SH2 domain-containing inositol-5-phosphatase 1 (SHIP1) [16], and to some degree activates ζ chain–associated protein kinase of 70 kD (ZAP-70) [17].

Downstream of the BCR signaling, activated SYK phosphorylates B cell linker protein (BLNK), which is also known as Src homology 2 (SH2) domain-containing leukocyte protein of 65 kDa (SLP-65). The phosphorylated BLNK in turn serves as a scaffold to mediate the formation of macromolecular complexes by recruiting several other SH2 domain-containing effector proteins including Bruton's tyrosine kinase (BTK) and phospholipase (PLC)-γ2 [18, 19]. BTK is a non-receptor tyrosine kinase belonging to the TEC family of tyrosine kinases, and consists of five structural domains including a pleckstrin homology domain (PH), a TEC domain, a Src homology 3 (SH3) domain, a SH2 domain and a SH1 or tyrosine kinase domain [20, 21]. Interaction between BLNK and BTK enables their translocation to specific membrane fractions and allow them to interact with activated SYK bound to the immunoreceptor tyrosine-based activation motif of BCR, resulting in SYK-mediated BTK phosphorylation at tyrosine 551 in its kinase domain and then auto phosphorylation at tyrosine 223 in the SH3 domain [22].

Activated BTK subsequently phosphorylates PLCγ2, and the activated PLCγ2 hydrolyzes phosphatidylinositol-4,5-bisphosphate (PIP2) to produce diacylglycerol (DAG) and inositol-1,4,5-trisphosphate (IP3), which in turn mobilizes intracellular calcium levels, triggers downstream RAS-RAF pathway, and activates MAP kinase and protein kinase C (PKC)-β [23, 24]. Activation of PKC-β leads to stimulation of the nuclear transcription factor NF-κB and induction of the expression of anti-apoptotic NF-κB-dependent genes such as *bcl-xL* and *bcl-2* [25].

BCR signaling can be activated in the absence of antigen, which is known as tonic BCR signaling and is known to be essential for the survival of mature B cells [5]. Tonic BCR signaling is independent of LYN-SYK phosphorylation, but mediated via the phosphoinositide 3-kinase (PI3K) pathway [26, 27]. When PI3K is activated, it phosphorylates phosphatidylinositol 4,5-bisphosphate (PI(4,5)P2) to generate phosphatidylinostital-3,4,5- triphosphate (PtdIns(3,4,5)P3), which results in the recruitment of PtdIns(3,4,5)P3-binding effectors such as BTK and AKT to the cellular membrane. Following the translocation to the cell membrane, AKT, the key effector of PI3K, is phosphorylated at Thr308 by protein kinase 1 (PDK1) and Ser473 by the mammalian target of rapamycin complex 2 (mTORC2) [28-31]. Activated AKT in turn phosphorylates a number of downstream targets crucial to B cell proliferation and survival of B cells including glycogen synthase kinase 3 (GSK3), Forkhead box O (FOXO) transcription factor and the mTROC1 inhibitor TSC2α [32-34].

In contrast to the unmutated type of B-CLL that derives from mature CD5-positive B cells, the mutated type of B-CLL that shows hyper mutation of the immunoglobulin heavy-chain variable gene segment is likely to arise from GC-derived memory B cells [35]. Regardless of the mutation status, BCRs derived from CLL patients are polyreactive, including reacting with antigens released by apoptotic cells [36-38]. Moreover, CLL-derived BCRs can be activated by the heavy-chain complementarity determining region (HCDR3)-mediated interactions with a variety of autoantigens, including a conserved epitope within the second framework region (FR2) of their own BCRs, to induce antigen-independent cell-autonomous signaling on BLNK activation [37, 39, 40]. Furthermore, when expressed in a cellular system designed to measure BCR signaling cascade activation, CLL-derived BCRs show signaling properties that are equivalent to those of the pre-BCR [39]. In addition, despite the general consensus on the absence of somatic mutation on both CD79A and CD79B in BCR, one study has reported mutations in CD79B [41]. Nonetheless, there is evidence for mutations in BTK and PLCγ2 in the downstream BCR signaling cascade that may confer resistance to BTK inhibition in CLL [42]. Overall, the mounting evidence demonstrates that, despite being structurally normal, BCR functions as an oncogene in CLL and is solely characterized by its autonomous signaling property.

1.2. Constitutive Activation of ERK Pathway in CLL

In CLL cells, several important signaling pathways, such as the activation of protein tyrosine kinase (PTK) via BCR, are defective. In particular, constitutive activation of extracellular signal-regulated kinase (ERK) pathway is commonly observed in CLL [43, 44]. The RAS-ERK pathway plays an essential role in the proliferative expansion of early B cells by transmitting signals from multiple cell surface receptors to transcription factors in the nucleus [45, 46]. In immature B cells, basal activation of the RAS-ERK pathway is controlled by tonic BCR signaling [47]. Tonic BCR signaling positively regulates the activity of the mitogen-activated protein kinase (MAPK) MEK-ERK pathway, which in turn mediates cell differentiation into the transitional/mature B-cell stages [47]. In the unmutated CLL subtype in which the proximal BCR signaling is intact, phosphorylation and activation of ERK are mediated by MEK in response to BCR stimulation [48, 49].

The magnitude and duration of ERK signaling have been shown to be important determinants of the cellular response in CLL. Transient ERK activation induces transcriptional activation of the *MYC* gene but fails to effectively increase MYC protein expression because it does not prevent MYC degradation [50, 51], whereas protracted ERK1/2 activation leads to increased *MYC* gene transcription and stabilization of MYC via phosphorylation [52, 53], suggesting the kinetics of ERK1/2 activation that is critical for regulation of MYC. However, blocking MEK activity reduces but does not abrogate MYC expression [44], suggesting other pathways may contribute to the optimal MYC expression in CLL. For example, it has been demonstrated that stimulation of the surface IgM of BCR induces the activation of NF-κB, and NF-κB may also contribute to MYC expression [54, 55]. The role of ERK in promoting B cell survival is associated with ERK mediated phosphorylation of BCL-2-interacting mediator of cell death (BIM; also known as BCL2L11), which prevents BIM from interacting with antiapoptotic MCL1 [56]. The BCR-ERK-BIM pathway has been documented in malignant cells from patients with unmutated B-CLL, which is relatively more responsive to BCR signaling as compared with mutated B-CLL, as well as a subset of mutated B-CLL associated with progressive disease [57].

1.3. PI3K/AKT Pathway in CLL

The PI3K/AKT pathway controls the expression and function of many proteins that are essential for the trafficking, survival, and proliferation of B cells [58]. The PI3K family comprises eight catalytic isoforms that are grouped into *three* main classes with distinct structure, cellular distribution, mechanism of action, and substrate preference [59]. Among the three classes of PI3K (I, II and III), only Class I PI3K isoforms are clearly implicated in cancer [60, 61]. The Class IA PI3Ks are activated by growth factor signaling through receptor tyrosine kinases (RTK), while Class IB PI3K (also known as PI3Kgamma) is activated by G protein-coupled receptors (GPCR) [62, 63]. The Class IA PI3Ks are heterodimeric kinases consisting of a p85 regulatory subunit and a p110 catalytic subunit. The regulatory p85 subunit exists in *three isoforms*—p85, p55, and p50, while the catalytic p110 subunit in *three isoforms* (α, β and δ) [64]. The p110δ isoform of Class IA PI3Ks (PI3Kδ) is the predominant form in leukocytes and crucially involved in the pathogenesis of CLL as it is the only p110 isoform with a lipid binding domain and can lead to cancerous transformation [65, 66]. Activation of p110δ results in the conversion of PI(4,5)P2 to PtdIns (3,4,5)P3, and subsequently triggers several downstream effects, many of which are mediated by AKT [67, 68].

Similar to the RAF/MEK/ERK pathway, the PI3K/AKT pathway control BCR-stimulated CLL cell survival by inducing expression of several important antiapoptotic proteins, including MCL-1, BCL-XL and X-linked inhibitor of apoptosis protein (XIAP) [69-71]. MCL-1 is a pro-survival member of the BCL-2 family of proteins that plays an important role in the survival of most normal and malignant tissues by regulating the intrinsic (mitochondrial) apoptotic cascade [72, 73]. Activation of AKT inhibits GSK-3 through inhibitory phosphorylation, whereas inhibition of AKT releases GSK-3 from this inhibition to phosphorylate MCL1 at serine 159, resulting in increased ubiquitination and proteasomal degradation of MCL1 [74]. Alternatively, AKT indirectly activates mTORC1 [75], leading to promotion of MCL1 translation through a GSK-3-independent mechanism [76]. XIAP is a prominent protein member of the inhibitor of apoptosis (IAP) with the ability to improve the survival of cancer cells through the inhibition of apoptosis [77, 78]. AKT is functionally associated with XIAP via a feedback loop in the pathogenesis in many cancers [78]. As a result, activation of AKT has been demonstrated to be involved in the protection of XIAP degradation by chemotherapeutic agents in malignant cells [71]. Aberrant expression of Bcl-2 is common in chronic lymphocytic leukemia (CLL) and is associated with poor prognosis and decreased overall survival [79]. BCL-XL is an antiapoptoic factor belonging to the BCL-2 family of apoptotic regulators [80]. Activated *AKT targets downstream* signaling substrates that are implicated in the regulation of apoptotic induction, proliferation, differentiation, and metabolism [81]. One of the downstream targets of AKT is IKKα, which phosphorylation induces the degradation of I-κB, leading to activation and nuclear translocation of the transcription factor *NFκB* and increase in expression of *NFκB* target gene, including *BCL-XL* [82, 83].

2. Chronic Myelogenous Leukemia

Chronic myelogenous leukemia (CML) is a myeloproliferative disorder characterized by the Philadelphia (Ph) chromosome, which results from a balanced *reciprocal translocation* between the long arms of *chromosomes 9* and *22* [i.e., t(9;22)(q34;q11) reciprocal translocation] [84]. The reciprocal (9:22) translocation fuses the breakpoint cluster region (*bcr*) gene on chromosome 22 to the Abelson-leukemia-virus (*abl*) gene on chromosome 9. The *abl* gene that encodes a tyrosine kinase becomes constitutively active when fused to the *bcl* gene. The *bcr-abl* oncogene generates the chimeric BCR-ABL fusion protein. Depending on the breakpoint within the *bcr* gene, the size of the fusion protein may vary [85]. In ~ 95% of patients with CML, the breakpoints within *BCR* map to a 5.8-kb area spanning from exon12 to exon 16 (formerly known as b1-b5. giving rise to fusion transcripts with either b2a2 or b3a2 junctions that generate a 210-kDa protein ($p210^{BCR-ABL}$) [86].

In rare cases of CML and two-thirds of patients with Ph-positive B-cell acute lymphoblastic leukemia (Ph_ B-ALL), the *BCR* breakpoint localizes to a 54.4-kb area between exons e2_ and e2 (minor breakpoint cluster region or m-*bcr*), which generates an e1a2 transcript that translates into the $p190^{BCR-ABL}$ isoform [87]. A third breakpoint cluster region generating the $p230^{BCR-ABL}$ isoform is not found in CML but in chronic neutrophilic leukemia [88]. Overall, the BCR-ABL fusion protein plays an essential role in human hematopoietic progenitor transformation in CML and in promoting the growth advantage of leukemic cells and maintaining the leukemia phenotype [89-92].

2.1. BCR-ABL Constructs and Autoregulation

The human BCR is composed of 1,271 amino acids (aa). Within the first 63 aa is a coiled-coil domain that mediates the formation of homotetramers [93]. Wildtype c-Abl consists of two isoforms (human types 1a and 1b, murine types I and IV), which are generated by alternative slicing of the first exon [93]. The kinase core of c-Abl protein contains an N-terminal cap region (N-cap), sequential regulatory Src homology (SH) 3 and SH2 domains, and a catalytic domain with tyrosine kinase activity [94-96]. The SH3 and SH2 domains are located between aa 42 and 101 and between 101 and 214, respectively, while the kinase domain is located between aa 214 and 474 [93]. The c-Abl SH3 domain comprises two short antiparallel β-sheets and binds to proline-rich peptides that adopt a polyproline type II (PPII) helical conformation [97]. The N-cap region of the Abl kinase core contains a signal sequence for myristoylation, which plays dual roles in regulation of kinase activity and in membrane localization [95].

In the downregulated state of c-Abl, the SH3 domain binds to the linker that connects the SH2 and kinase domains and forms a PPII helix. Regulatory domain interactions are stabilized by binding of the N-terminal myristic acid group to a deep hydrophobic pocket in the C-terminal lobe (C-lobe) of the kinase domain, which induces a bend in C-lobe helix αI, allowing the SH2 domain to dock onto the C-lobe of the kinase domain [98]. Since interaction of the myristoylated N-cap with the C-lobe is critical to maintenance of the downregulated state of c-Abl, mutations of the myristoylation signal sequence or mutations that perturb any of the intramolecular interactions would lead to aberrant activation of the kinase domain [99]. In CML, BCR-ABL fusion protein is 210-kDa containing either the first 927 or 902 aa of BCR. Relative to wildtype c-ABL, the BCL-ABL oncoprotein retains the ABL SH3 domain but lacks *abl* exon 2 *sequences* and myristoylation and gains a coiled-coil oligomerization domain [100].

It has been demonstrated that oligomerization through the BCR coiled-coil domain constitutively dysregulates the ABL kinase, whereas BCR-ABL fusion protein without the N-terminal coiled coil domain fails to induce CML in a murine model, suggesting disruption of BCR-ABL oligomerization as therapeutic strategy for CML [101, 102]. However, complete deletion of the SH3 domain of the ABL kinase can restore cell transformation by BCR-ABL lacking he coiled-coil domain [103]. The possible mechanism is that mutations in the Abl SH3 domain blocks binding of SH3 to a single proline (Pro242 in type 1b/IV c-Abl) in the SH2-CD linker, thereby dysregulating ABL kinase activity [94, 104, 105].

In addition to eliciting kinase activity through the formation of homotetrameric complexes mediated by the BCR coiled-coil domain [106], BCR-ABL also has kinase-independent functions that involve phosphorylation of *tyrosine* 177 in the BCR domain. In fact, phosphorylation of Tyr177 of BCR-ABL is a crucial event for BCR-ABL-mediated genesis of CML, whereas mutation of Tyr177 to phenylalanine (Tyr177Phe) mutant of BCR–ABL diminishes CML disease [101, 107, 108].

2.2. Downstream BCR-ABL Oncogenic Pathway

The presence of many protein-protein interaction domains enables BCR-ABL to form numerous stable and inducible associations with signaling intermediates that engage downstream pathways [98, 109]. Many of those signal transduction pathways play a pivotal role in regulating important cellular functions, including cell differentiation, proliferation and survival. For example, the binding of BCR–ABL to the growth factor receptor-bound protein 2 (GRB2) adaptor is important for activation of the RAS and PI3K pathways, while direct phosphorylation of STAT5 by BCR–ABL leads to the activation of STAT5.

2.2.1. Activation of the RAS Pathway

The mitogenic and transforming activities of BCR-ABL involve stimulation of the RAS pathway, which involves the interaction of BCR-ABL with cytoplasmic proteins that mediate Ras activation. Such cytoplasmic proteins include GRB2, which comprises a single Src homology 2 (SH2) domain flanked by two SH3 domains [110], and the 66, 52 and 46 kDa Shc proteins which possess an SH2 domain in their carboxy-terminus [111]. *Phosphorylation of BCR-ABL* at BCR *Tyr177* is essential to RAS activation. The phosphorylated Tyr177 residue of BCR serves as a docking site for growth factor receptor bound protein 2 (GRB2), which has no catalytic function but serves as an adaptor protein to form signaling protein complexes through one SH2 domain and two SH3 domains [112].

The SH2 domain of GRB2 recognizes specific phosphotyrosine-containing motifs on BCR-ABL [113, 114]. The two SH3 domains of GRB2 bind to proline-rich motifs on the guanine nucleotide releasing factor son-of-sevenless (SOS) and the scaffold adapter protein Grb2-associated binder (GAB2) [115, 116]. As a consequence, the GRB2/GAB2/SOS complex stimulates conversion of the inactive GDP-bound form of Ras to its active GTP-bound state, leading to constitutive activation of RAS downstream mitogen-activated protein kinase (MAPK) and other signaling pathways [117, 118]. Alternatively, GRB2 and SOS could then bind to membrane-bound Shc rather than directly to the receptor. In addition, BCR-ABL upregulates granulocyte–macrophage colony-stimulating factor receptor β common (IL-3Rβc) and IL-3 receptor β (IL-3Rβ) chains, which have been shown to interact with SHC and GRB2 adaptors, leading to RAS-MAPK activation [119].

2.2.2. Activation of the PI3K Pathway

PI3K is a heterodimeric protein composed of a p85 regulatory subunit and a p110 Catalytic subunit. The phosphorylated PI3K p85 subunit forms complexes with BCR-ABL through interaction with CBL and CRKL [120]. CBL, which was originally discovered as the cellular homologue of the transforming gene of the murine Cas-NS1 retrovirus capable of causing pre-B cell lymphomas and fibroblast transformation [121], is a major target of rapid tyrosine phosphorylation upon stimulation of multiple receptor types, including the antigen receptors for T cells [122] and B cells [123, 124], Fc receptors [125], and various RTKs, such as epidermal growth factor (EGF), colony-stimulating factor-1 (CSF-1), and platelet-derived growth factor (PDGF) [126]. CRKL is a 39-kDa SH2, SH3 domain-containing adapter protein that is related to the *CRK* oncogene of the avian sarcoma virus, CT10 [127]. Both CBL and CRKL act as key downstream signaling intermediates of the BCR-ABL pathway [120, 128-130]. In addition to CBL and CRK, GAB2 that is recruited to Tyr177 of BCR-ABL through a GRB2/GAB2 complex is a prominent factor linking BCR-ABL to PI3K activation [131].

Upon the activation of PI3K, the downstream effector AKT becomes active and exerts its cellular functions through phosphorylation of multiple AKT downstream substrates, including mTOR, Bad, caspase 9, ASK1, MDM2, and the forkhead transcription factor (FAKRL1) [132]. In addition to CBL and CRKL, activation of IL-3Rβc and IL-3Rβ chains by BCR-ABL has been shown to turn on the PI3K/AKT pathway, leading to the development of more aggressive leukemia [119].

2.2.3. Activation of the JAK-STAT Pathway

Growth of normal haematopoietic cells is controlled by cytokines. In nornal myeloid cells, cell growth and differentiation are regulated by two cytokins, i.e., granulocyte-moncyte colony stimulating factor (GM-CSF) and interleukin 3 (IL-3) [133, 134]. Nuclear translocation of STATs occurs exclusively after cytokine binding to receptors and is mediated by activation of the receptor-associated JAK kinase [135, 136]. In CML cells, BCR-ABL fusion protein has been shown to either constitutively activates the JAK-STAT pathway via activation of JAK2 and phosphorylation of STAT1, STAT3 and

STAT5 [137-141]. Interestingly, activation of JAK2 in BCR-ABL positive cells does not involve phosphorylation of JAK2 by the BCR-ABL but the interaction of BCR-ABL with the IL-3 receptor β (IL-3Rβ) chains [142]. BCR-ABL may directly activate STAT5 independent of JAK2, suggesting that JAK2 may not be necessary for CML disease maintenance [143].

2.2.4. Wnt/β-Catenin Signaling Pathway

Wnt/β-catenin signaling pathway is crucial to maintenance of hematopoeitic stem cells, including CML stem cells (also known as leukemic stem cells or LSC), with β-catenin being a central mediator of the Wnt signaling [144-146]. In normal cells, a number of proteins including adenomatous polyposis coli (APC), axin, glycogen synthase kinase 3 (GSK3), and casein kinase alpha (CK1α) form the destruction complex with β-catenin [147, 148]. In the absence of an activating signal, phosphorylation of β-catenin by the Axin/GSK-3/CK1/APC complex causes β-catenin to interact with the ligase β-transducin repeat-containing protein (β-TrCP), resulting in its ubiquitination and degradation, executed by proteasome [147].

BCR-ABL signaling is known to directly activate the Wnt/β-catenin pathway through its involvement in β-catenin activation. BCR-ABL mediated phosphorylation of β-catenin at Y86 and Y654 impairs its association with Axin and promotes its protein stabilization and nuclear translocation and TCF4 binding [149]. The WNT-activated Frizzled-LRP5/LRP6 receptors provide additional mechanisms by which Axin can be seized from cytosolic β-catenin thereby blocking its proteasome degradation [150, 151]. Since the Wnt/β-catenin signaling pathway is pivotal to LSC survival, genetic and pharmacological inhibition of β-catenin activity has been shown to synergize with TKI to eradicate LSC, thereby delaying recurrence of CML [152]. In contrast, treatment with TKI alone induces the upregulation of CD70 ligand-induced CD27 signaling, resulting in β-catenin nuclear translocation and activation of Wnt target genes, including NOTCH and c-MYC [153, 154]. Alternatively, TKI exposure induces β-catenin-independent noncanonical Wnt/Ca^{2+} pathway mediated through NFAT signaling, which is able to maintain BCR-ABL^+ CML cells despite BCR-ABL inhibition [155].

2.3. BCR-ABL Independent Hedgehog Signaling Pathway

Hedgehog (Hh) signaling pathway has been implicated in the pathogenesis of various haemopoietic malignancies [156-159]. Accumulating evidence has indicated that Hh signaling is increased in BCR-ABL^+ progenitor cells and is one of the major pathways influencing the maintenance and proliferation of CML stem cells LSC [160-163]. The Hh protein is activated by undergoing an autocatalytical processing in which the Hh protein is also modified at its N- and C-termini by palmitoyl and cholesterol adducts, respectively [164]. The receptor of Hh is Patched (Ptc), which is is a negative receptor because it keeps the Hh pathway inactivated in its unliganded state [165]. In the absence of Hh, Ptc suppresses the activity of Smoothened (SMO), which is the transducing molecule of the extracellular signal Hh following its interaction with Ptc.

Experiments using murine models of CML have demonstrated that Hh signaling was upregulated in a pMSCV/Bcr-Abl/IRES-GFP retroviral vector murine model of CML through upregulation of SMO [163]. *Smo* deletion or pharmacological inhibition results in reduced LSC but has not effect on HSC, and reduces greatly the capacity of LSC to recrudesce the disease in secondary hosts [162, 163]. In fact, binding of Hh to Ptc activates SMO that in turn activates the transcription factor GLI1, leading to reduced expression of NUMB, a Hedgehog-pathway inhibitor, and increased MDM2-mediated degradation of the p53 protein, and suppressed apoptotic responses and/or cell-cycle arrest through repression of p53 targets [166, 167].

Conclusion

Major strides have been made in our understanding of molecular bases of CLL and CML. In CLL, much progression has been made to pinpoint the prominent signaling pathways downstream of the B-cell receptor that affect B cell survival. With the advent of new technologies such as whole-genome, whole-exome and whole-transcriptome sequencing, phosphoproteomics and single-cell analysis approaches, our understanding of the whole landscape of driver mutations and mutational signatures involved in B cell transformation and malignant B cell survival will continue to evolve, and should provide further insights into signaling pathways that are truly essential for the clinical phenotype of CLL and facilitate the discovery of therapeutic compounds that specifically target relevant aspects of the leukaemogenic pathway. In CML, the constitutively activated *bcr-abl* tyrosine kinase is the central pathogenetic event activating multiple signaling pathways and leading to dysregulation of oncogenes during leukemic cell progenitor expansion.

The development of BCR-ABL inhibitors, including imatinib, dasatinib and nilotinib, has considerably changed the standard of care for CML. Since long-term survival has become a reality for many patients with BCR-ABL positive CML, one would assume that there might be much less demand for new therapies. However, acquired resistance to BCR-ABL inhibitors that eventually leads to patient relapse remains a daunting *challenge*. The cause of acquired resistance to BCR-ABL inhibitors is likely to be multifactorial. Further investigation into the underlying mechanisms of the resistance is mandatory in order to develop appropriate molecular therapies to combat the resistance.

REFERENCES

[1] Weissman IL. Stem cells: units of development, units of regeneration, and units in evolution. *Cell.* 2000;100(1):157-168.

[2] Kelly LM, Gilliland DG. Genetics of myeloid leukemias. *Annu Rev Genomics Hum Genet.* 2002;3:179-198.

[3] Chiorazzi N, Rai KR, Ferrarini M. Chronic lymphocytic leukemia. *The New England journal of medicine.* 2005;352(8):804-815.

[4] De Silva NS, Klein U. Dynamics of B cells in germinal centres. *Nature reviews Immunology.* 2015;15(3):137-148.

[5] Lam KP, Kuhn R, Rajewsky K. In vivo ablation of surface immunoglobulin on mature B cells by inducible gene targeting results in rapid cell death. *Cell.* 1997;90(6):1073-1083.

[6] Kraus M, Alimzhanov MB, Rajewsky N, Rajewsky K. Survival of resting mature B lymphocytes depends on BCR signaling via the Igalpha/beta heterodimer. *Cell.* 2004;117(6):787-800.

[7] Treanor B. B-cell receptor: from resting state to activate. *Immunology.* 2012;136(1):21-27.

[8] Gatto D, Brink R. The germinal center reaction. *The Journal of allergy and clinical immunology.* 2010;126(5):898-907; quiz 908-899.

[9] Chaudhuri J, Alt FW. Class-switch recombination: interplay of transcription, DNA deamination and DNA repair. *Nature reviews Immunology.* 2004;4(7):541-552.

[10] Honjo T, Muramatsu M, Fagarasan S. AID: how does it aid antibody diversity? *Immunity.* 2004;20(6):659-668.

[11] Kato L, Begum NA, Burroughs AM, et al. Nonimmunoglobulin target loci of activation-induced cytidine deaminase (AID) share unique features with immunoglobulin genes. *Proceedings of the National Academy of Sciences of the United States of America.* 2012;109(7):2479-2484.

[12] Wang LD, Clark MR. B-cell antigen-receptor signalling in lymphocyte development. *Immunology.* 2003;110(4):411-420.

[13] Herzog S, Reth M, Jumaa H. Regulation of B-cell proliferation and differentiation by pre-B-cell receptor signalling. *Nature reviews Immunology.* 2009;9(3):195-205.

[14] Pierce SK, Liu W. The tipping points in the initiation of B cell signalling: how small changes make big differences. *Nature reviews Immunology.* 2010;10(11):767-777.

[15] Kurosaki T, Shinohara H, Baba Y. B cell signaling and fate decision. *Annual review of immunology.* 2010;28:21-55.

[16] Turner M, Gulbranson-Judge A, Quinn ME, Walters AE, MacLennan IC, Tybulewicz VL. Syk tyrosine kinase is required for the positive selection of

immature B cells into the recirculating B cell pool. *The Journal of experimental medicine.* 1997;186(12):2013-2021.
[17] Gobessi S, Laurenti L, Longo PG, Sica S, Leone G, Efremov DG. ZAP-70 enhances B-cell-receptor signaling despite absent or inefficient tyrosine kinase activation in chronic lymphocytic leukemia and lymphoma B cells. *Blood.* 2007;109(5):2032-2039.
[18] Fu C, Turck CW, Kurosaki T, Chan AC. BLNK: a central linker protein in B cell activation. *Immunity.* 1998;9(1):93-103.
[19] Chiu CW, Dalton M, Ishiai M, Kurosaki T, Chan AC. BLNK: molecular scaffolding through 'cis'-mediated organization of signaling proteins. *The EMBO journal.* 2002;21(23):6461-6472.
[20] Tsukada S, Rawlings DJ, Witte ON. Role of Bruton's tyrosine kinase in immunodeficiency. *Curr Opin Immunol.* 1994;6(4):623-630.
[21] Mohamed AJ, Yu L, Backesjo CM, et al. Bruton's tyrosine kinase (Btk): function, regulation, and transformation with special emphasis on the PH domain. *Immunological reviews.* 2009;228(1):58-73.
[22] Baba Y, Hashimoto S, Matsushita M, et al. BLNK mediates Syk-dependent Btk activation. *Proceedings of the National Academy of Sciences of the United States of America.* 2001;98(5):2582-2586.
[23] Poli A, Mongiorgi S, Cocco L, Follo MY. Protein kinase C involvement in cell cycle modulation. *Biochemical Society transactions.* 2014;42(5):1471-1476.
[24] Follo MY, Manzoli L, Poli A, McCubrey JA, Cocco L. PLC and PI3K/Akt/mTOR signalling in disease and cancer. *Adv Biol Regul.* 2015;57:10-16.
[25] Petro JB, Rahman SM, Ballard DW, Khan WN. Bruton's tyrosine kinase is required for activation of IkappaB kinase and nuclear factor kappaB in response to B cell receptor engagement. *The Journal of experimental medicine.* 2000;191(10):1745-1754.
[26] Srinivasan L, Sasaki Y, Calado DP, et al. PI3 kinase signals BCR-dependent mature B cell survival. *Cell.* 2009;139(3):573-586.
[27] Schmitz R, Young RM, Ceribelli M, et al. Burkitt lymphoma pathogenesis and therapeutic targets from structural and functional genomics. *Nature.* 2012;490(7418):116-120.
[28] Alessi DR, Cohen P. Mechanism of activation and function of protein kinase B. *Current opinion in genetics & development.* 1998;8(1):55-62.
[29] Moore SF, Hunter RW, Hers I. mTORC2 protein complex-mediated Akt (Protein Kinase B) Serine 473 Phosphorylation is not required for Akt1 activity in human platelets [corrected]. *The Journal of biological chemistry.* 2011;286(28):24553-24560.
[30] Chen X, Zhang Y, Wang Y, et al. PDK1 regulates platelet activation and arterial thrombosis. *Blood.* 2013;121(18):3718-3726.

[31] Dangelmaier C, Manne BK, Liverani E, Jin J, Bray P, Kunapuli SP. PDK1 selectively phosphorylates Thr(308) on Akt and contributes to human platelet functional responses. *Thrombosis and haemostasis.* 2014;111(3):508-517.

[32] Ruvolo PP, Qiu Y, Coombes KR, et al. Phosphorylation of GSK3alpha/beta correlates with activation of AKT and is prognostic for poor overall survival in acute myeloid leukemia patients. *BBA Clin.* 2015;4:59-68.

[33] Hay N. Interplay between FOXO, TOR, and Akt. *Biochimica et biophysica acta.* 2011;1813(11):1965-1970.

[34] Szydlowski M, Jablonska E, Juszczynski P. FOXO1 transcription factor: a critical effector of the PI3K-AKT axis in B-cell development. *International reviews of immunology.* 2014;33(2):146-157.

[35] Seifert M, Sellmann L, Bloehdorn J, et al. Cellular origin and pathophysiology of chronic lymphocytic leukemia. *The Journal of experimental medicine.* 2012;209(12):2183-2198.

[36] Sthoeger ZM, Wakai M, Tse DB, et al. Production of autoantibodies by CD5-expressing B lymphocytes from patients with chronic lymphocytic leukemia. *The Journal of experimental medicine.* 1989;169(1):255-268.

[37] Herve M, Xu K, Ng YS, et al. Unmutated and mutated chronic lymphocytic leukemias derive from self-reactive B cell precursors despite expressing different antibody reactivity. *The Journal of clinical investigation.* 2005;115(6):1636-1643.

[38] Chu CC, Catera R, Zhang L, et al. Many chronic lymphocytic leukemia antibodies recognize apoptotic cells with exposed nonmuscle myosin heavy chain IIA: implications for patient outcome and cell of origin. *Blood.* 2010;115(19):3907-3915.

[39] Duhren-von Minden M, Ubelhart R, Schneider D, et al. Chronic lymphocytic leukaemia is driven by antigen-independent cell-autonomous signalling. *Nature.* 2012;489(7415):309-312.

[40] Iacovelli S, Hug E, Bennardo S, et al. Two types of BCR interactions are positively selected during leukemia development in the Emu-TCL1 transgenic mouse model of CLL. *Blood.* 2015;125(10):1578-1588.

[41] Payelle-Brogard B, Magnac C, Mauro FR, Mandelli F, Dighiero G. Analysis of the B-cell receptor B29 (CD79b) gene in familial chronic lymphocytic leukemia. *Blood.* 1999;94(10):3516-3522.

[42] Woyach JA, Furman RR, Liu TM, et al. Resistance mechanisms for the Bruton's tyrosine kinase inhibitor ibrutinib. *The New England journal of medicine.* 2014;370(24):2286-2294.

[43] Petlickovski A, Laurenti L, Li X, et al. Sustained signaling through the B-cell receptor induces Mcl-1 and promotes survival of chronic lymphocytic leukemia B cells. *Blood.* 2005;105(12):4820-4827.

[44] Krysov S, Dias S, Paterson A, et al. Surface IgM stimulation induces MEK1/2-dependent MYC expression in chronic lymphocytic leukemia cells. *Blood.* 2012;119(1):170-179.

[45] Chang F, Steelman LS, Shelton JG, et al. Regulation of cell cycle progression and apoptosis by the Ras/Raf/MEK/ERK pathway (Review). *International journal of oncology.* 2003;22(3):469-480.

[46] Chang F, Steelman LS, Lee JT, et al. Signal transduction mediated by the Ras/Raf/MEK/ERK pathway from cytokine receptors to transcription factors: potential targeting for therapeutic intervention. *Leukemia.* 2003;17(7):1263-1293.

[47] Rowland SL, DePersis CL, Torres RM, Pelanda R. Ras activation of Erk restores impaired tonic BCR signaling and rescues immature B cell differentiation. *The Journal of experimental medicine.* 2010;207(3):607-621.

[48] Richards JD, Dave SH, Chou CH, Mamchak AA, DeFranco AL. Inhibition of the MEK/ERK signaling pathway blocks a subset of B cell responses to antigen. *J Immunol.* 2001;166(6):3855-3864.

[49] Piatelli MJ, Doughty C, Chiles TC. Requirement for a hsp90 chaperone-dependent MEK1/2-ERK pathway for B cell antigen receptor-induced cyclin D2 expression in mature B lymphocytes. *The Journal of biological chemistry.* 2002;277(14):12144-12150.

[50] Sears RC. The life cycle of C-myc: from synthesis to degradation. *Cell cycle.* 2004;3(9):1133-1137.

[51] Vervoorts J, Luscher-Firzlaff J, Luscher B. The ins and outs of MYC regulation by posttranslational mechanisms. *The Journal of biological chemistry.* 2006;281(46):34725-34729.

[52] Murphy LO, Blenis J. MAPK signal specificity: the right place at the right time. *Trends in biochemical sciences.* 2006;31(5):268-275.

[53] Meloche S, Pouyssegur J. The ERK1/2 mitogen-activated protein kinase pathway as a master regulator of the G1- to S-phase transition. *Oncogene.* 2007;26(22):3227-3239.

[54] Bernal A, Pastore RD, Asgary Z, et al. Survival of leukemic B cells promoted by engagement of the antigen receptor. *Blood.* 2001;98(10):3050-3057.

[55] Hewamana S, Alghazal S, Lin TT, et al. The NF-kappaB subunit Rel A is associated with in vitro survival and clinical disease progression in chronic lymphocytic leukemia and represents a promising therapeutic target. *Blood.* 2008;111(9):4681-4689.

[56] O'Reilly LA, Kruse EA, Puthalakath H, et al. MEK/ERK-mediated phosphorylation of Bim is required to ensure survival of T and B lymphocytes during mitogenic stimulation. *J Immunol.* 2009;183(1):261-269.

[57] Paterson A, Mockridge CI, Adams JE, et al. Mechanisms and clinical significance of BIM phosphorylation in chronic lymphocytic leukemia. *Blood.* 2012;119(7):1726-1736.

[58] Ortiz-Maldonado V, Garcia-Morillo M, Delgado J. The biology behind PI3K inhibition in chronic lymphocytic leukaemia. *Ther Adv Hematol.* 2015;6(1):25-36.

[59] Engelman JA, Luo J, Cantley LC. The evolution of phosphatidylinositol 3-kinases as regulators of growth and metabolism. *Nature reviews Genetics.* 2006;7(8):606-619.

[60] Vadas O, Burke JE, Zhang X, Berndt A, Williams RL. Structural basis for activation and inhibition of class I phosphoinositide 3-kinases. *Science signaling.* 2011;4(195):re2.

[61] Jia S, Liu Z, Zhang S, et al. Essential roles of PI(3)K-p110beta in cell growth, metabolism and tumorigenesis. *Nature.* 2008;454(7205):776-779.

[62] Liu P, Cheng H, Roberts TM, Zhao JJ. Targeting the phosphoinositide 3-kinase pathway in cancer. *Nature reviews Drug discovery.* 2009;8(8):627-644.

[63] Condliffe AM, Davidson K, Anderson KE, et al. Sequential activation of class IB and class IA PI3K is important for the primed respiratory burst of human but not murine neutrophils. *Blood.* 2005;106(4):1432-1440.

[64] Davids MS, Brown JR. Phosphoinositide 3'-kinase inhibition in chronic lymphocytic leukemia. *Hematol Oncol Clin North Am.* 2013;27(2):329-339.

[65] Kang S, Denley A, Vanhaesebroeck B, Vogt PK. Oncogenic transformation induced by the p110beta, -gamma, and -delta isoforms of class I phosphoinositide 3-kinase. *Proceedings of the National Academy of Sciences of the United States of America.* 2006;103(5):1289-1294.

[66] Vanhaesebroeck B, Welham MJ, Kotani K, et al. P110delta, a novel phosphoinositide 3-kinase in leukocytes. *Proceedings of the National Academy of Sciences of the United States of America.* 1997;94(9):4330-4335.

[67] Bae YS, Cantley LG, Chen CS, Kim SR, Kwon KS, Rhee SG. Activation of phospholipase C-gamma by phosphatidylinositol 3,4,5-trisphosphate. *The Journal of biological chemistry.* 1998;273(8):4465-4469.

[68] Vivanco I, Sawyers CL. The phosphatidylinositol 3-Kinase AKT pathway in human cancer. *Nature reviews Cancer.* 2002;2(7):489-501.

[69] Longo PG, Laurenti L, Gobessi S, Sica S, Leone G, Efremov DG. The Akt/Mcl-1 pathway plays a prominent role in mediating antiapoptotic signals downstream of the B-cell receptor in chronic lymphocytic leukemia B cells. *Blood.* 2008;111(2):846-855.

[70] Kitada S, Andersen J, Akar S, et al. Expression of apoptosis-regulating proteins in chronic lymphocytic leukemia: correlations with In vitro and In vivo chemoresponses. *Blood.* 1998;91(9):3379-3389.

[71] Dan HC, Sun M, Kaneko S, et al. Akt phosphorylation and stabilization of X-linked inhibitor of apoptosis protein (XIAP). *The Journal of biological chemistry.* 2004;279(7):5405-5412.

[72] Strasser A, Cory S, Adams JM. Deciphering the rules of programmed cell death to improve therapy of cancer and other diseases. *The EMBO journal.* 2011;30(18):3667-3683.

[73] Perciavalle RM, Opferman JT. Delving deeper: MCL-1's contributions to normal and cancer biology. *Trends Cell Biol.* 2013;23(1):22-29.

[74] Maurer U, Charvet C, Wagman AS, Dejardin E, Green DR. Glycogen synthase kinase-3 regulates mitochondrial outer membrane permeabilization and apoptosis by destabilization of MCL-1. *Molecular cell.* 2006;21(6):749-760.

[75] Manning BD, Cantley LC. AKT/PKB signaling: navigating downstream. *Cell.* 2007;129(7):1261-1274.

[76] Mills JR, Hippo Y, Robert F, et al. mTORC1 promotes survival through translational control of Mcl-1. *Proceedings of the National Academy of Sciences of the United States of America.* 2008;105(31):10853-10858.

[77] Hussain AR, Uddin S, Ahmed M, et al. Prognostic significance of XIAP expression in DLBCL and effect of its inhibition on AKT signalling. *The Journal of pathology.* 2010;222(2):180-190.

[78] Hussain AR, Bu R, Ahmed M, et al. Role of X-Linked Inhibitor of Apoptosis as a Prognostic Marker and Therapeutic Target in Papillary Thyroid Carcinoma. *The Journal of clinical endocrinology and metabolism.* 2015;100(7):E974-985.

[79] Schimmer AD, Munk-Pedersen I, Minden MD, Reed JC. Bcl-2 and apoptosis in chronic lymphocytic leukemia. *Curr Treat Options Oncol.* 2003;4(3):211-218.

[80] Xerri L, Hassoun J, Devilard E, Birnbaum D, Birg F. BCL-X and the apoptotic machinery of lymphoma cells. *Leukemia & lymphoma.* 1998;28(5-6):451-458.

[81] Nicholson KM, Anderson NG. The protein kinase B/Akt signalling pathway in human malignancy. *Cellular signalling.* 2002;14(5):381-395.

[82] Suzuki H, Matsuda S, Terauchi Y, et al. PI3K and Btk differentially regulate B cell antigen receptor-mediated signal transduction. *Nature immunology.* 2003;4(3):280-286.

[83] Song J, Salek-Ardakani S, Rogers PR, Cheng M, Van Parijs L, Croft M. The costimulation-regulated duration of PKB activation controls T cell longevity. *Nature immunology.* 2004;5(2):150-158.

[84] Nowell PC. The minute chromosome (Phl) in chronic granulocytic leukemia. *Blut.* 1962;8:65-66.

[85] Shtivelman E, Lifshitz B, Gale RP, Roe BA, Canaani E. Alternative splicing of RNAs transcribed from the human abl gene and from the bcr-abl fused gene. *Cell.* 1986;47(2):277-284.

[86] Faderl S, Talpaz M, Estrov Z, O'Brien S, Kurzrock R, Kantarjian HM. The biology of chronic myeloid leukemia. *The New England journal of medicine.* 1999;341(3):164-172.

[87] Pardanani A, Tefferi A, Litzow MR, et al. Chronic myeloid leukemia with p190BCR-ABL: prevalence, morphology, tyrosine kinase inhibitor response, and kinase domain mutation analysis. *Blood.* 2009;114(16):3502-3503.

[88] Pane F, Frigeri F, Sindona M, et al. Neutrophilic-chronic myeloid leukemia: a distinct disease with a specific molecular marker (BCR/ABL with C3/A2 junction). *Blood.* 1996;88(7):2410-2414.

[89] Daley GQ, Van Etten RA, Baltimore D. Induction of chronic myelogenous leukemia in mice by the P210bcr/abl gene of the Philadelphia chromosome. *Science.* 1990;247(4944):824-830.

[90] Heisterkamp N, Jenster G, ten Hoeve J, Zovich D, Pattengale PK, Groffen J. Acute leukaemia in bcr/abl transgenic mice. *Nature.* 1990;344(6263):251-253.

[91] Kelliher MA, McLaughlin J, Witte ON, Rosenberg N. Induction of a chronic myelogenous leukemia-like syndrome in mice with v-abl and BCR/ABL. *Proceedings of the National Academy of Sciences of the United States of America.* 1990;87(17):6649-6653.

[92] Melo JV, Barnes DJ. Chronic myeloid leukaemia as a model of disease evolution in human cancer. *Nature reviews Cancer.* 2007;7(6):441-453.

[93] Renshaw MW, McWhirter JR, Wang JY. The human leukemia oncogene bcr-abl abrogates the anchorage requirement but not the growth factor requirement for proliferation. *Molecular and cellular biology.* 1995;15(3):1286-1293.

[94] Barila D, Superti-Furga G. An intramolecular SH3-domain interaction regulates c-Abl activity. *Nature genetics.* 1998;18(3):280-282.

[95] Pluk H, Dorey K, Superti-Furga G. Autoinhibition of c-Abl. *Cell.* 2002;108(2):247-259.

[96] Brasher BB, Van Etten RA. c-Abl has high intrinsic tyrosine kinase activity that is stimulated by mutation of the Src homology 3 domain and by autophosphorylation at two distinct regulatory tyrosines. *The Journal of biological chemistry.* 2000;275(45):35631-35637.

[97] Pisabarro MT, Serrano L, Wilmanns M. Crystal structure of the abl-SH3 domain complexed with a designed high-affinity peptide ligand: implications for SH3-ligand interactions. *J Mol Biol.* 1998;281(3):513-521.

[98] Nagar B, Hantschel O, Young MA, et al. Structural basis for the autoinhibition of c-Abl tyrosine kinase. *Cell.* 2003;112(6):859-871.

[99] Hantschel O, Nagar B, Guettler S, et al. A myristoyl/phosphotyrosine switch regulates c-Abl. *Cell.* 2003;112(6):845-857.

[100] Gross AW, Zhang X, Ren R. Bcr-Abl with an SH3 deletion retains the ability To induce a myeloproliferative disease in mice, yet c-Abl activated by an SH3 deletion

induces only lymphoid malignancy. *Molecular and cellular biology.* 1999;19(10):6918-6928.
[101] Zhang X, Subrahmanyam R, Wong R, Gross AW, Ren R. The NH(2)-terminal coiled-coil domain and tyrosine 177 play important roles in induction of a myeloproliferative disease in mice by Bcr-Abl. *Molecular and cellular biology.* 2001;21(3):840-853.
[102] He Y, Wertheim JA, Xu L, et al. The coiled-coil domain and Tyr177 of bcr are required to induce a murine chronic myelogenous leukemia-like disease by bcr/abl. *Blood.* 2002;99(8):2957-2968.
[103] Maru Y, Witte ON, Shibuya M. Deletion of the ABL SH3 domain reactivates de-oligomerized BCR-ABL for growth factor independence. *FEBS letters.* 1996;379(3):244-246.
[104] Van Etten RA, Debnath J, Zhou H, Casasnovas JM. Introduction of a loss-of-function point mutation from the SH3 region of the Caenorhabditis elegans sem-5 gene activates the transforming ability of c-abl in vivo and abolishes binding of proline-rich ligands in vitro. *Oncogene.* 1995;10(10):1977-1988.
[105] Brasher BB, Roumiantsev S, Van Etten RA. Mutational analysis of the regulatory function of the c-Abl Src homology 3 domain. *Oncogene.* 2001;20(53):7744-7752.
[106] McWhirter JR, Galasso DL, Wang JY. A coiled-coil oligomerization domain of Bcr is essential for the transforming function of Bcr-Abl oncoproteins. *Molecular and cellular biology.* 1993;13(12):7587-7595.
[107] Pear WS, Miller JP, Xu L, et al. Efficient and rapid induction of a chronic myelogenous leukemia-like myeloproliferative disease in mice receiving P210 bcr/abl-transduced bone marrow. *Blood.* 1998;92(10):3780-3792.
[108] Chu S, Li L, Singh H, Bhatia R. BCR-tyrosine 177 plays an essential role in Ras and Akt activation and in human hematopoietic progenitor transformation in chronic myelogenous leukemia. *Cancer research.* 2007;67(14):7045-7053.
[109] Nagar B, Hantschel O, Seeliger M, et al. Organization of the SH3-SH2 unit in active and inactive forms of the c-Abl tyrosine kinase. *Molecular cell.* 2006;21(6):787-798.
[110] Lowenstein EJ, Daly RJ, Batzer AG, et al. The SH2 and SH3 domain-containing protein GRB2 links receptor tyrosine kinases to ras signaling. *Cell.* 1992;70(3):431-442.
[111] Pelicci G, Lanfrancone L, Grignani F, et al. A novel transforming protein (SHC) with an SH2 domain is implicated in mitogenic signal transduction. *Cell.* 1992;70(1):93-104.
[112] Pawson T, Scott JD. Signaling through scaffold, anchoring, and adaptor proteins. *Science.* 1997;278(5346):2075-2080.

[113] Pendergast AM, Quilliam LA, Cripe LD, et al. BCR-ABL-induced oncogenesis is mediated by direct interaction with the SH2 domain of the GRB-2 adaptor protein. *Cell.* 1993;75(1):175-185.

[114] Puil L, Liu J, Gish G, et al. Bcr-Abl oncoproteins bind directly to activators of the Ras signalling pathway. *The EMBO journal.* 1994;13(4):764-773.

[115] Buday L, Downward J. Epidermal growth factor regulates p21ras through the formation of a complex of receptor, Grb2 adapter protein, and Sos nucleotide exchange factor. *Cell.* 1993;73(3):611-620.

[116] Egan SE, Giddings BW, Brooks MW, Buday L, Sizeland AM, Weinberg RA. Association of Sos Ras exchange protein with Grb2 is implicated in tyrosine kinase signal transduction and transformation. *Nature.* 1993;363(6424):45-51.

[117] Baltensperger K, Kozma LM, Cherniack AD, et al. Binding of the Ras activator son of sevenless to insulin receptor substrate-1 signaling complexes. *Science.* 1993;260(5116):1950-1952.

[118] Gale NW, Kaplan S, Lowenstein EJ, Schlessinger J, Bar-Sagi D. Grb2 mediates the EGF-dependent activation of guanine nucleotide exchange on Ras. *Nature.* 1993;363(6424):88-92.

[119] Guthridge MA, Stomski FC, Thomas D, et al. Mechanism of activation of the GM-CSF, IL-3, and IL-5 family of receptors. *Stem cells.* 1998;16(5):301-313.

[120] Sattler M, Salgia R, Okuda K, et al. The proto-oncogene product p120CBL and the adaptor proteins CRKL and c-CRK link c-ABL, p190BCR/ABL and p210BCR/ABL to the phosphatidylinositol-3' kinase pathway. *Oncogene.* 1996;12(4):839-846.

[121] Langdon WY, Hartley JW, Klinken SP, Ruscetti SK, Morse HC, 3rd. v-cbl, an oncogene from a dual-recombinant murine retrovirus that induces early B-lineage lymphomas. *Proceedings of the National Academy of Sciences of the United States of America.* 1989;86(4):1168-1172.

[122] Donovan JA, Ota Y, Langdon WY, Samelson LE. Regulation of the association of p120cbl with Grb2 in Jurkat T cells. *The Journal of biological chemistry.* 1996;271(42):26369-26374.

[123] Cory GO, Lovering RC, Hinshelwood S, MacCarthy-Morrogh L, Levinsky RJ, Kinnon C. The protein product of the c-cbl protooncogene is phosphorylated after B cell receptor stimulation and binds the SH3 domain of Bruton's tyrosine kinase. *The Journal of experimental medicine.* 1995;182(2):611-615.

[124] Kim TJ, Kim YT, Pillai S. Association of activated phosphatidylinositol 3-kinase with p120cbl in antigen receptor-ligated B cells. *The Journal of biological chemistry.* 1995;270(46):27504-27509.

[125] Ota Y, Samelson LE. The product of the proto-oncogene c-cbl: a negative regulator of the Syk tyrosine kinase. *Science.* 1997;276(5311):418-420.

[126] Miyake S, Mullane-Robinson KP, Lill NL, Douillard P, Band H. Cbl-mediated negative regulation of platelet-derived growth factor receptor-dependent cell proliferation. A critical role for Cbl tyrosine kinase-binding domain. *The Journal of biological chemistry.* 1999;274(23):16619-16628.
[127] Mayer BJ, Hamaguchi M, Hanafusa H. A novel viral oncogene with structural similarity to phospholipase C. *Nature.* 1988;332(6161):272-275.
[128] ten Hoeve J, Arlinghaus RB, Guo JQ, Heisterkamp N, Groffen J. Tyrosine phosphorylation of CRKL in Philadelphia+ leukemia. *Blood.* 1994;84(6):1731-1736.
[129] de Jong R, ten Hoeve J, Heisterkamp N, Groffen J. Crkl is complexed with tyrosine-phosphorylated Cbl in Ph-positive leukemia. *The Journal of biological chemistry.* 1995;270(37):21468-21471.
[130] Bhat A, Kolibaba K, Oda T, Ohno-Jones S, Heaney C, Druker BJ. Interactions of CBL with BCR-ABL and CRKL in BCR-ABL-transformed myeloid cells. *The Journal of biological chemistry.* 1997;272(26):16170-16175.
[131] Sattler M, Pride YB, Quinnan LR, et al. Differential expression and signaling of CBL and CBL-B in BCR/ABL transformed cells. *Oncogene.* 2002;21(9):1423-1433.
[132] Komatsu N, Watanabe T, Uchida M, et al. A member of Forkhead transcription factor FKHRL1 is a downstream effector of STI571-induced cell cycle arrest in BCR-ABL-expressing cells. *The Journal of biological chemistry.* 2003;278(8):6411-6419.
[133] Warren MK, Rose WL, Beall LD, Cone J. CD34+ cell expansion and expression of lineage markers during liquid culture of human progenitor cells. *Stem cells.* 1995;13(2):167-174.
[134] Baines P, Truran L, Bailey-Wood R, et al. Haemopoietic colony-forming cells from peripheral blood stem cell harvests: cytokine requirements and lineage potential. *British journal of haematology.* 1994;88(3):472-480.
[135] Ihle JN, Kerr IM. Jaks and Stats in signaling by the cytokine receptor superfamily. *Trends in genetics : TIG.* 1995;11(2):69-74.
[136] Schindler C, Darnell JE, Jr. Transcriptional responses to polypeptide ligands: the JAK-STAT pathway. *Annu Rev Biochem.* 1995;64:621-651.
[137] Wilson-Rawls J, Xie S, Liu J, Laneuville P, Arlinghaus RB. P210 Bcr-Abl interacts with the interleukin 3 receptor beta(c) subunit and constitutively induces its tyrosine phosphorylation. *Cancer research.* 1996;56(15):3426-3430.
[138] Xie S, Wang Y, Liu J, et al. Involvement of Jak2 tyrosine phosphorylation in Bcr-Abl transformation. *Oncogene.* 2001;20(43):6188-6195.
[139] Xie S, Lin H, Sun T, Arlinghaus RB. Jak2 is involved in c-Myc induction by Bcr-Abl. *Oncogene.* 2002;21(47):7137-7146.

[140] Shuai K, Halpern J, ten Hoeve J, Rao X, Sawyers CL. Constitutive activation of STAT5 by the BCR-ABL oncogene in chronic myelogenous leukemia. *Oncogene.* 1996;13(2):247-254.

[141] Carlesso N, Frank DA, Griffin JD. Tyrosyl phosphorylation and DNA binding activity of signal transducers and activators of transcription (STAT) proteins in hematopoietic cell lines transformed by Bcr/Abl. *The Journal of experimental medicine.* 1996;183(3):811-820.

[142] Tao WJ, Lin H, Sun T, Samanta AK, Arlinghaus R. BCR-ABL oncogenic transformation of NIH 3T3 fibroblasts requires the IL-3 receptor. *Oncogene.* 2008;27(22):3194-3200.

[143] Hantschel O, Warsch W, Eckelhart E, et al. BCR-ABL uncouples canonical JAK2-STAT5 signaling in chronic myeloid leukemia. *Nature chemical biology.* 2012;8(3):285-293.

[144] Reya T, Duncan AW, Ailles L, et al. A role for Wnt signalling in self-renewal of haematopoietic stem cells. *Nature.* 2003;423(6938):409-414.

[145] Reya T, Clevers H. Wnt signalling in stem cells and cancer. *Nature.* 2005;434(7035):843-850.

[146] Zhao C, Blum J, Chen A, et al. Loss of beta-catenin impairs the renewal of normal and CML stem cells in vivo. *Cancer cell.* 2007;12(6):528-541.

[147] Novak A, Dedhar S. Signaling through beta-catenin and Lef/Tcf. *Cellular and molecular life sciences : CMLS.* 1999;56(5-6):523-537.

[148] Akiyama T. Wnt/beta-catenin signaling. *Cytokine & growth factor reviews.* 2000;11(4):273-282.

[149] Coluccia AM, Vacca A, Dunach M, et al. Bcr-Abl stabilizes beta-catenin in chronic myeloid leukemia through its tyrosine phosphorylation. *The EMBO journal.* 2007;26(5):1456-1466.

[150] Davidson G, Wu W, Shen J, et al. Casein kinase 1 gamma couples Wnt receptor activation to cytoplasmic signal transduction. *Nature.* 2005;438(7069):867-872.

[151] Zeng X, Tamai K, Doble B, et al. A dual-kinase mechanism for Wnt co-receptor phosphorylation and activation. *Nature.* 2005;438(7069):873-877.

[152] Heidel FH, Bullinger L, Feng Z, et al. Genetic and pharmacologic inhibition of beta-catenin targets imatinib-resistant leukemia stem cells in CML. *Cell Stem Cell.* 2012;10(4):412-424.

[153] Schurch C, Riether C, Matter MS, Tzankov A, Ochsenbein AF. CD27 signaling on chronic myelogenous leukemia stem cells activates Wnt target genes and promotes disease progression. *The Journal of clinical investigation.* 2012;122(2):624-638.

[154] Riether C, Schurch CM, Flury C, et al. Tyrosine kinase inhibitor-induced CD70 expression mediates drug resistance in leukemia stem cells by activating Wnt signaling. *Science translational medicine.* 2015;7(298):298ra119.

[155] Gregory MA, Phang TL, Neviani P, et al. Wnt/Ca2+/NFAT signaling maintains survival of Ph+ leukemia cells upon inhibition of Bcr-Abl. *Cancer cell.* 2010;18(1):74-87.

[156] Dierks C, Grbic J, Zirlik K, et al. Essential role of stromally induced hedgehog signaling in B-cell malignancies. *Nature medicine.* 2007;13(8):944-951.

[157] Lin TL, Wang QH, Brown P, et al. Self-renewal of acute lymphocytic leukemia cells is limited by the Hedgehog pathway inhibitors cyclopamine and IPI-926. *PloS one.* 2010;5(12):e15262.

[158] Queiroz KC, Ruela-de-Sousa RR, Fuhler GM, et al. Hedgehog signaling maintains chemoresistance in myeloid leukemic cells. *Oncogene.* 2010;29(48):6314-6322.

[159] Irvine DA, Copland M. Targeting hedgehog in hematologic malignancy. *Blood.* 2012;119(10):2196-2204.

[160] Radich JP, Dai H, Mao M, et al. Gene expression changes associated with progression and response in chronic myeloid leukemia. *Proceedings of the National Academy of Sciences of the United States of America.* 2006;103(8):2794-2799.

[161] Sengupta A, Banerjee D, Chandra S, et al. Deregulation and cross talk among Sonic hedgehog, Wnt, Hox and Notch signaling in chronic myeloid leukemia progression. *Leukemia.* 2007;21(5):949-955.

[162] Zhao C, Chen A, Jamieson CH, et al. Hedgehog signalling is essential for maintenance of cancer stem cells in myeloid leukaemia. *Nature.* 2009;458(7239):776-779.

[163] Dierks C, Beigi R, Guo GR, et al. Expansion of Bcr-Abl-positive leukemic stem cells is dependent on Hedgehog pathway activation. *Cancer cell.* 2008;14(3):238-249.

[164] Briscoe J, Therond PP. The mechanisms of Hedgehog signalling and its roles in development and disease. *Nature reviews Molecular cell biology.* 2013;14(7):416-429.

[165] Ingham PW, Taylor AM, Nakano Y. Role of the Drosophila patched gene in positional signalling. *Nature.* 1991;353(6340):184-187.

[166] Di Marcotullio L, Ferretti E, Greco A, et al. Numb is a suppressor of Hedgehog signalling and targets Gli1 for Itch-dependent ubiquitination. *Nature cell biology.* 2006;8(12):1415-1423.

[167] Liu L, Lanner F, Lendahl U, Das D. Numblike and Numb differentially affect p53 and Sonic Hedgehog signaling. *Biochemical and biophysical research communications.* 2011;413(3):426-431.

In: Frontiers in Leukemia Pharmacotherapy
Editor: Lunawati L. Bennett
ISBN: 978-1-53614-960-9

Chapter 4

LEUKEMIA PHARMACOLOGY

Lunawati L. Bennett*, PhD, PharmD
Union University, College of Pharmacy, Jackson, Tennessee, US

ABSTRACT

Cancer drug development continues to expand fast since 1964 when there were only 12 drugs marketed for the treatment. Besides the increase in the number of drugs available to treat cancer, there is fundamentally a changed in how oncologists and researchers prescribe and develop drugs. Drugs are now formulated to be narrower indicated to target cancer cells specifically and to prevent undesirable adverse events to the normal cells. The basis of the success or failure of the drug therapy is to match the instrinsic sensitivity of the cancer. The drug with perfect, narrow match and suitable concentration to kill cancer cells without severe adverse events affecting the normal cells will be the desire of every scientists to develop.

This chapter highlight drugs that have been used traditionally either as monotherapy or in combination, new small synthetic molecules, and biologics such as monoclonal antibodies (mAbs) or mAbs that are conjugated to toxins. Combination therapy known as VAMP (vincristine, aminopterin, 6-mercaptopurine, and prednisone) regimens and others will be mentioned briefly. Chapters 6-13 describes in detail the dosing and dose on how chemotherapeutic drug (s) is/are being administered.

Keywords: lenalidomide, L-asparaginase, rituximab, CD20, CD33, FLT3, FLAG, HiDAC, FCR, VAMP, methotrexate, cytarabine, 6-mercaptopurine, vincristine, bendamustine, fludarabine, cyclophosphamide, all-trans retinoic acid, arsenic trioxide, gemtuzumab, chloroambucil

* Corresponding Author Email: llbennett@uu.edu.

ABBREVIATIONS

CD	cluster differentiation
IL	interleukin
MDS	myelodysplastic syndrome
MM	multiple myeloma
ALL	acute lymphocytic leukemia
AML	acute myeloid leukemia
CML	chronic myeloid leukemia
CLL	chronic lymphocytic leukemia
APL	acute promyelocytic leukemia
FDA	Food and Drug Administration
CNS	central nervous system
FLAG	fludarabine, cytarabine, filgrastim regimen
HiDAC	high dose cytarabine
FCR	fludarabine, cyclophosphamide, rituximab regimen
VAMP	vincristine, aminopterin, 6-mercaptopurine, prednisone regimen
BR	bendamustine and rituximab regimen
IDH	isocitrate dehydrogenase
ATRA	all-trans retinoic acid
ATO	arsenic trioxide
DNA	deoxyribose nucleic acids
RNA	ribonucleic acids
DMTI	DNA methyl transferase inhibitor
6-MP	6-mercapto purine
MTX	methotrexate
TPMT	thiopurine S-methyl transferase
FGM	filgrastim
mAbs	monoclonal antibodies
i.v.	intravenous
s.c.	subcutaneous
L-ASP	L-asparaginase
5-FU	5 fluoro uracil

INTRODUCTION

For successful cancer therapy, drugs with less severe adverse events and better delivery to the cancer cells with high efficacy to prevent and minimize relapse is the desire of every scientists when develop the drugs. Understanding the linkage between drug actions (pharmacodynamics, PD) and drug delivery (pharmacokinetic, PK) continues to be a major challenge in leukemia pharmacology. In leukemia pharmacology, the basis for success or failure of drug therapy is the ability to find a treatment that is matched to the intrinsic sensitivity of the cancer cells. The perfect match can still fail if the drug is not delivered to the cancer cells at the correct concentration to kill the cells nor if high concentrations are needed but cause severe toxicities [1]. Besides PK and PD, pharmacogenomics (PG) profile of the patients is another important factor that need to be considered. PG contributes to how individual responds to drugs. There are a subset of patients who respond as fast metabolizers, intermediate/extensive or poor metabolizers which can cause sub-, correct-, or supra-therapeutics outcomes, respectively.

Many cancers require combination drugs to be effective. It is rare to use a single drug in cancer treatment. Within a combinational chemotherapy regimen, the drugs are intended to interact at PD level with non-overlapping toxicities. Most combinations are used based on a preexisting scientific rationale or by an addition of a new agent to an established regimen [1].

In choosing the drug regimen, several factors need to be considered such as volume of distribution and protein binding to determine drug formulation, half-life to determine dose interval, bioavailability to determine the concentration of the drug that reach systemic circulation, the patient's organ function, drug-drug or drug food interactions. Intravenous (i.v.) route is the predominant route of administration in cancer therapy. Drug is titrated based on the patient's body weight and body surface area. Intravenous administration will continue to be important regimens or if the drug can't be delivered *via* oral route. Many of the new drugs which are under development, especially for chronic daily dosing, are projected to be in oral formulations [2].

VAMP and Hyper CVAD Regimens

The intent of induction therapy in acute lymphocytic leukemia (ALL) is to reduce the initial leukemic cells to more than 99% eradication. The routine therapy is using VAMP (vincristine, aminopterin, 6-mercaptopurine, and prednisone) [3-4]. Although the regimen have evolved over time, the majority of adult and pediatric ALL regimens are still include antracycline (doxorubicin, daunorubicin), corticosteroids (prednisone, dexamethasone), vincristine, cyclophosphamide, methotrexate, etoposide, cytarabine and 6-mercaptopurine. The most common regimen is hyper-CVAD which contains 8 alternatives i.v. cycles as regimen A and B. Regimen A includes cyclophosphamide, vincristine, doxorubicin, and dexamethasone, while regimen B includes methotrexate and cytarabine [3-4].

FLAG AND FLAG-IDA REGIMENS

Fludarabine, cytarabine and filgrastim (FLAG) regimen has become popular for post remission therapy in acute myeloid leukemia (AML) or high risk myelodysplastic syndrome (MDS) [5-7]. The clinical effects of cytarabine is highly dependent on the intracellular conversion of cytarabine to its active metabolite ARA-C-5-triphosphate (ARA-CTP) which is then incorporated into deoxyribonucleic acid (DNA) resulting in leukemic cell death. The accumulation of ARA-CTP can be increased with the addition of fludarabine. Granulocyte colony stimulating factor (G-CSF) such as filgrastim is usually added as prophylactic for patients at high-risk experiencing febrile neutropenia [5-8]. Addition of idarubicin to FLAG regimen (FLAG-IDA) have also been tried with tolerable toxicity in younger patient. Lower dose of FLAG-IDA regimen also showed promising results [8-9].

FCR REGIMEN

Fludarabine, cyclophosphamide and rituximab (FCR) have been used as standard cares for younger, physically fit patients with previously untreated chronic lymphocytic leukemia (CLL). Rituximab can be given as i.v. or subcutaneous (s.c.) to improve patient's convenience. The s.c. dose of rituximab is formulated at 12 fold more concentrated than i.v. [10]. The s.c. formulation of rituximab has recombinant human hyaluronidase to cause C_{trough} concentration of rituximab after administration similar or higher than i.v. formulation [10-11]. As oral fludarabine and cytarabine are already available, and with s.c. rituximab, this represent important advancement in leukemia chemotherapy for patient's convenience [12].

FLUDARABINE

Fludarabine (Fludara ®, Oforta®) is a purine analog that is rapidly dephosphorylated to 2-fluoro-arabino furanosyl adenosine, which is then phosphorylated intracellularly by deoxycytidine kinase to the triphosphate. The triphosphate is then incorporated into DNA causing inhibition of DNA synthesis and functions [13-15]. It is also works as a potent immunosuppressant with inhibitory effects on CD4 and CD8 T cells. This drug is mainly used for non-Hodgins's lymphoma and CLL in combination with others. The main dose limiting toxicity is myelosuppression [13-16]. The drug induces more complete remission (CR) than other chemotherapeutic agents [15]. Because of possible risk of developing infection by *Pneumocystis Jirovecii* pneumonia (PCP), patients should receive prophylaxis with trimethoprim sulfamethoxazole for three times weekly and continue for up to 1 year after stopping chemotherapy [16]. Although it has been used with cytarabine, some studies showed that the combination is similar to fludarabine monotherapy [15].

CYTARABINE

Cytarabine (Depocyt®) or arabinosylcytosine is a deoxycytidine analog that has been on the market for over 50 years [4]. It is an antimetabolite known as 4-amino-1-B-D arabinofuranosyl-2 (1H)-pyrimidone that is converted and metabolized to the main cytotoxic metabolite, ara - cytarabine triphosphate, which cause inhibition of DNA polymerase or chain prolongation causing termination of the leukemic cells [17-19]. This drug also causes inhibition of Akt-mTOR pathway which is dysregulated in cancer cells [20-21]. Cytarabine can be given as s.c, intramuscular (i.m.), or i.v. High dose administration (greater than 500 mg/mL) *via* i.v. over a 5-7 day period shown serum level of 10^5 mol/L that is correlated with death of leukemic cells [17-19]. Normal cytarabine is usually given at the dose of 100 – 200 mg/m^2 every 12 hours. An alternative therapy using high dose cytarabine (HiDAC) at 1000 – 3000 mg/m^2 every 12 hours thought to cause higher intracellular level of the drug that can help overcome minimal residual disease (MRD) and preventing drug resistance. However, the benefit of HiDAC as compare to the normal dose is still controversial issue due to the questionable survival benefits and toxicity complications [22].

Cytarabine is distributed widely to the tissue. The drug has half-life of 10 minutes. Primary metabolism occurs in the liver follow by excretion in the urine [20]. Adverse events include nausea, vomiting, diarrhea, myelosuppression, and severe neurotoxicity with fever like symptoms, ocular, irregular heartbeat, dyspnea, and respiratory distress [17-19]. Myelosuppression that requires platelet transfusions and cause prolonged hospitalization are seen in patients older than 60 years; therefore, this drug should be avoided in this age group [20]. Primary care providers must check hepatic function of the patient prior to the administration and modify dosage schedules based on the peak extracellular concentration.

ANTRACYCLINES - DOXORUBICIN, DAUNORUBICIN, IDARUBICIN MITOXANTRONE

Several drugs belong to the family of antracyclines, an antibiotic isolated from *Streptomyces peucetius var caesius* [19]. These drugs are: doxorubicin, daunorubicin, idarubicin, epirubicin and mitoxantrone. The antracyclines exert their cytotoxic action through 4 major mechanisms: 1) DNA intercalation blocking transcription and replication of DNA and RNA (ribonucleic acids); 2) inhibition of topoisomerase II activity by binding to the DNA-topoisomerase II α complex; 3) production of free radicals and reactive oxygen species (ROS) which affect metabolic process of the cells; and 4) alteration of cellular membrane fluidity and ion transport of the cancer cells [19, 23-25].

Doxorubicin (Adriamycin®, Doxil®) is a very important anticancer drug with activity against cancers of breast, liver, lung, endometrial, ovarian, testicular, thyroid, stomach, multiple myeloma, bone, brain, and ALL [19, 23-25]. Doxorubicin has been found to work better as a combination therapy rather than as a monotherapy. A retrospective study found that there were no differences between monotherapy of doxorubin and combination therapy with overall survival (OS) the same, but most studies suggested combination therapy had a better response rate, longer time of treatment failure, longer period of recurrence, lower treatment-related death and cancer-related death than the monotherapy [26]. Combination therapy usually includes cyclophosphamide, cisplatin, and 5 fluorouracil (5-FU) [19]. Because the toxicity of doxorubicin in causing heart failure at the cumulative dose of 550 mg/m^2, the use of smaller or divided dose can decrease the likelihood of developing heart failure [27].

Daunorubicin (DaunoXome ®) was the first drug of the anthracyclines family to be clinically isolated, which is still used for AML, but has limited use in solid cancer [19]. For decades, the standard care for AML has been combination of cytarabine and daunorubicin as a combination of 7+3. Recently, a liposomal-encapsulated combination ratio of daunorubicin at 1 molar and cytarabine at 5 molar was approved by the FDA as Vyxeos ® for the treatment of therapy-related AML (tAML) and AML with myelodysplasia (MDS) [28].

Idarubicin is a semisynthetic glycose analog of daunorubicin which when being combined with cytarabine appears to be better producing CR and improving survival of AML patients better than daunorubicin [19]. This is thought due to idarubicin is less sensitive to p-glycoprotein mediated drug efflux than daunorubicin [19]. Unlike other antracyclines, idarubicin can be given as oral [29].

Mitoxantrone (Novantrone ®) is anthracene that resemble anthracycline ring. It works by binding to DNA of leukemic cells to produce strand break and to inhibit DNA and RNA synthesis. It is also works as topoisomerase II inhibitor. Dose limiting toxicity are nausea, vomiting, mucositis, alopecia, and myelosuppression. Acute and chronic cardiac toxicity is similar like doxorubicin. In addition, drugs that work as topoisomerase II inhibitors including mitoxantrone, etoposide and doxorubicin are linked to cause the development of tAML with chromosomal rearrangement at band 11q23 and acute promyelocytic leukemia with t(15:17) rearrangement [30].

Antracyclines are susceptible to resistance due to cancer cells can repair their DNA and continue to survive [31-33]. Antracyclines cause myelosuppression, mucosititis and cardio toxicity showing as arrhythmias, dilated cardiomyopathy with heart failure, which can occur even 24 hours after a single dose or can happen years later due to the generation of ROS within myocardium [30-33].

ETOPOSIDE

Etoposide (VePesid®, Etopophos®) is a topoisomerase II inhibitor that works by blocking the coiling and uncoiling of the DNA helix, therefore causing DNA strand to break. Topoisomerase II are essential enzymes that modulate DNA under- and over winding, knotting and tangling by introducing transient double stranded breaks into the genetic material, transporting an intact double helix (T segment) through the cleaved DNA gate (G segment) and resealing the original break [34-35]. In order to maintain genomic integrity while the G-segment is cleaved, topoisomerase II covalently attaches the newly DNA forming cleavage of complex [36]. Proposed mechanism of etoposide is depicted in Figure 1 [31]. Pendleton et al. proposed that "if the level of topoisomerase II-mediated DNA cleavage decreases below threshold levels, cells are not able to untangle daughter chromosomes and ultimately die of mitotic failure (left). If the level of cleavage becomes too high (right), the action of DNA tracking systems can convert these transient complexes to permanent double-stranded breaks. The resulting DNA breaks and the inhibition of essential DNA process, initiate recombination/repair pathways and generate chromosome translocation and other DNA aberration. If the strand breaks overwhelm the cell, they can trigger cell death [31].

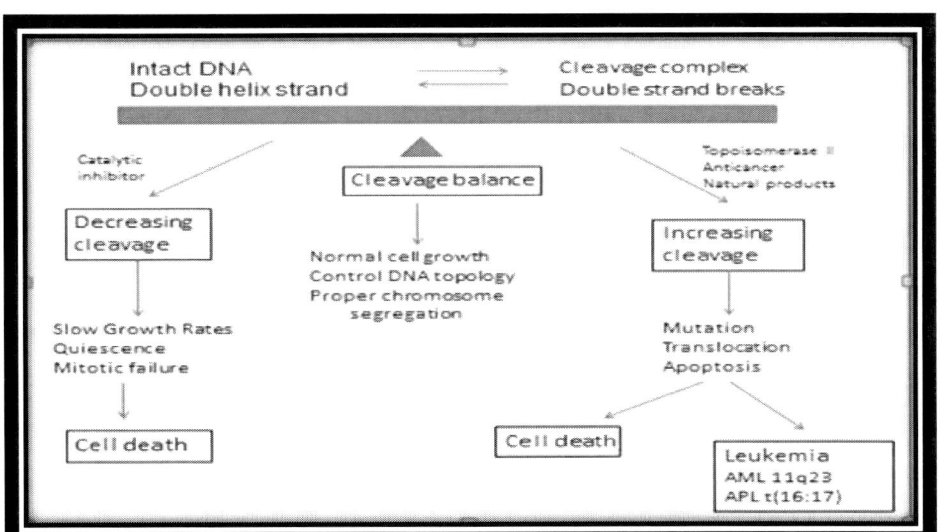

Figure 1. Schematic mechanism of topoisomerase II causing malignant formation [31].

Alkylating Agents - Cyclophosphamide, Bendamustine, Busulfan

Cyclophosphamide (Cytoxan ®, Neosar ®) is an alkylating drug that exerts its toxicity by transferring its alkyl groups to cancer cells forming DNA cross-links resulting in inhibition of DNA synthesis and function [19]. It is inactive as a parent drug and needs liver microsomal to convert to active forms 4-hydroxycyclophosphamide and aldophosphamide which are delivered to cancer and normal cells for further cleavage to cytotoxic form of phosphoramide mustard and acrolein. Adverse events are bone myelosuppression, malignancy, sterility, and hemorrhagic cystitis (bladder toxicity) which can be prevented by Mesna and adequate hydration [19].

Bendamustine (Treanda ®) is a multifunctional alkylating drug that is used for the treatment of CLL and B cell non-Hodgins's lymphoma. Although the mechanism of action have not fully understood, it works as bifunctional alkylator that crosslinks DNA causing single and double strand breaks. Bendamustine is metabolized into two metabolites monohydroxy-bendamustine (HP1) and dihydroxy-bendamustine (HP2) [37]. Despite the extensive clinical experience with bendamustine, its overall pharmacokinetics or pharmacodynamics relationships, and drug–drug interactions have not been fully understood [38]. Systemic effect of bendmustine is similar in adults and pediatric because this drug is given as an i.v. based on body's surface are (BSA). Adverse events are increased risk of nausea and infection [39].

Busulfan (Myleran ®, Busulfex ®) is a bifunctional alkylating agent that contains 2 labile methane sulfonate groups attached to opposite ends of a 4-carbon alkyl chain. After busulfan is hydrolyzed, the methane sulfonate groups are released and carbonium ions are produced which then alkylating DNA producing guanine-adenine intrastrand crosslinks at guanine N7 and causing interference of DNA replication and RNA transcription. Sign of overdose includes allergic reaction, unusual bleeding or bruising, sudden weakness or unusual fatigue, persistent cough, congestion or shortness of breath, flank, stomach or joint pain, pronounced nausea, vomiting, diarrhea, dizziness, confusion, darkening of the skin, chills, fever, collapse, and loss of consciousness [40].

Vinca Alkaloids

Vincristine (Oncovin®) is a vinca alkaloid derived from the plant *Catharanthus roseues* (periwinkle) that works as anticancer by interfering microtubules of the mitotic spindle at the metaphase stage of leukemic cells causing death [41]. Vincristine has unpredictable pharmacologic characteristics such as variation in half-life, volume distribution and clearance, and narrow therapeutic index. It causes peripheral neuropathy and nerve damage with symptoms of muscle weakness, neuropathic pain, sensory loss which is more prevalent in Caucasian race, or patients using high dose, or in older patients [42]. Other adverse events are neurotoxicity, syndrome of inappropriate antidiuretic hormone secretion, myelosuppression, and alopecia [43-44].

METHOTREXATE

Methotrexate (Otrexup®, Rosuvo®) is a folate analog that has become a pioneering anticancer drugs for childhood ALL for more than half a century ago [45]. Methotrexate is converted into methotrexate polyglutamate (MTX-PG) by the enzyme polyglutamyl transferase that enhance methotrexate intracellularly. MTX-PG then inhibits dihydrofolate reductase, the enzyme responsible to reduce folates to their bioactive tetrahydrofolate [46]. Methotrexate can be given as i.v., intrathecal or as oral route. Oral bioavailability is saturable and erratic at dose greater than 25 mg/m^2 and usually used for treatment of rheumatoid arthritis, inflammatory bowel disease and other auto immune diseases. Methotrexate is excreted renally and need dose adjustment in renal dysfunction. [45-46]. At high dose, it can cause myelosuppression, mucositis, hepatic, renal and pulmonary toxicity, hand foot syndrome, and others [47]. Leucovorin, which is the active enantiomer of folate, should be used when high dose of MTX is used to prevent toxicity to normal cells.

6-THIOPURINES

6-mercaptopurine (Purinetho®, Purixan®, 6-MP) is mainly used for childhood acute leukemia. It is metabolized into 3 major pathways: 1) 6-thiouric acid, inactive metabolite by the enzyme xanthine oxidase through first pass metabolism; 2) 6 thioguanine (6T-G), an active metabolite through a multistep process involving hypoxanthine guanine phosphoribosyl transferase; and 3) 6-methyl mercaptopurine (6-MMP) inactive metabolite catalyzed by the enzyme thiopurine S-methyl transferase (TPMT) [48-50]. Patients with TPMT polymorphism can significantly diminished enzyme activity and increased risk of myelosuppresion. Approximately 10% patients have heterozygous TPMT with intermediate activity [51]. In patients with homozygous TPMT deficiency, dose reduction for up to 90% are sometimes needed with frequent monitoring to prevent 6-MP toxicities [52]. Therefore, it is important to check patients' TPMT variants to decide the correct dosing [53-54]. Over 24 low-functioning TPMT variants have been identified with TPMT*2 and TPMT*3 causing 95% of defective genes. Although the anti-leukemic mechanism of 6-MP and methotrexate are not completely understood, their benefits on ALL chemotherapy are well proven. There is no international consensus on the dosing of methotrexate and 6-MP due to significant interindividual and intraindividual variations in drug disposition (polymorphism among patients) [47, 54].

ARSENIC TRIOXIDE

Arsenic trioxide (ATO, $As_2 O_3$, Trisenox ®) is a traditional Chinese medicine that is used for the treatment of various cancers and acute promyelocytic leukemia (APL). ATO works by causing degradation of chimeric PML/RAR-α protein (fusion gene on chromosome 15 and 17, [t (15; 170(q24; q21) which disrupts the gene for nuclear receptor for retinoic acid that fuses with PML gene) [55-56]. It also induces apoptosis through a mitochondrial dependent process resulting in release of cytochrome C and activation of caspases. [56-57]. The main toxicities are QT prolongation and arrhythmias. Adverse events are fatigue, fever dyspnea, skin rash, fluid retention and weight gain. Even at low dose, ATO can cause development of secondary cancer, but the underlying mechanism of this effect remains unclear [55-56]. Therefore, many studies are tried to use at lower dose ATO to decrease the toxicity or to be used in combination with all trans retinoic acid [55-58].

ALL TRANS RETINOIC ACID

All- *trans*-retinoic acid (ATRA, Tretinoin®) works by binding to PML/RARA-α inducing a conformational change, allowing the differentiation dissociation of co-repressors and activation of gene transcription and cellular differentiation [59]. ATRA also induces PML-RARA α degradation through recruitment of proteases, caspase, proteasomes [59-61]. ATRA causes serious adverse events similar to toxicity due to excess vitamin A. These symptoms are headache, fever, dry skin, skin rash, pruritis, conjunctivitis, leukocytosis, dyspnea, weight gain, pulmonary and pleural pericardial effusions [62]. The combination of ATO and ATRA, which cause synergistic destruction of the PML/RARA-α protein in high risk APL, has benefit of causing complete response in 90%-100% of these patients [55]. The differentiation syndrome (DS) also known as retinoic syndrome or cytokine storm is adverse events after ATRA and/or ATO therapy and can be fatal if not quickly reversed [62]. DS is thought due to the release of inflammatory cytokines causing capillary leak, edema and hypotension. Symptoms include fever, weight gain, hypoxemia, edema, acute respiratory distress, and hypotension and multi organ dysfunction. Corticosteroids have been used to prevent this syndrome [62].

L-Asparaginase

The anti-proliferative of L -asparaginase on leukemic cells was first identified and characterized in human clinical trials in 1970. Leukemic cells require large amount of L-asparagine to maintain their malignant growth. The leukemic cells obtain non-acidic hydrophilic amino acids from blood serum and able to synthesize the amino acids asparagine themselves, but in a limited amount [63]. Leukemic cells are unable to synthesize L-asparagine *de novo* due to their lacking or having low level of enzyme asparagines synthase. By giving L-asparaginase as a drug, this enzyme catalyzes the hydrolysis of asparagine into aspartic acids and ammonia. The depletion of circulating pools of asparagine (due to formation of aspartic acids and ammonia) from the blood cause leukemic cells to die. The low level of asparagine only affects the cancerous cells without disturbing normal cells [64].

The transformation of L asparagine to aspartic acid (L-aspartate) and ammonia involves a double displacement or "ping pong" mechanism in which the nucleophilic group of the enzymes attack the Cγ of the substrate asparagine forming a tetrahedral intermediate that breaks down to form an acyl-enzyme intermediate, follow by elimination of ammonia. A second nucleophile causing formation of aspartic acid, followed by the regeration of free enzyme [65-66]. Furthermore, L asparaginase result in metabolic shutdown of the leukemic cells via the reduction of glycolysis and oxidative phosphorylation that cause damage to the mitochondria of cancer cells [67].

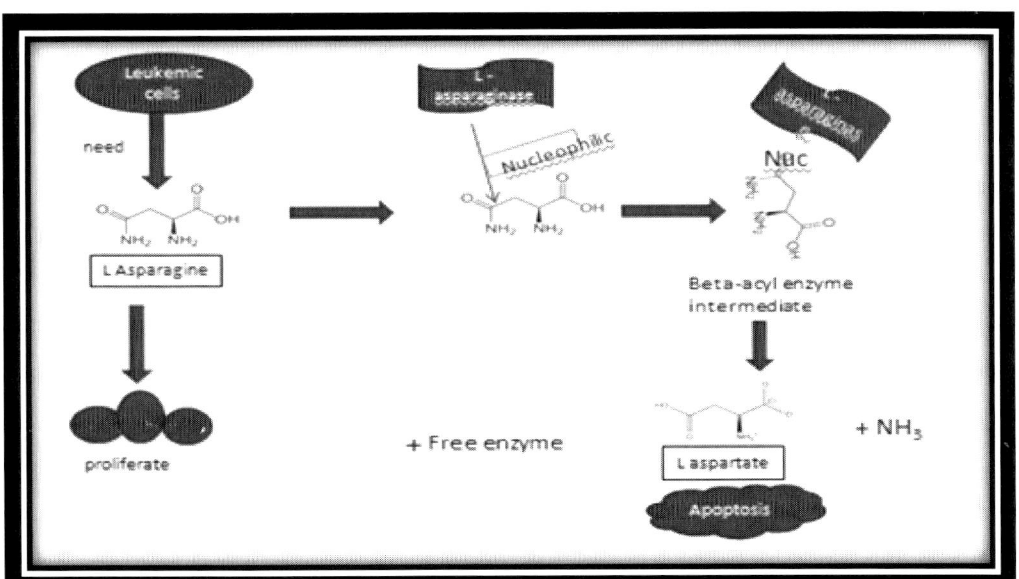

Figure 2. Schematic mechanism of action of L-asparaginase.

L-Asparaginase are indicated for ALL, pediatric ALL, AML, late stage CLL and non-Hodgkin lymphoma. Currently in the USA, there are 3 asparaginase preparations available: 1) native *E. coli* asparaginase (Elspar®), 2) Pagasparagase (Oncaspar®), and 3) Erwinase®; while different countries use different names such as Medac®, Crasnitin®, Leunase® and others. The common adverse events of L-asparaginase are leucopenia, CNS problems (seizures, hallucination, agitation), anaphylaxis, coagulation abnormalities (venous thrombosis, cerebral thrombotic complications), pancreatitis (vomiting, abdominal pain, back pain, anorexia), eye problems (blurred vision, ocular pain, corneal toxicity), development of myocardial infraction and secondary leukemia. About 2% to 8% patients develop anti-asparaginase antibodies requiring discontinuation of the therapy [68].

Several methods have been tried to decrease the immunogenic complications, to reduce resistance, to increase half-life of asparaginase by addition of poly ethylene glycol (PEG), dextran, or silk fibroin (to decrease immunogenicity), or acylation (to make the drug become hydrophobic), or addition of palmitoyl (to prolonged half-life without acute toxicity). Other important method is to prevent resistance to L-asparaginase. Cancer cells can response to the depletion of amino acid by induction of autophagy. Autophagy is a degradation process of proteins and organelles by the cancerous cells that provide metabolic intermediates and reduce oxidative stress renders leukemic cells become resistance. Therefore, L-asparaginase are often combined with vincristine, prednisone, and chloroquine to prevent autophagy [67].

LENALIDOMIDE

Lenalidomide (Revlimid®) is an immunomodulatory drugs (IMiDs), a derivative of thalidomide. Due to severe adverse events of thalidomide for causing congenital malformation in pregnant patients, lenalidomide was synthesized. It is used for myelodysplastic syndrome (MDS), multiple myeloma (MM), or other cancers but with less toxicities and adverse events. Lenalidomide contains two enantiomers S (-) and R (+) with optical rotation of zero produced from the racemic mixture [69-70]. One oxy group was removed from the phthaloyl ring of the structure of thalidomide and was replaced with an amine at the 4th position of the same ring system. With this minor change, lenalidomide became 100-1000 times more potent in stimulating T cell proliferation, interferon (IFN-γ) and IL-2 production, than thalidomide [69-70].

Although lenalidomide is a more efficacious than that of the parent drug thalidomide, the mechanism of action is still unclear. Lenalidomide has pleotropic and anti-inflammatory activities. The primary mechanism of action of the drug is thought through the secretion of pro-inflammatory cytokines from activated monocytes, macrophages and other cells [71-73]. Lenalidomide costimulates CD28 on T cells and causes transcription activation and expression of IL-2 and IFN-γ producing more T cells and natural killer cells (NK) [74-78]. Lenalidomide has been shown to increase antibody-dependent cell-mediated cytotoxicity (ADCC) in breast cancer cells that express HER-2 and Non-Hodgkin's lymphoma cell lines that express CD20 coated with antibodies [79]. Lenalidomide can target 5q deletion in MDS. Patients who respond to lenalidomide had increased expression of the genes involved in erythroid cell maturation and differentiation [80].

Lenalidomide is given as an oral dose at 2.5 to 25 mg/day. Maximal efficacy is seen after 0.5-4 hours with half-life ($t_{1/2}$) of about 3 hours. Lenalidomide is excreted in the urine 70% with 30% of the drug bound to protein. Further renal damage can occur in patients who have renal impairment. Lenalidomide is not metabolized by specific CYP enzymes; therefore, administration with other drugs may not cause problems [81-82]. Common adverse events are neutropenia, thrombocytopenia, fatigue, constipation, diarrhea, rash, peripheral edema, muscle aches, and somnolence [74, 83-84]. Pregnancy category is X, and has box warning of causing hematological toxicity, embryo-fetal toxicity, and venous thromboembolism. Patients taking lenalidomide should be advised to take weekly blood counts for the first eight weeks [84-86]. Lenalidomide should not be used for the treatment of chronic lymphocytic leukemia (CLL) due to tumor flare reactions were seen in about 53% of patients [68]. Prolonged exposure to lenalidomide can cause secondary malignancies [85-87].

Lenalidomide in combination with dexamethasone has been studied in several clinical trials. However, dexamethasone at higher doses appears to antagonize the immune response produced by lenalidomide by inhibiting IL-2 production in T cells and by inhibiting IFN-γ in NK cells; however, when used in low doses dexamethasone and lenalidomide have shown positive therapeutic effects due to their synergistic effect as compared to lenalidomide alone [69].

FDA approved use of lenalidomide in combination with dexamethasone in MDS with deletion of 5q, MM, relapse MCL and Hodgkin's lymphoma. In the United States, lenalidomide use requires registration and adherence with REM (Risk Evaluation and Mitigation) program (RevAssit at www.revlimid.com) to prevent pregnant patient taking lenalidomide accidently.

FLT3 INHIBITORS

About 25%-30% mutated gene in AML is due to FLT3 that lead to poor prognosis and resistance. FLT3 involves in 3 main signaling pathways such as Ras/MAPK, JAK/p-stat5, and P13K-Akt [88-90]. FLT3 is a surface receptor that consists of extracellular ligand-binding domain, transmembrane domain, a juxtamembrane domain, and two tyrosine kinase (TK) domain. The most common FLT3 mutation is an internal tandem duplication (ITD) in the juxtamembrane domain (FLT3-ITD) [90-91]. FLT3 inhibitors is the largest family of the targeted chemotherapy agents. This class is divided into first and second generations. First generations include sorafenib (Nexavar ®), lestaurtinib, midostaurin (Rydapt®), sunitinib (Sutent ®), and tandutinib. The second generation drugs have better potency than first generation and cause less adverse events. These drugs are crenolanib, quizartinib and cabozantinib (Cabometyx ®).

Sorafenib and quizartinib inhibit only FLT3-ITD, while midostaurin, crenolanib, and gilteritinib inhibit both FLT3-ITD and FLT3 TKD (tyrosine kinase domain). Sorafenib and midostaurin are multi kinase inhibitors that are also active against KIT, vascular endothelial growth factor receptor (VEGFR) and platelet derived growth factor receptor (PDGFR) [92]. Some of these drugs are still investigated in several clinical trials, while others are approved as orphan drugs by the FDA [92-93]. Figure 3 shows FLT3 kinase signaling pathway and sites blocked by the FLT3 inhibitors.

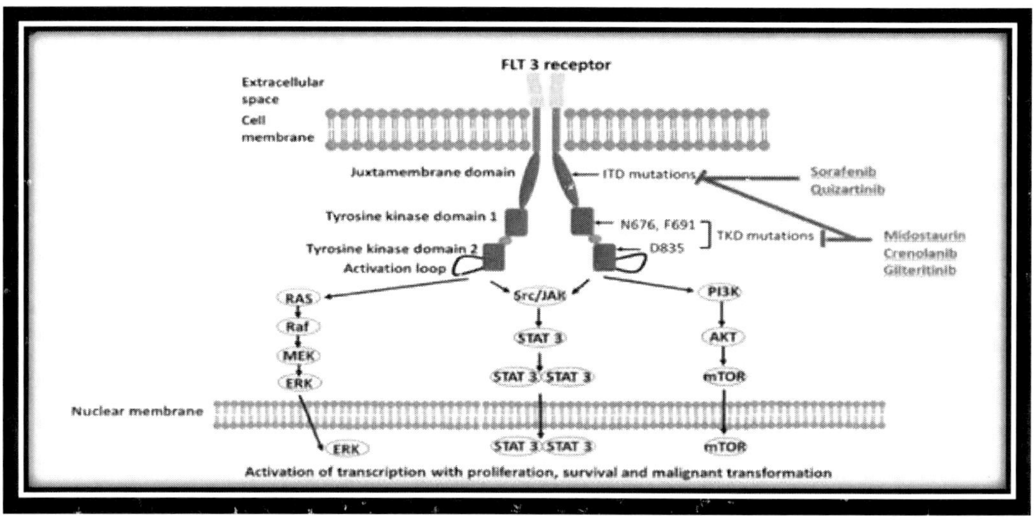

Figure 3. FLT3 kinase signaling pathway and sites blocked by FLT3 inhibitors. Sorafenib and quizartinib inhibit only FLT3-ITD mutations, while midostaurin, crenolanib, and gilteritinib inhibit both FLT3-ITD and FLT3TKD mutations [92].

BCL2 INHIBITOR

Venotoclax (Venckexta ®) is an oral small molecule that inhibits the anti-apoptotic BCl2 protein. This drug also induce rapid apoptosis of CLL cells and approved by the FDA for CLL with or without 17p deletion [94]. Adverse events include tumor lysis syndrome, neutropenia, thrombocytopenia, nausea, fatigue, and anemia. BCl2 overexpression disrupts normal regulation of the mitochondrial membrane, antagonizes apoptosis and contributes to chemotherapy resistance [95]. This drug is also in development for AML use and in combination with low dose cytarabine or hypomethylating agents in previously untreated older AML who were not eligible for intensive induction chemotherapy [96].

Phosphoinositide 3-Kinase (PI3K) Inhibitor

Idelalisib (Zydelig®) is an oral kinase inhibitor of delta isoform PI3K, which is the predominant PI3K isoform in B lymphoma-CLL. As an inhibitor of PI3K signaling downstream in CLL, it also interfering with chemokines such as CXCR4, CD40, and CD49d [97]. This drug is indicated for relapse CLL in combination with rituximab and for relapsed B cell non-Hodgkin lymphoma. It causes diarrhea, fatigue, pneumonia, pyrexia, cough, and nausea. Black box warning includes intestinal perforation and hepatoxicity. It may cause fetal harm [98]. It is metabolized by CYP450 3A4 which interact with strong inducers or inhibitors. Prophylaxis use of antibiotics to prevent infections by herpes simplex, *Pneumocystis Jirovecii* pneumonia, and cytomegalovirus are recommended for all patients on idelalisib [98].

Isocitrate Dehydrogenase (IDH) Inhibitors

Enasidenib (Idhifa ®) is the first FDA approved drug used to treat relapsed AML with specific mutations of isocitrate dehydrogenase 1 (IDH1) and IDH2, and for MDS patients. IDH1 and IDH2 genes encode for NADP dependent-IDH located in the cytosol and mitochondria [91]. Mutations in IDH1/2 have been detected in 15-20% of AML with normal karyotype. IDH mutations occur early in leukemogenesis and act to disturb DNA and histone methylation in hematopoietic stem cells through the production of an abnormal metabolite isocitrate to α-ketoglutarate (α-KG) [99]. Enasidenib induced differentiation of leukemic blast into normal neutrophils [96]. Adverse events are nausea, diarrhea, fatigue, anorexia, hyperbilirubinemia without hepatic transaminase elevation. Black box warning is differentiation syndrome showing as acute respiratory distress, dyspnea, hypoxia, plural effusion, lymphadenopathy and renal impairment which can be fatal if left untreated. Other IDH1 inhibitor ivosidenib (Tibsovo ®) is on clinical trial phase 1 or 2, while several others are in the pipelines [100].

DNA METHYL TRANSFERASE INHIBITORS (DMTIS)

Azacitidine (Vidaza ®) and decitabine (Dacogen ®) are pyrimidine nucleoside analog that cause direct cytotoxicity to abnormal bone marrow cells *via* DNA methyl transferase hypo methylation and causing cell death. Mutation in DNA methylation occurs in 20% of AML, with frequency increases with age and is associated with poor clinical outcome [101-102]. These drugs have been used as monotherapy or in combination with low dose cytarabine for AML and MDS. The patients' response to the therapy may take several months. Most patients will experience one episode of neutropenic fever requiring hospitalization during treatment [101]. Common adverse events are cytopenia, injection site reactions, fever, fatigue, skin rash, dizziness, peripheral edema, nausea, vomiting, constipation, weakness and cough [103].

Guadecitabine (SGI-110), another DMTIs was approved by FDA as an orphan drug for resistance AML. Unlike azacitidine and decitabine, it is resistance to degradation by cytidine deaminase.

MONOCLONAL ANTIBODIES TARGETING CD20

Cluster differentiation (CD) 20 is glycosylated transmembrane phospho protein expressed on the surface of malignant B cells. Mature B cells or B cell progenitor usually do not express this protein; therefore, depleting B cells at the development stages using anti CD-20 monoclonal antibodies (mAbs) does not usually cause permanent adverse events [105]. Rituximab (Rituxan ®) is a chimeric mouse and human mAb that was the top selling oncology drug for nearly a decade. It was approved in 1997 and has improved the outcomes of B cell non-Hodgkin lymphoma (NHLs), Burkitt lymphoma, mantle cell lymphoma, follicular lymphoma, hairy cell leukemia, and chronic lymphocytic leukemia (CLL) [105]. Rituximab also used in treating wide variety of autoimmune disease by reducing the adaptive immune response against self-such as rheumatoid arthritis (RA), myasthenia gravis, and others [106].

Figure 4 depicts different kind of mAbs, while Figure 5 shows the mechanism of action of rituximab [105, 107-108]. The FDA approved rituximab based on phase 2 trials in patients receiving i.v. at 125, 250, or 375 mg/m^2 weekly for 4 weeks [109]. The now standard therapy is using 375 mg/m^2. In CLL patients who are young, fit and lack deletion of 17p or TP53, current treatment guidelines recommend chemotherapy known as FCR (Fludarabine, cyclophosphamide, and rituximab) based on several clinical trials result [110].

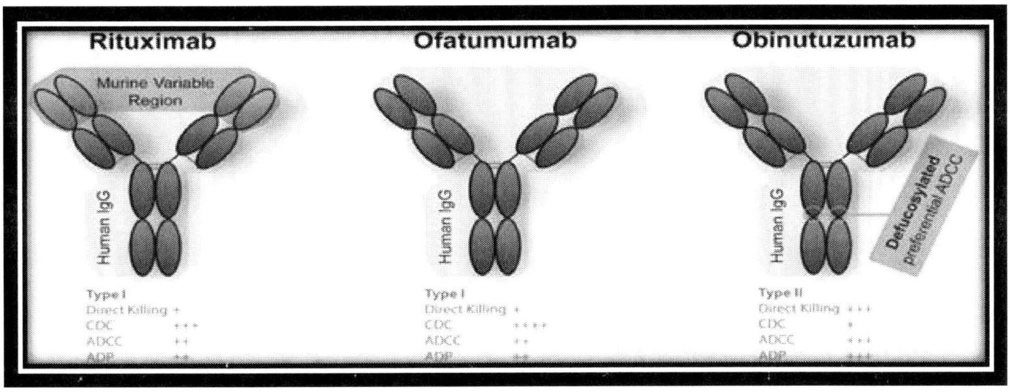

Figure 4. Engineered differences between FDA approved anti CD20 monoclonal antibodies. Rituximab is a chimeric mAb that is partially humanized, that has a human Fc portion but retains the murine variable regions that recognize CD20. Both ofatumumab and obinutuzumab are fully humanized mAbs, which reduces unintended immune response against therapies. Oftumumab also has glycoengineered Fc region which results in better binding with immune effector cells [107-108].

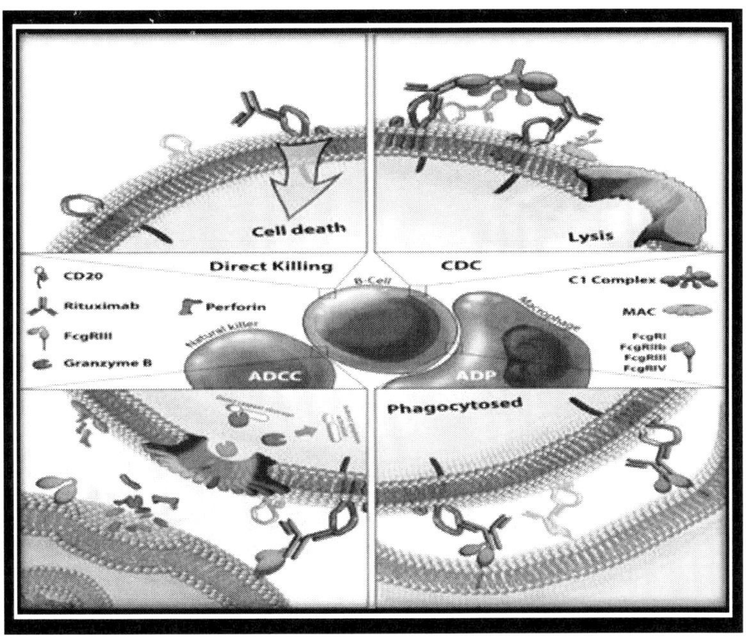

Figure 5. Rituximab-mediated cell killing of CD20 expressing B cells. Top Left- Binding of rituximab to CD20 can directly trigger apoptosis through both caspase-dependent and independent mechanisms that are still not fully characterized. Top Right- Bound rituximab can recruit the C1 complex triggering the classical complement cascade that lead to insertion of membrane attack complex (MAC) and lead to cell lysis, also known as complement-dependent cytotoxicity (CDC). Bottom Left- Bound rituximab can recruit natural killer cells via recognition by FcyRIII leading to antibody-dependent cell mediated cytotoxicity (ADCC). This facilitates release of perforin, which assembles into membrane compromising pores in the target cell and granzyme B, which enters the target cells and triggers apoptosis by cleaving caspases and other methods. Bottom Right- Macrophages recognize CD20 bound rituximab through various Fcy receptors, which lead to antibody-dependent phagocytosis (ADP) of the target cells. With permission [105].

FDA has approved s.c. formulation of rituximab, which is combined with recombinant hyaluronidase. Addition of hyaluronidase increased the dispersion and absorption of molecule and allows very small highly concentrated volumes to be injected as s.c. Rituxan Hycela®, the s.c. formulation, should be given after patients undergoes 1 cycle of i.v. follow by s.c. injection every 21 days for up to a total of 7 cycles. [111]. The most common adverse events are increased risk of infection, low white blood count, nausea, low platelet count, fever, vomiting and injection site redness [112].

In the past decades, two new anti-CD20 mAbs have been approved: ofatumumab (Arzerra®) and obinutuzumab (Gazvya®). Ofatumumab binds not only the small loop of CD20 like rituximab, but it also binds to large extracellular loop of CD20 which is more proximal to the cell membrane and can increase the CDC activity than rituximab [108]. Ofatumumab is approved for the treatment of CLL that is refractory to fludarabine or alemtuzumab therapies [113].

Obinutuzumab became the first glycoengineered mAb using two glycosylation enzymes MGAT III and Golgi Mannosidase II which resulted in better binding to effector immune cells and caused a more efficacious response by inducing antibody-dependent cell-mediated cytotoxicity (ADCC) and complement dependent cytotoxicity (CDC) [107, 114]. Direct comparison between rituximab, ofatumumab and obinutuzimab is difficult to be evaluated, due to in the clinical trials rituximab was given at a lower dose than the other two [115].

OTHER MONOCLONAL ANTIBODIES

Besides mAb targeting CD20, other antibodies known as bispecific T cell engager (BiTE) such as blinutuzumab and conjugated mAb such as inotuzumab ozogamicin (IO), gemtuzumab ozogomicin (GO) and others are now available. mAbs such as rituximab or obinutuzumab that don't bind to specific chemicals, are also called "naked" mAb regardless the CDs they bind. They are a few drugs targeting CD on the B-lineage leukemic cells such as CD 19, CD 20, CD 52 and CD 33 [116-117].

Alemtuzumab (Campath®) target CD52 that are expressed in 70% of T-ALL and Pre-B-ALL. The drug is given as s.c. The drug is also used for cutaneous T cell lymphoma and multiple sclerosis. Adverse events are increased risk of neutropenia and cause death which limit further development of alemtuzumab [117].

Over 90% of B-cells are positive for CD 19, making it an attractive target to form "immunologic synapse" between cytotoxic T cells (CTLs) and malignant cells resulting in activation of immune system and destruction of malignant clones. However, the drug is known to internalize upon binding to antibody, making it unsuitable target for naked mAbs. Blinatumomab (Blincyto ®) is a bispecific T-cell engaging antibody (BiTE) construct that binds to CD3 on CTLs and CD19 on B cells, causes lysis of CD19 by releasing cytokines such as interleukin (IL) 2, IL6, IL10, tumor necrosis factor and interferon γ and pore-forming perforin system [116-117]. Besides blinatumomab, disulfide-stabilized form of BiTE is also under active development [117].

Inotuzumab ozogamicin (IO, Besponsa®) is an antibody drug conjugate (ADC) that has calicheamicin (a potent DNA-binding cytotoxic) attached to an engineered humanized mAb immunoglobulin G4 antibody that target CD 22. CD 22 is a transmembrane sialoglycoprotein that regulate B-cell migration, survival, signal transduction, homing and cell adhesion [117-119]. Calicheamicin binds to the minor DNA grove causing double strand DNA cleavage and cell apoptosis [117-119]. It is used for relapse ALL-B cell [120]. Adverse events are hepatoxicity, hepatic veno occlusive disease (VOD), increased risk of post-hematopoietic stem cell transplant; none relapse mortality, myelosuppression, QT prolongation, and infusion related reactions [119-121]. Several clinical studies of inotuzumab ozogamicin in combination with standard chemotherapy such as cyclophosphamide, doxorubicin or study in older patients with ALL, or study on older patients with Philadelphia chromosome negative CD22+B cell precursor ALL are ongoing. For information see www.clinicaltrials.gov.

Gemtuzumab ozogomicin (GO, Mylotarg®) is a CD33 mAb that also bind to calicheamicin approved for the treatment of CD33 positive AML in newly diagnosed or relapsed patient. In 2010, because of it causing the risk of hepatic sinusoidal obstructive syndrome at dose 9 mg/m^2, FDA recommend that GO is withdrawn from the market [91]. However, if the drug is used at 3 mg/m^2, several studies showed dose and schedule play a significant role in the optimal use of GO. In 2017, FDA gave full approval for GO based on significant reduction in relapse rate and improve overall survival at 3 mg/m^2 [96]. Adverse events include fever, nausea, vomiting, constipation and increase in AST and ALT [96].

Chimeric Antigen Receptor T Cell (CARTs)

Genetically engineered immunotherapy of the T cells such as CAR-T has the potential to cure patients with highly resistant ALL. The structure of the first generation CART is composed of three domains: 1) the extracellular region which codes for a single chain variable fragment (scFv) of an antibody against the antigen present in the cancer cells, which has spacer/hinge domain derived from CD8 and from IgG sequences that affects CAR function and scFv flexibility; 2) the CAR transmembrane (TM) domain which is derived from T-cell molecules, such as CD3ζ, CD4, CD8a, or CD28, links the extracellular domain; and 3) the intracellular domain which activates T cells and is composed of CD3ζ T cell receptor [122].

The second and third generation CART has one or two intracellular signaling domains with costimulatory molecules such as CD28 or 4-IBB [123-126]. The CAR construct is then inserted to a viral vector follow by transduction unto autologous or allogenic T cells to express the CAR on their cell surface [123, 127-128]. The CAR that expressed T cells is then infused directly unto the patient, where it specifically target cancer cells expression recognized by the scFv [123].

FDA approved i.v. tisagenlecleucel (Kymriah ®) as the first gene transfer therapy for patients under 26 years old that has relapsed or refractory B-cell ALL. A Risk Evaluation and Mitigation Strategy (REMS) program is mandated by FDA to ensure education and training of complication such as cytokine release syndrome (CRS) [123]. Other adverse events are CAR T encephalopathy syndrome (CRES), confusion, delirium, tremor, agitation and hallucination [123]. FDA approved over 40 certified treatment centers, under REMS program, that can administer Kymriah ®.

CONCLUSION

Leukemia treatment therapy has changed over the last few decades. Besides the increased in the number of drugs available to treat cancer, there are now many mAbs with specific targets that are routinely use with traditional chemotherapeutic agents. Recent trends for the development of new leukemia drugs are narrow indication, oral formulation, and targeting specific biomarkers of leukemia.

ACKNOWLEDGMENT

The author thank Maxwell Nell, pharmacy 2nd year student for writing a portion of lenolidomide.

REFERENCES

[1] Collins JM. Cancer Pharmacology. In *Abeloff's Clinical Oncology*. Ed; Niederhuber et al, 5th ed. Elsevier Saunders, Philadelphia, PA 2014.

[2] http://www.acessdata.fda.gov/scripts/cder/drugsatfda/.

[3] Freireich EJ, Frei E. Recent advances in acute leukemia. *Prog Hematol* 1964;4:187-202.

[4] Lichtman MA. A historical perspective on the development of cytarabine (7 days) and daunorubicin (3 days) treatment regimen for acute myelogenous leukemia:

2013 the 40th anniversary of 7+3. *Blood, Cells, Molecules and Diseases* 2013;50:119-130.

[5] Ossenkoppele GJ, Graveland WJ, Sonneveld P, et al. The value of fludarabine in addition to ARA-C and G-CSF in the treatment of patients with high-risk myelodysplastic syndromes and AML in elderly patients. *Blood* 2004; 103:2908-2913

[6] Estey E, Gandhi V, Plunkett W, et al. Fludarabine and arabinosylcytosine therapy of refractory and relapsed acute myelogenous leukemia. *Leuk Lymphoma.* 1993;9:343-350.

[7] Estey E, Thall P, Andreeff M, et al. Use of G-CSF before during and after fludarabine plus cytarabine induction therapy of newly diagnosed acute myelogenous leukemia of myelodysplastic syndromes: comparison with fludarabine plus cytarabine without G-CSF. *J Clin Oncol.* 1994;12:671- 67.

[8] Rubia de la, Regadera A, Martin F, et al. FLAG-IDA regimen (fludarabine, cytarabine, idarubicin and G-CSF) in the treatment of patients with high-risk myeloid malignancies. *Leuk Res* 2002;26(8):725-730.

[9] Kim H, Lee JH, Joo JD, et al. Prospective, multicenter, phase II study on reducing the dosage of idarubicin and FLAG for patients younger than 65 years with resistant acute myeloid leukemia: a comparison with a higher dosage trial. *Acta Haematol* 2014;132 (1): 87-96.

[10] Assouline S, Buccher V, Delmer A, et al. Pharmacokinetic and safety of subcutaneous rituximab plus fludarabine and cyclophosphamide for patients with CLL. *Bri J of Clin Pharmacol* 2015; 80(5): 1001-1009.

[11] Frost GI. Recombinant human hyaluronidase (rHuPH20): an enabling platform for subcutaneous drug and fluid administration. *Expert Opin Drug Deliv* 2007;4:427-440.

[12] Davies A, Merli F, Mihaljevic B, et al. Pharmacokinetics, safety, and efficacy of subcutaneous rituximab in follicular lymphoma (SABRINA): stage I analysis of randomized phase 3 study. *Lancet Oncol* 2014;15:343-352.

[13] Plunkett W, Gandhi V, Huanf P et al. Fludarabine: pharmacokinetics, mechanisms of action, and rationales for combination therapies. *Semin Oncol* 1993;20:2-12.

[14] Rai KR, Peterson BL, Appelbaum FR, et al. Fludarabine compared with chlorambucil as primary therapy for chronic lymphocytic leukemia. *N Engl J Med* 2000:343:1750-1757.

[15] Hallek M. Chronic lymphocytic leukemia: 2017 update on diagnosis, risk stratification, and treatment. *Am J Hematol* 2017;92 (9): 946-965.

[16] Anaissie EJ, Kontoyiannis DP, O'brien S et al. Infections in patients with chronic lymphocytic leukemia treated with fludarabine. *Ann Intern Med* 1998;129:5559-566.

[17] Betcher DL, Burnham N. Cytarabine. *J of Ped Oncol Nursing.* 1990:7(4), 154-157. doi:10.1177/104345429000700406.

[18] Ohtake S, Miyawaki S, Fujita H, et al. Randomized study of induction therapy comparing standard-dose idarubicin with high-dose daunorubicin in adult patients with previously untreated acute myeloid leukemia: The JALSG AML201 Study. *Blood.* 2010;117(8): 2358-2365.

[19] Chu E. Cancer Chemotherapy. In: Katzung BG. eds. *Basic & Clinical Pharmacology.* http://accesspharmacy.mhmedical.com/content.aspx?bookid=2249 &sectionid=175224452. Accessed July 12, 2018. doi:10.1182/blood-2010-03-2732 43.

[20] Chen L, Guo P, Zhang Y, et al. Autophagy is an important event for low-dose cytarabine treatment in acute myeloid leukemia cells. *Leukemia Research.* 2017;60:44-52. 15. doi:10.1016/j.leukres.2017.06.007.

[21] Cheong JW, Kim Y, Eom HK, Jeung YH. Enhanced autophagy in cytarabine arabinoside-resistant U937 leukemia cells and its potential as a target for overcoming resistance. *Mol. Med. Rep.* 2016;13(4): 3433–3440.

[22] Lowenberg B, Pabst T, Vellenga E, et al. Cytarabine in acute myeloid leukemia. *N Engl J Med* 2011;364 (11): 1027.

[23] Silva EF, Bazoni RF, Ramos EB, Rocha MS. DNA doxorubicin interaction: New insights and peculiarities. *Biopolymers.* 2017:107(3)22998.

[24] Jeon K, Yu HV, Kwon Y. Hyperactivated m-calpain affects acquisition of doxorubicin resistance in breast cancer cells. Biochimica et Biophysica Acta (BBA) - General Subjects, 2018; 1862(5): 1126–1133.

[25] Hajra S, Patra AR, Basuetal A.Prevention of doxorubicin (DOX)-induced genotoxicity and cardiotoxicity: Effect of plant derived small molecule indole-3-carbinol (I3C) on oxidative stress and inflammation. *Biomedicine & Pharmacotherapy.* 2018;101:228–243.

[26] McGowan JV, Chung R, Maulik A. Anthracycline Chemotherapy and Cardiotoxicity. *Cardiovascular Drugs and Therapy.* 2017;31(1): 63–75.

[27] Vokkova M, Russell R. Anthracycline cardiotoxicity: prevalence, pathogenesis and treatment. *Curr Cardio Rev* 2011;7(4):214-220.

[28] Chen EC, Fathi AT, Brunner AM. Reformulating acute myeloid leukemia: liposomal cytarabine and daunorubicin (CPX-351 as an emerging therapy for secondary AML. *Onco Targets Thers* 2018;11:3425-3434.

[29] Minotti G, Menna P, Salvatorelli E, Cairo G, Gianni L. "Anthracyclines: molecular advances and pharmacology developments in antitumor activity and cardiotoxicity," *Pharmacological Reviews.* 2004: 56(2);185–229.

[30] Nielsen D, Maare C, Skovsgaard T. Cellular resistance to anthracyclines. *General Pharmacology: The Vascular System.* 1996: 27(2); 251–255.

[31] Pendleton MJ, Linsdsey RH, Felix CA et al. Topoisomerase II and leukemia. *Ann NY Acad Sci* 2014;1310:98-110.

[32] DenBoer ML, Pieters R, Veerman AJP. Mechanisms of cellular anthracycline resistance in childhood acute leukemia. *Leukemia*. 1998;12(11):1657–1670.

[33] Cutts SM, Swift LP, Rephaeli A, Nudelman A, Phillips DR. Recent advances in understanding and exploiting the activation of anthracyclines by formaldehyde. *Current Med Chemi-Anti-Cancer Agents*. 2005;5(5):431– 447.

[34] Liu Z, Deibler RW, Chen HS. The why and how of DNA unlinking. *Nucleic Acids Rec* 2009;37:661-671.

[35] McClendon AK, Osheroff N. DNA topoisomerase II, genotoxicity, and cancer. *Mutant Res* 2007;623:83-97.

[36] Zeihiedrich EL, Christiansen K, Andersen AH et al. Double-stranded DNA cleavage/relegation reaction of eukaryotic topoisomerase II: evidence for anicked DNA intermediate. *Biochemistry* 1989;28:6229-6236.

[37] Teva Branded Pharmaceutical Products R&D, Inc (2013) *TREANDA® prescribing information.* http://treandahcp.com/PDF/TREANDAfinal_PI.pdf.

[38] Darwish M, Bond M, Hellriegel E, et al. Pharmacokinetic and pharmacodynamics profile of bendamustine and its metabolites. *Cancer Chemother Pharmacol.* 2015;75(6):1143-1154.

[39] Darwish M, Megason G, Bond M, et al. Population pharmacokinetics and pharmacokinetic/pharmacodynamics of bendamustine in pediatric patients with relapsed/refractory acute leukemia. *Curr Med Res Opin.* 2014;30(11):2305–2315. doi: 10.1185/03007995.2014.941976.

[40] Galaup A, Paci A. Pharmacology of dimethanesulfonate alkylating agents: busulfan and treosulfan. *Expert Opin Drug Metab Toxicol* 2013;9(3):333-347.

[41] Coccia PF, Altman J, Bhatia S, et al. Adolescent and young adult oncology clinical practice guidelines in oncology. *JNCCN J Nat Compr Cancer Net* 2012;10:1112-1150.

[42] van del Velde ME, Kaspers GL, Abbink FCH, et al. Vincristine-induced peripheral neuropathy in children with cancer: a systemic review. *Critical Reviews in Oncology/Hematology* 2017;114:114-130.

[43] Haggard ME, Fernbach DJ, Holcomb TM., et al.Vincristine in acute leukemia of childhood. *Cancer*. 1968; 22: 438–444.

[44] Tsujita Y, Iwao N, Makino S, Ohsawa N. Syndrome of inappropriate secretion of antidiuretics hormone and neurotoxicity induced by vincristine and alkylating agents during chemotherapy for malignant lymphoma of thyroid gland. *Gan To Kagaku Ryoho* (Japanese) 1998;25:757-760.

[45] Farber S, Diamond LK, Mercer RD, et al. Temporary remissions in acute leukemia in children produced by folic acid antagonist 4-aminopteroylglutamic acid (aminopterin). *N Engl J Med*. 1948;238:787–793.

[46] Chabner BA, Allegra CJ, Curt GA, et al. Polyglutamation of methotrexate. Is methotrexate a prodrug? *J Clin Invest.* 1985;76:907–912.
[47] Schmiegelow K, Nielsen SN, Frandsen TL, Nersting J. Mercaptopurine/ methotrexate maintenance therapy of childhood acute lymphoblastic leukemia: clinical facts and fiction. *J Pediatr Hematol Oncol* 2014;36(7):503-517
[48] Zimm S, Collins JM, Riccardi R, et al. Variable bioavailability of oral mercaptopurine. Is maintenance chemotherapy in acute lymphoblastic leukemia being optimally delivered? *N Engl J Med.* 1983;308:1005–1009.
[49] Hedeland RL, Hvidt K, Nersting J, et al. DNA incorporation of 6-thioguanine nucleotides during maintenance therapy of childhood ALL and non-Hodgkin lymphoma. *Cancer Chemother Pharmacol.* 2010;66:485–491.
[50] Relling MV, Gardner EE, Sandborn WJ, et al. Clinical pharmacogenetics implementation consortium guidelines for thiopurine methyltransferase genotype and thiopurine dosing: 2013 update. *Clin Pharmacol Ther.* 2013;93:324–325.
[51] Evans WE, Hon YY, Bomgaars L et al. Preponderance of thiopurine S-methyltransferase deficiency and heterozygosity among patients intolerant to mercaptopurine or azathipprine. *J Clin Oncol* 2001;19(8):2293-2301.
[52] Andersen JB, Szumlanski C, Weinshilboum RM, et al. Pharmacokinetics, dose adjustments, and 6-mercaptopurine/methotrexate drug interactions in two patients with thiopurine methyltransferase deficiency. *Acta Paediatr* 1998;87(1):108-111.
[53] Schmiegelow K. Advances in individual prediction of methotrexate toxicity: a review. *Br J Haematol.* 2009;146:489–503.
[54] Kim H, Kang HJ, Kim HJ, et al. Pharmacogenetic analysis of pediatric patients with acute lymphoblastic leukemia: a possible association between survival rate and ITPA polymorphism. *PLoS One.* 2012;7:e45558.
[55] McCulloch D, Brown C, Illand H. Retinoic acid and arsenix trioxide in the treatment of acute promyelocytic leukemia: current perspective. *Onco Tarets Ther.* 2017;10:1585-1601. doi: 10.2147/OTT.S100513.
[56] Rowley JD, Golomb HM, Dougherty C. 15/17 translocation, a consistent chromosomal change in APL. *Lancet.* 1977;1(8010):549–550.
[57] Zhang X, Yu D, Geng H, et al. Dual effects of arsenic trioxide on tumor cells and the potential underlying mechanisms. *Oncol Lett* 2018;16(3): 3812-3820.
[58] Chen GQ, Shi XG, Tang W, et al. Use of arsenic trioxide (As2O3) in the treatment of acute promyelocytic leukemia (APL): I. As2O3 exerts dose-dependent dual effects on APL cells. *Blood.* 1997;89:3345–3353.
[59] Wang Z-Y, Chen Z. Acute promyelocytic leukemia: from highly fatal to highly curable. *Blood.* 2008;111(5):2505–2515.
[60] Raelson J, Nervi C, Rosenauer A, et al. The PML/RAR alpha oncoprotein is a direct molecular target of retinoic acid in acute promyelocytic leukemia cells. *Blood.* 1996;88(8):2826–2832.

[61] Nervi C, Ferrara FF, Fanelli M, et al. Caspases mediate retinoic acid-induced degradation of the acute promyelocytic leukemia PML/RARalpha fusion protein. *Blood.* 1998;92(7):2244–2251.

[62] Sanz MA, Montesinos P. How we prevent differentiation syndrome in patients with acute promyelocytic leukemia. *Blood* 2014;123:2777-2782.

[63] Narta UK, Kanwar SS, Azmi W. Pharmacological and clinical evaluation of L-asparaginase in the treatment of leukemia. *Crit. Rev. Oncol Hematol* 2007; 61:208-221.

[64] Alu U, Naveed M, Ullah A, et al. L-asparaginase as a critical component to combat acute lymphoblastic leukemia: a novel approach to target ALL. *Eur J Pharmacol.* 2016;771:199-210.

[65] Ehrman M, Cedar H, Schwartz JH. L-asparaginase II of E Coli studies on the enzymatic mechanism of action. *J Biol Chem* 1971;246:88-94.

[66] Rohm KH, Van Etten RL. The 180 isotope effect in 13C nuclear magnetic resonance spectroscopy: mechanistic studies on asparaginase from *E Coli. Arch Biochem Biophys* 1986; 244:128-136.

[67] Takahashi H, Inoue J, Sakaguchi K, et al. Autophagy is required for cell survival under L-asparaginase-induced metabolic stress in acute lymphoblastic leukemia cells. *Oncogene* 2017; 36:4267-4276.

[68] Strullu M, Corradini N, Audrain M, et al. Silent hypersensitivity to E coli asparaginase in children with acute lymphoblastic leukemia. *Leuk Lymphoma* 2010;51:1464-1472.

[69] Ghosh N, Grunwald MR, Fasan O, Bhutani M. Expanding role of lenalidomide in hematologic malignancies. *Cancer Management and Research* 2015;&:105-119.

[70] Kotla V, Goel S, Nischal S, et al. Mechanism of action of lenalidomide in hematological malignancies. *Journal of Hematology & Oncology*. 2009;2:1–10. doi:10.1186/1756-8722-2-36.

[71] Hideshima T, Chauhan D, Shima Y, et al. Thalidomide and its analogs overcome drug resistance of human multiplemyeloma cells to conventional therapy. *Blood.* 2000; 96 :2943-2950.

[72] Moreira Al, Sampaio Ep, Zmuidzinas A, et al. Thalidomide exerts its inhibitory action on tumor necrosis factor alpha by enhancing mRNA degradation. *J. Exp Med.* 1993;177(6):1675-1680.

[73] Corral LG, Haslett Pa, Muller GW, et al. Differential cytokinase modulation and T cell activiation by two distinct classes of thalidomide analogues that are potent inhibitors of TNF-*a*. *J Immunol.* 1999;163: 380-386.

[74] Bartlett JB, Dredge K, Dalgleish AG. The evolution of thalidomide and its IMiD derivatives as anticancer agents. *Nature Reviews Cancer*. 2004;4:314-322. doi:10. 1038/nrc1323

[75] Leblanc R, Hideshima T, Catley LP, et al. Immunomodulatory drug costimulates T cells via the B7-CD28 pathway. *Blood* 2004;103(5):1787-1790. doi:10.1182/blood-2003-02-0361.

[76] Davies Fe, Raje N, Hideshima T, et al. Thalidomide and immunodulatory derivatives augment natural killer cell cytotoxicity in multiple myeloma. *Blood.* 2001;98(1):210-216. 210-216. doi:10.1182/blood.v98.1.210.

[77] Tai Y, LI X, Catley L, et al. Immunomodulatory drug lenalidomide (CC-5013, IMiD3) augments anti-CD40 SGN-40-induced cytotoxicity in human multiple myeloma: clinical implications. *Cancer Research.* 2005;65(24):17712-11720. doi:10.1158/0008-5472.can-05-1657.

[78] Stirling D. Thalidomide: a novel template for anticancer drugs. *Seminars in Oncology.* 2001;28(6):602-606. doi:10.1053/sonc.2001.28595.

[79] Saloura V, Grivas PD, Lenalidomide: a synthetic compound with an evolving role in cancer management. *Hematology* 2010;15(5):318–331.

[80] McGraw KL, Bassiorka AA, Johnson JO, et al. Lenaliodmide induces lipid raft assembly to enhance erythroprotein receptor signaling in myelodysplastic syndrome progenitors. *PLoS One* 2014;9: e114149.

[81] Mitsiades CS, Mitsiades N. CC-5013 (Celgene). *Curr Opin Investig Drugs* 2004; 5(6): 635-647.

[82] Tep S, Oliver J, Harden D, Stirling D, Thoms S, Scheffler M. A phase I, single blind, placebo-controlled, ascending angle oral dose, safety, tolerability, and pharmacokinetics study of CD-501, a novel immunomodulatory-oncologic agent, in health male subjects with a comparison of fed and fasted. *Clinical Pharmacology Therapy.* 2002;71(2):93.

[83] Fajardo S, Zook F, Dotson E, Specialty pharmacy for hematologic malignancies. *American Journal of Health-System Pharmac*y 2016;73(11):797–809. doi:10.2146/ajhp150749.

[84] Zonder JA, Crowley J, Hussein MA et al. Lenalidomide and high-dose dexamethasone compared with dexamethasone as initial therapy for multiple myeloma: a randomized Southwest Oncology trial (SO232). *Blood* 2010;116 (26):5838-5841.

[85] Kastritis E, Dimopoulos MA. The evolving role of lenalidomide in the treatment of hematologic malignancies. *Expert Opinion on Pharmacotherapy.* 2007;8(4):497–509. doi:10.1517/14656566.8.4.497.

[86] Anderson KC. Lenalidomide and Thalidomide: Mechanisms of Action—Similarities and Differences. *Seminars in Hematology.* 2005;42. doi:10.1053/j.seminhematol.2005.10.001.

[87] Davies F, Baz R, Lenalidomide mode of action: linking bench and clinical findings. *Blood Reviews* 2010;24. doi:10.1016/s0268-960x(10)70004-7.

[88] Mizuki M, Fenski R, Halfter H et al. FLT3 mutations from patients with acute myeloid leukemia induce transformation of 32D cells mediated by the Ras and STAT5 pathways. *Blood* 2000; 96(12):3907-3914.
[89] Choudhary C, Schwable J, Brandts C et al. AML associated FLT3 kinase domain mutations show signal transduction differences compared with FLT3 ITD mutations. *Blood* 2005: 106(1): 265-273.
[90] Moreno I, Martin G, Bolufer P et al. Incidence and prognostic value of FLT3 internal tandem duplication and D835 mutations in acute myeloid leukemia. *Hametologica* 2003: 88(1):19-24.
[91] Lin M, Chen B. Advances in the drug therapies of acute myeloid leukemia (except acute promyelocytic leukemia). *Drug Design, Develop Ther* 2018;12:1009-1017.
[92] Lim SH, Duvielecka PM, Raghunathan VM. Molecular targeting in acute myeloid leukemia. *J Transl Med* 2017; 15:183.
[93] Annesley CE, Brown P. Novel agents for the treatment of childhood acute leukemia. *Ther Adv Hematol* 2015;6(2) 61-79.
[94] Shustik C, Bence-bruckler I, Delage R et al. Advances in the treatment of relapsed/refractory chronic lymphocytic leukemia. *Ann Hematol* 2017;96:1185-1196.
[95] Wei A, Strickland SA, Roboz GJ et al. Safety and efficacy of venotoclax plus low-dose cytarabine in treatment-naïve patients aged greater than 65 years with acute myeloid leukemia. *Blood* 2016;128:102.
[96] Perl AE. The role of targeted therapy in the management of patients with AML. *Blood Advances* 2017;54-65.
[97] Yang Q, Modi P, Newcomb T et al. Idelilisib: first in class PI3K delta inhibitor for the treamtne of chronic lymphoblastic leukemia, small lymphoblastic leukemia, and follicular lymphoma. *Clin Cancer Res* 2015;21:1537-1542.
[98] Zydelig® Prescribing information. Gilead Sciences, Inc. 2018. Foster City, CA.
[99] Shlush LI, Zandi S, Mitchell A et al. HALT Pan- Leukemia Consortium. Identification of pre-leukemic hematopoietic stem cells in acute leukemia. *Nature* 2014;506 (7488): 328-333.
[100] DiNardo CD, de Botton S, Stein EM et al. Determination of IDH1 mutational burden and clearance via next-generation sequencing in patients with IDH1 mutation-positive hematologic malignancies receiving AG-120, a first-class inhibitor of mutant IDH1. *Blood* 2016;28 (22): 1070.
[101] Azacitidine. Lexi-Drugs. *Lexicomp*. Wolters Kluwer Health, Inc. Riverwoods, IL. Available at: http://online.lexi.com. Accessed May 24, 2018.
[102] Ley TJ, Ding L, Walter MJ et al. DNMT3A mutations in acute myeloid leukemia. *N Eng J Med* 2010; 363:2424-2433.
[103] Fenaux P, Mufti GJ, Hellstrom-Lindberg E, et al. Efficacy of azacitidine compared with that of conventional care regimens in the treatment of higher-risk

myelodysplastic syndromes: a randomised, open-label, phase III study. *Lancet Oncol* 2009;10:223–232.

[104] Issa JP, Roboz G, Rizzieri D et al. Safety and tolerability of guadecitabine (SGI-110) in patients with MDS and AML: a multicenter, randomized, dose escalation phase 1 study. *Lancet Oncol* 2015;16:1099-1110.

[105] Pierpont TM, Limper CB, Richards KL. Past, present, and future of rituximab-the world's first oncology antibody therapy. *Front Oncol* 2018; 4;8:163. doi: 10.3389/fonc.2018.00163. eCollection 2018.

[106] Schioppo T, Ingegnoli F. Current perspective on rituximab in rheumatic diseases. *Drug Des Devel Ther* 2017; 11:2891–904.10.2147/DDDT.S139248.

[107] Al-Sawaf O, Fischer K, Engelke A, et al. Obinutuzumab in chronic lymphocytic leukemia: design, development and place in therapy. *Drug Des Devel Ther* (2017) 11:295–304.10.2147.

[108] Rafiq S, Butchar JP, Cheney C et al. Comparative assessment of clinically utilized CD20-directed antibodies in chronic lymphocytic leukemia cells reveals divergent NK cell, monocyte, and macrophage properties. *Journal Immunol* (2013) 190:2702.

[109] Maloney DG, Grillo-López AJ, Bodkin DJ, et al.IDEC-C2B8: results of a phase I multiple-dose trial in patients with relapsed non-Hodgkin's lymphoma. *J Clin Oncol* 1997; 15:3266 74.10.1200/JCO.1997.15.10.3266.

[110] Collett L, Howard DR, Munir T, et al. Assessment of ibrutinib plus rituximab in front-line CLL (FLAIR trial): study protocol for a phase III randomised controlled trial. *Trials* 2017; 18:387.10.1186/s13063-017-2138-6.

[111] https://www.rituxanhycela.com/.

[112] Cang S, Mukhi N, Wang K, Liu D. Novel CD20 monoclonal antibodies for lymphoma therapy. *J Hematol Oncol* 2012; 5:64.10.1186/1756-8722-5-64

[113] Hallek M. Chronic lymphocytic leukemia: 2017 update on diagnosis, risk stratification, and treatment. *Am J Hematol* 2017; 92:946–65.10.1002/ajh.24826.

[114] Pottier J, Chastang R, Dumet C, Watier H. Rethinking the INN system for therapeutic antibodies. *MAbs* 2016; 9:5

[115] Cartron G, de Guibert S, Dilhuydy MS, et al. Obinutuzumab (GA101) in relapsed/refractory chronic lymphocytic leukemia: final data from the phase 1/2 GAUGUIN study. *Blood* 2014; 124:2196–202.10.1182/blood-2014-07-586610.

[116] Buie LW, Pecoraro JJ, Horvat TZ, et al. Blinatumomab: A First-in-Class Bispecific T-Cell Engager for Precursor B-Cell Acute Lymphoblastic Leukemia. *Ann Pharmacother* 2015;49(9):1057–1067.

[117] Wei G, Wang J, Huang H, Zhao Y. Novel immunotherapies for adult patients with B-lineage acute lymphoblastic leukemia. *J Hematol and Oncol*. 2017;10:150.

[118] Wu J, Fu J, Zhang M, Liu D. Blinatumomab: a bispecific T cell engager (BiTE) antibody against CD 19/CD3 for refractory acute lymphoid leukemia. *J Hematol Oncol* 2015;8: 104.

[119] Le Jeune C, Thomas X. Potential for bispecific T-cell engagers: role of blinatumomab in acute lymphoblastic leukemia. *Drug Des Devel Ther*. 2016;10:757-765.

[120] Fan D, Li W, Yang Y et al. Redirection of CD4+ and CD8+T lymphocyte via an anti-CD3 X anti CD-19 bi-specific antibody combined with cytosine arabinoside and the efficient lysis of patient-derived B-ALL cells. *J Hematol Oncol* 2015; 8:108.

[121] https://www.pfizermedicalinformation.com/en-us/besponsa.

[122] Dai H, Wang Y, Lu X, Han W. Chimeric Antigen Receptors Modified T-Cells for Cancer Therapy. *J Natl Cancer Inst*. 2016 Jul;108(7).

[123] Forsberg MH, Das A, Saha K, Capitini CM. The potential of CART therapy for relapsed or refractory pediatric and young adult B-cell All. *Ther Clin Ris Management* 2018;1573-1584.

[124] Finney HM, Lawson AD, Bebbington CR, Weir AN. Chimeric receptors providing both primary and costimulatory signaling in T cells from a single gene product. *J Immunol.* 1998;161(6):2791–2797.

[125] Hombach A, Wieczarkowiecz A, Marquardt T, et al. Tumor-specific T cell activation by recombinant immunoreceptors: CD3 zeta signaling and CD28 costimulation are simultaneously required for efficient IL-2 secretion and can be integrated into one combined CD28/CD3 zeta signaling receptor molecule. *J Immunol.* 2001;167(11):6123–6131.

[126] Tammana S, Huang X, Wong M, et al. 4-1BB and CD28 signaling plays a synergistic role in redirecting umbilical cord blood T cells against B-cell malignancies. *Hum Gene Ther*. 2010;21(1):75–86.

[127] Hu WS, Pathak VK. Design of retroviral vectors and helper cells for gene therapy. *Pharmacol Rev*. 2000;52(4):493–511.

[128] Levine BL, Miskin J, Wonnacott K, Keir C. Global manufacturing of CAR T cell therapy. *Mol Ther Methods Clin Dev*. 2017;4:92–101.

In: Frontiers in Leukemia Pharmacotherapy
Editor: Lunawati L. Bennett
ISBN: 978-1-53614-960-9

Chapter 5

THE ROLE OF TYROSINE KINASE INHIBITORS IN LEUKEMIA

***Michelle D. Lesé*[*], PharmD**
Former Palm Beach Atlantic University School of Pharmacy Faculty,
West Palm Beach, Florida, US

ABSTRACT

Tyrosine kinase inhibitors (TKIs) have dramatically improved management of chronic myeloid leukemia (CML). Kinases are enzymes that transfer a phosphate group to a protein. Most protein kinases promote cell proliferation, survival, and migration. TKIs are constitutively overexpressed and are associated with carcinogenesis and metastases in various types of cancer.

This chapter aims to highlight the different category of TKIs, to discuss in depth first, second, and third generation TKIs currently available and their drug-drug and Cytochrome p450 interactions.

Keywords: chronic myeloid/myelogenous leukemia, tyrosine kinase, tyrosine kinase inhibitors, BCR-ABL mutations, imatinib, dasatinib, nilotinib, bosutinib, ponatinib

ABBREVIATIONS

TKIs	tyrosine kinase inhibitors
TK	tyrosine kinase
RTKs	receptor tyrosine kinases

[*] Corresponding Author Email: mssoigne@gmail.com.

NRTKs	non-receptor tyrosine kinases
BCR-ABL	break point cluster-Abelson murine leukemia
CNS	central nervous system
CML	chronic myeloid leukemia
FDA	Food and Drug Administration
Ph^+	Philadelphia chromosome positive
CP	chronic phase
AP	accelerated phase
BP	blast phase
ATP	adenosine triphosphate
CCyR	complete cytogenetic response
MMR	major molecular response
Mabs	monoclonal antibodie

INTRODUCTION

Chronic myelogenous leukemia (CML) is a myeloproliferative neoplasm that arises from a clonal hematopoietic stem cell disorder characterized by a reciprocal translocation that involves fusion of the Abelson oncogene (ABL) located in chromosome 9q34 with the breakpoint cluster region (BCR) located on chromosome 22q11.2 [1-2]. This translocation results in the formation of BCR-ABL1, a fusion oncoprotein constitutively active tyrosine kinase; therefore, causing stimulation of hematopoietic transformation, continuous cell growth, and proliferation [1-2]. The reciprocal translocation t(9;22)(q34;q11.2) that forms an abnormal chromosome 22 is referred to as the Philadelphia positive (Ph^+) chromosome [1-2]. The Ph^+ chromosome is considered the hallmark of CML and is a characteristic cytogenetic abnormality observed in 90 to 95% of patients with CML and 15 to 30% of patients with acute lymphoblastic leukemia (ALL) [1-3]. Typically, patients who receive the diagnosis of CML present in the indolent chronic-phase (CP) of the disease when they are asymptomatic or have minimal symptoms (e.g., fatigue, night sweats, malaise, weight loss) [4]. Patients will usually have elevated white blood cell counts and occasionally have thrombocytosis and splenomegaly [4].

Without medical intervention, after four to five years, chronic-phase CML (CP-CML) will invariably evolve into the more aggressive accelerated phase (AP) and blast phases (BP) or blast crisis (BC) of the disease which are associated with high mortality usually related to infection and hemorrhage [4]. Prior to the development of targeted therapies, therapeutic interventions for CML consisted of conventional, non-specific cytotoxic chemotherapies using busulfan, hydroxyurea, interferon alfa (Ifα), and cytarabine, and allogenic hematopoietic stem cell transplantation (HSCT). Unfortunately, treatment with IFα was associated with poor tolerability and progressive disease [5].

Although allogenic HSCT is a proven curative treatment for CML, lack of suitable donors, advanced age (greater than 60 years), and high morbidity and mortality associated with graft-versus-host disease limit its widespread use [5-6]. This dilemma led researchers to develop novel, small molecules with target-specific mechanisms as potential therapeutic options for cancers [7-8].

TYROSINE KINASES

Protein kinases are a group of enzymes that are essential components of signal transduction pathways regulating cellular processes such as proliferation and differentiation and adaption to the extracellular environment [9]. These enzymes catalyze the transfer of the terminal gamma phosphate from adenosine triphosphate (ATP) via covalent bonding to one or more amino acid residues in a protein substrate side chain [3, 10]. The category of a protein kinase is determined by the residue to which the phosphate is transferred. Protein kinases can be classified into three different kinase groups: kinases that phosphorylate tyrosine residues (most common), kinases that phosphorylate serine and threonine residues, and kinases with activity toward all three residues [9, 11].

Based upon their relationship with the cell membrane, tyrosine kinases (TKs) can be further subdivided into receptor tyrosine kinases (RTKs) and nonreceptor tyrosine kinases (NRTKs) [12-14]. Of the 90 tyrosine kinase genes identified, there are 58 RTKs and 32 NRTKs [12]. Some examples of subfamilies of RTKs include EGFR, ERBB2 (also known as HER-2), PDGFR, VEGFR, FGFR, whereas examples of NRTKs include Src, ABL, FAK, and Janus kinase (JaK) [12, 15]. At least 45 TKs have been implicated in playing a key role in the development of many malignancies [16]. When TKs cease to function normally, oncogenic activation can occur in several ways: gene mutations or deletions, gene amplification and/or overexpression of protein tyrosine kinases such as EGFR), genomic rearrangements, chromosomal translocation, or autocrine-paracrine stimulation by overexpression of ligands [16-17].

BCR-ABL TYROSINE KINASE INHIBITORS

Targeted therapies in oncology are broadly classified as either monoclonal antibodies (MAbs) or small molecules [18]. MAbs, which are typically water soluble and large molecule, recognize antigens expressed on the surface of cancer cells or target growth factors responsible for tumor proliferation [18]. They directly exert their therapeutic effects by binding to cell surface receptors and cellular antigens leading to antibody-dependent apoptosis of malignant cells [19]. MAbs also exert their anticancer effects indirectly via various mechanisms that involve the host immune system, resulting in tumor cell toxicity by mediating antibody-dependent cellular cytoxicity (ADCC) or complement dependent cytotoxicity (CDC) [20].

Small molecules of interest in oncology are protein kinases because when protein kinases fail to function appropriately due to genetic mutations, abnormal signaling, loss of autoregulatory processes, or overexpression malignancies may occur [15, 18]. Because protein kinases play such a critical role in cellular function, they have become an important therapeutic target for the treatment of many cancers [7]. In particular, aberrant ABL NRTK activity leading to disruption of regulation of the cell cycle has been implicated in the etiology of CML [3].

In contrast to MAbs, TKIs are mostly hydrophobic and able to penetrate the cell membrane where they can interact with intracellular receptors and signaling molecules effectively blocking receptor signaling and interfering with discrete downstream intracellular pathways [21-22]. Because these agents exert pharmacologic specificity, normal cells are spared and their toxicity profile is more favorable than that of traditional cytotoxic agents [3]. Currently, there are five commercially available BCR-ABL-TKI compounds that have been developed to selectively target and inhibit NRTKs involved in the pathobiology of CML (Table 1).

Table 1. Current FDA-Approved TKIs for Leukemia [from 10, 23, 32-35]

Drug	Trade	Target TKs	FDA-Approval Date	Indication(s)
Imatinib	Gleevec®	BCR-ABL, c-KIT, PDGFR-α and -β	May 2001	CML, ALL, GIST, MDS, MPD, ASM, HES, CEL, DFSP
Dasatinib	Sprycel®	BCR-ABL, Src, c-KIT, PDGFR-β	June 2006	CML, ALL
Nilotinib	Tasigna®	BCR-ABL, c-KIT, PDGFR-α and -β	October 2007	CML
Bosutinib	Bosulif®	BCR-ABL, Src	September 2012	CML
Ponatinib	Iclusig®	BCR-ABL, Src, VEGFR, FGFR, PDGFR-α and -β, EPH	December 2012	CML with T315I mutation, ALL

Abbreviation: ALL: acute lymphoblastic leukemia; ASM: aggressive systemic mastocytosis; BCR-ABL: breakpoint cluster region-Abelson oncogene; c-kit: stem cell growth factor receptor; CEL: chronic eosinophilic leukemia; CML: chronic myelogenous leukemia; DFSP: dermatofibrosarcoma protuberans; EPH: ephrin; FGFR: fibroblast growth factor receptor; GIST: gastrointestinal stromal tumor; HES: hypereosinophilic syndrome; MDS/MPD: myelodysplastic/myeloproliferative disorder; PDGFR: platelet-derived growth factor receptor; Src: sarcoma family of nonreceptor tyrosine kinase inhibitors; VEGFR: vascular endothelial growth factor receptor.

Imatinib

In 2001, the Food and Drug Administration (FDA) approved imatinib, the first oral TKI, for the management of CML (Table 1) [23]. The International Randomized Study of Interferon and ST1571 (IRIS) study was the pivotal phase III open-label, randomized, multicenter crossover clinical trial that compared imatinib to IFα plus cytarabine in patients newly diagnosed with CP-CML [24]. At a median follow-up of 18 months, a complete cytogenetic response (CCyR), an absence of Ph^+ cells in metaphase, was observed in 76% of imatinib versus 15% of IFα/cytarabine patients.

Imatinib demonstrated superiority, improved overall and event-free survival, and reduced rates of transformation from CP-CML to AP- or BP-CML [24]. In addition, imatinib demonstrated a much more favorable toxicity profile than cytotoxic chemotherapies previously used. The results of this landmark study solidified imatinib as the standard of care in CML treatment. At a median follow-up of 60 months, patients who received continuous treatment with imatinib as initial therapy for their CP-CML had durable responses in overall and event-free survival of 89 and 83 percent, respectively [25]. Furthermore, patients who responded to imatinib had a low overall risk of disease progression (i.e., 97% of patients had not progressed to the AP or BC [25]. These overall outcomes and conclusions have remained durable with 8 years of follow-up of the IRIS study [26].

Imatinib inhibits autophosphorylation of BCR-ABL tyrosine kinase, the constitutive abnormal gene product of the Ph^+ chromosome in CML [5]. Inhibition of this enzyme suppresses proliferation and tumor formation of BCR-ABL expressing myeloid cells with minimal harm to normal cells (Figure 1). In addition to BCR-ABL, imatinib effectively inhibits phosphorylation of c-KIT, the tyrosine kinase receptor for stem cell factor, and the receptor kinase platelet-derived growth factor (PDGF) [27]. Imatinib is very effective for inducing cytogenetic responses in up to 90% of patients with CML, but many patients experience relapse within months of treatment [9, 25, 28]. However, imatinib is less potent than the second-generation TKIs such as dasatinib, nilotinib, or bosutinib [29].

While TKIs are not cytotoxic chemotherapy and are generally well tolerated, most patients will experience some adverse events such as myelosuppression; anemia; fluid retention such as periorbital and peripheral edema; muscle cramps; gastrointestinal disturbances such as nausea, vomiting, diarrhea, and abdominal pain; musculoskeletal pain; rash; fatigue; joint pain; and headache [24]. Dosing recommendations and pharmacokinetic properties for BCR-ABL TKIs approved for leukemias are detailed in Tables 2 and 3, respectively [23, 30-36].

Dasatinib

Dasatinib is a second generation TKI with dual ABL/SRC inhibition that demonstrates a 325-fold higher potency *in vitro* in comparison to imatinib [37]. Dasatinib binds to the active and inactive conformations of the ABL kinase domain and has activity against the majority of the kinase domain mutations; however, it cannot overcome the threonine-to-isoleucine mutation at position 315 (T315I) [38]. The T315I mutation, often referred to as the gatekeeper mutation, is present in up to 20% of patients with resistance to TKIs [39]. In 2006, dasatinib was initially FDA-approved for chronic, accelerated, or blast phase CML patients with resistance or intolerance to prior therapy (e.g., imatinib) as well as Ph^+ acute lymphoblastic leukemia (ALL) with resistance or intolerance to prior therapy [32]. The phase III randomized, open-label, multinational trial Dasatinib versus Imatinib Study in Treatment-Naïve CML Patients (DASISION) was conducted to compare the efficacy and safety of dasatinib vs. imatinib in patients with newly diagnosed CP-CML [37]. The primary objective of DASISION was to determine whether patients who received dasatinib had a higher rate of CCyR compared to the first-line therapy, imatinib [37]. After 12 months, dasatinib met its primary end point and demonstrated superior efficacy compared to imatinib in patients experiencing higher rates of CCyR [37]. At 24 months, the cumulative CCgR and major molecular response (MMR) such as reduction in BCR-ABL transcript levels rates were still higher for dasatinib [40].

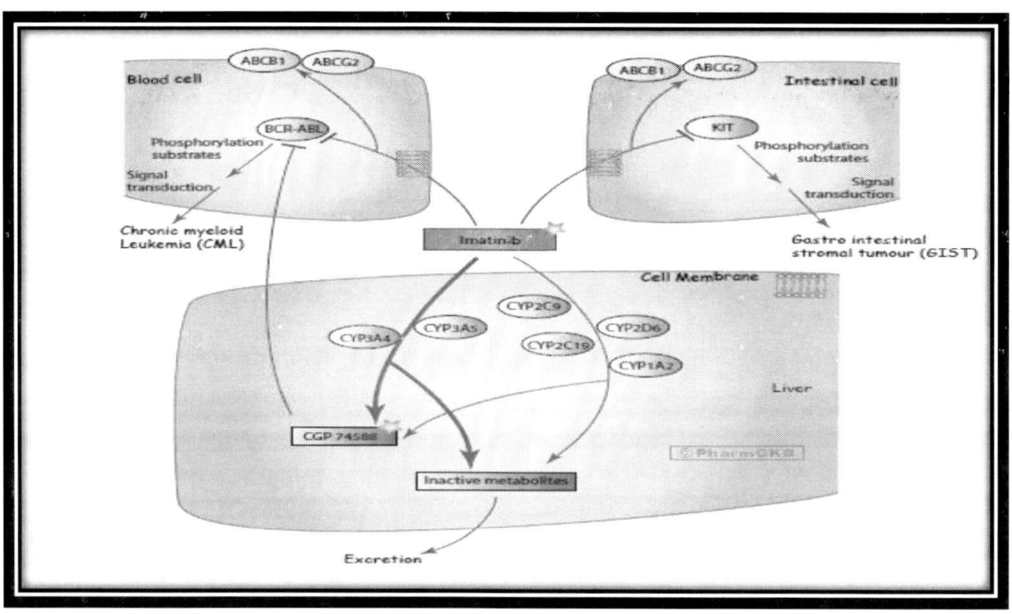

Figure 1. Imatinib metabolism pathway. Permission from PharmGKB and Stanford University [27].

Table 2. Dosing recommendations of TKIs for CML [23, 32-36]

Drug	Dose	Administration Recommendations	Dose Adjustment in Renal Impairment	Dose Adjustment in Hepatic Impairment
Imatinib	400 mg QD	With food	Yes; ↓ starting dose 50%	Yes; 300 mg QD
Dasatinib	100 mg QD	With or without food	No	No
Nilotinib	300 mg BID	Empty stomach	No	Yes; 200 mg BID
Bosutinib	500 mg QD	With food	Yes; 300QD	Yes; 200 mg QD
Ponatinib	45 mg QD	With or without food	No	Yes; 30 mg QD

Abbreviation: QD: once daily; BID: twice daily.

Table 3. Pharmacokinetic of TKIs [Ref 23, 30-36]

Drug	Bioavailability (oral, %)	Food Effect on Bioavailability	Metabolism	Elimination $t_{1/2}$	Serum Protein Binding (%)	Elimination
Imatinib	98	No effect	CYP3A4 CYP2C9 CYP2D6 CYP3A5	~ 18 (imatinib); ~ 40 metabolite (N-desmethyl metabolite)	95	~ 81% feces
Dasatinib	< 34	↑ AUC 14%	CYP3A4	3-5	93 - 96	~ 85% feces
Nilotinib	Unknown	↑ C_{max} 112%; ↑ AUC 82%	CYP3A4 CYP2C8 CYP2C9 CYP2D6	17	98	~ 93% feces
Bosutinib	34	No effect	CYP3A4	22	94 - 96	~ 91% feces
Ponatinib	Unknown	No effect	CYP3A4 CYP2C8 CYP2D6 CYP3A5	24 (12-66)	> 99	~ 87% feces

Abbreviation: TKI: tyrosine kinase inhibitors; CYP: cytochrome P450.

In addition, only 2.3% of dasatinib patients versus 5.0% of imatinib patients transformed to either AP- or BP-CML [40]. Results of the DASISION trial led to the additional approval of dasatinib for treatment of newly diagnosed patients with Ph$^+$ CP-CML. Common non-hematologic drug-related adverse events for dasatinib included: fluid retention, musculoskeletal pain, rash, headache, and diarrhea; however, these events occurred less frequently than patients being treated with imatinib [37]. However, pleural effusion was reported only in patients taking dasatinib. Furthermore, thrombocytopenia occurred with greater frequency in patients taking dasatinib compared to imatinib [37].

Dasatinib is well absorbed after oral administration; however, a neutral gastric pH significantly reduces its bioavailability [41]. Therefore, concomitant administration of histamine-antagonists such as famotidine, protein pump inhibitors such as omeprazole, or antacids should be avoided 2 hours before or after dasatinib administration [31-32, 42]. Dasatinib has been associated with a low incidence of pulmonary hypertension that usually improves upon treatment cessation; however, it is not always reversible [43].

Overall, BCR-ABL TKIs approved for the clinical management of leukemias have long half-lives with the exception of dasatinib which has a half-life of 3 – 5 hours [31].

Nilotinib

Nilotinib is a second generation that is a more potent and selective inhibitor of the BCR-ABL protein TK than imatinib and is effective against imatinib-resistant ABL kinase domain mutations [44-45]. In 2007, nilotinib was initially FDA-approved for treatment of CP and AP of Ph^+ CML in patients resistant or intolerant to imatinib [33]. The phase III study known as Evaluating Nilotinib Efficacy and Safety in Clinical Trials – Newly Diagnosed Patients (ENESTnd) was a randomized, open-label, multicenter trial conducted in patients diagnosed with CP-CML [46]. Patients were assigned to a 1:1:1 ratio to receive nilotinib at a dose of 300 mg or 400 mg twice daily or imatinib 400 mg once daily [46]. Patients in both nilotinib arms of the study demonstrated a significant improvement in the time to progression to either the AP or BP, as compared to patients in the imatinib arm [46]. Results of this study led to the added label indication of nilotinib for management of patients with newly diagnosed Ph^+ CP-CML.

Three-year follow-up analysis of ENESTnd continued to show high rates of MMR and low rates of progression to both AP- or BP-CML [47]. Unlike the other BCR-ABL inhibitors, the bioavailability of nilotinib increases significantly when taken concomitantly with a high-fat meal; therefore, nilotinib should be taken on an empty stomach (2 hours before or 1 hour after meals) to reduce the increased risk of toxicities such as QT interval prolongation [48-49]. Nilotinib displays pH-dependent aqueous solubility, thus it should not be co-administered with agents that inhibit gastric acid secretion such as proton pump inhibitors because elevated gastric pH levels may decrease its bioavailability [31]. However, use of short-acting antacids such as aluminum hydroxide, magnesium hydroxide, or simethicone have not been shown to alter the pharmacokinetics of nilotinib; therefore, antacids may be taken 2 hours before or 2 hours after administration of nilotinib [33, 42].

Common non-hematologic toxicities of nilotinib include headache and dermatologic reactions such as rash, alopecia, and pruritus. Imatinib was associated with higher rates of neutropenia and anemia, whereas nilotinib was associated with a higher frequency of thrombocytopenia [46]. Patients who develop thrombocytopenia on nilotinib therapy can be effectively managed with dose interruption or reductions that do not typically result in permanent discontinuation of therapy [50]. Nilotinib has been shown to prolong the QTc interval in some patients; therefore, careful monitoring for cardiac events and arrhythmias should be performed and medications like amiodarone, methadone, or moxifloxacin that may prolong the QTc interval should be avoided [51]. In addition, hypokalemia and hypomagnesemia should be corrected prior to nilotinib administration to minimize the potential for QT interval prolongation [50]. Although it is a rare phenomenon, cases of elevated serum lipases and pancreatitis have been reported with nilotinib use and warrant clinical monitoring, particularly in patients with a history of pancreatitis [52].

Bosutinib

Bosutinib is a second generation dual BCR-ABL/SRC inhibitor that is more potent than imatinib [2]. It has demonstrated activity against cell lines that are resistant to imatinib due to different mutations and BCR-ABL overexpression; however, the T315I mutation usually resistant to bosutinib [2]. The phase III study Bosutinib Efficacy and Safety in Newly Diagnosed CML (BELA) was a randomized, open-label, multinational clinical trial that compared bosutinib to imatinib in patients newly diagnosed with CP-CML [53]. The primary efficacy end point was CCgR at 12 months. Bosutinib did not demonstrate a superior CCyR at 12 months versus imatinib, thus it did not achieve its primary endpoint [53]. However, at 12 months the MMR rate, a secondary end point of the study, was higher with bosutinib compared to imatinib [53]. In 2012, bosutinib was FDA-approved for the management of CP, AP or BP- Ph^+ CML in patients with resistance or intolerance to prior therapy [34]. Similar to nilotinib, bosutinib is an agent with pH-dependent solubility. To avoid a reduction in bosutinib drug levels, it should not be co-administered with pH-altering medications such as proton pump inhibitors; however, short-acting antacids may be taken if concomitant administration is separated by 2 hours [34].

The most common non-hematologic adverse events associated with bosutinib include nausea, vomiting, diarrhea, abdominal pain, rash, and increases in aminotransferase levels [53]. Diarrhea associated with bosutinib use is frequently experienced by patients in the first 2 – 4 weeks of therapy and can be effectively controlled with anti-diarrheal medications such as loperamide or diphenoxylate and atropine [53]. Perhaps due to the minimal inhibition of c-KIT, bosutinib is associated with lower rates of neutropenia and anemia compared to imatinib [53].

Ponatinib

Ponatinib, a highly potent third generation BCR-ABL TKI, demonstrates activity against an extensive spectrum of kinase domain mutations, including the T315I mutation [54-56]. Imatinib and the second generation TKIs are unable to overcome the T315I gatekeeper mutation which functions by blocking access of an agent to the enzyme's ATP-binding site and results in drug-resistance in approximately 15 – 20% of patients with CML [56-58]. Based on the result from the phase II, Ponatinib Ph^+ Acute Lymphoblastic Leukemia [ALL] and CML Evaluation (PACE) trial, the FDA in 2012 granted ponatinib accelerated approval for the treatment of CML or Ph^+ ALL in patients resistant or intolerant to prior TKI therapy [35, 59].

Patients who developed resistance to, or experienced unacceptable adverse events from dasatinib or nilotinib therapy, or with the T315I mutation were eligible to be enrolled in the PACE study, an open-label, multinational, single-arm clinical trial [59]. The primary efficacy end point was a major cytogenetic response (Mcg) within the first 12 months in CP-CML and MCg at any time within the first 6 months in AP-CML, BP-CML, or Ph^+ -ALL [59]. In patients with CP-CML, ponatinib efficacy resulted in 56% Mcg response, 46% CCgR, and 34% MMR, respectively [59]. Seventy percent of patients with CP-CML with the T315I mutation achieved a Mcg response [59].

Ponatinib demonstrated activity against all single BCR-ABL mutations and 91% of patients achieved a sustained Mcg response for at least 12 months, and in AP-CML and BP-CML, 55% and 31% achieved Mcg responses, respectively [59]. Commonly reported non-hematologic adverse events included rash, dry skin, and abdominal pain [59]. Commonly reported hematologic adverse events were thrombocytopenia, neutropenia, and anemia [59]. Pancreatitis was the most common treatment-related serious adverse event; however, all cases were reversible (most resolved within 1 week) and only 1 patient discontinued treatment because of pancreatitis [59]. Serious-grade arterial thrombotic adverse events such as cardiovascular, cerebrovascular, and peripheral vascular were observed in 9% of ponatinib-treated patients, of which 3% were attributed to study treatment [59]. The Evaluation of Ponatinib versus Imatinib in CML (EPIC) study was a phase III randomized, open-label, international trial designed to assess the efficacy and safety of ponatinib compared to imatinib in patients newly diagnosed with CP-CML [60-61]. The primary efficacy end point was MMR at 12 months [60-61]. Amidst safety concerns regarding the benefit versus risk related to vascular events that continued to be reported in the previously ponatinib-treated population, the trial was terminated early and efficacy could not be established [60-61].

Postmarketing safety reports showed that at least 27% of ponatinib-treated patients from the phase I and II trials experienced arterial and venous vascular occlusion events. In October 2013, the manufacturer complied with the FDA's request to suspended marketing and sales of ponatinib after continued safety monitoring and follow-up data revealed a high frequency of serious adverse vascular events [62]. In December 2013, marketing of ponatinib was resumed with requirements from the FDA requiring more restrictive drug labeling and updated information on safety risks associated with ponatinib use [62]. The labeled indications for ponatinib have been narrowed to include treatment for CP-, AP-, or BP-CML in patients who are T315I-positive, or for whom no other TKI therapy is indicated, and for Ph^+ ALL who are T315I-positive or for whom no other TKI is indicated [35, 62].

Drug Interactions and the CYP450

Because TKIs are primarily metabolized via the cytochrome P450 system, potential drug interactions exist [42]. Although all BCR-ABL TKIs are primarily metabolized *via* the CYP3A4 liver microsomal enzyme, other cytochrome P450 enzymes such as CYP2C8, CYP2C9, CYP2D6, and CYP3A5 play minor roles in the metabolism of the BCR-ABL TKIs with the exception of dasatinib and bosutinib [31, 42]. Patients should be closely monitored for clinically relevant drug or food interactions related to the co-administration of TKIs and strong CYP3A4 inhibitors and inducers [63].

The use of strong CYP3A4 inhibitors may elevate TKI plasma concentrations and result in increased toxicities; therefore, concomitant use should be avoided [31]. Examples of strong CYP3A4 inhibitors include: azole antifungals ketoconazole, itraconazole; macrolides clarithromycin, telithromycin; HCV protease inhibitors boceprevir, telaprevir; HIV protease inhibitors indinavir, ritonavir; nefazodone; and grapefruit juice [50]. If concomitant use of a strong CYP3A4 inhibitor cannot be avoided, TKI dose reduction or discontinuation (with a washout period of 1 week) should be considered [50]. Concomitant use of strong CYP3A4 inducers may result in reduced TKI efficacy and should be avoided unless the benefit outweighs the risk of reduced TKI exposure. Clinicians should consider alternative therapeutic agents with little or no CYP3A4 enzyme induction potential. Examples of strong CYP3A4 inducers include: anticonvulsants carbamazepine, phenytoin, and phenobarbital; dexamethasone; rifampin; and St. John's wort [50]. Because of strong CYP3A4 inhibition, concomitant administration of dasatinib or imatinib with simvastatin, an HMG-CoA reductase inhibitor with a narrow therapeutic index, may result in an increased simvastatin maximum concentration and area under curve; therefore, combination treatment should be used with caution or avoided, but pravastatin or rosuvastatin may be initiated [23, 31-32, 35, 42]. Because warfarin is a substrate of both CYP2C9 and CYP3A4, concomitant use with imatinib should be avoided; alternatively, patients who require anticoagulation should be initiated on low-molecular weight or standard heparin therapy [23, 30-31].

Conclusion

Imatinib, the first TKI approved to block kinase activity of BCR-ABL, was developed over a decade ago and has since revolutionized the treatment management of CML [64]. Prior to the advent of TKI therapies, the prognosis for patients diagnosed with CP-CML was poor with median survival of 5 – 7 years [5]. TKIs used for the management of leukemias differ from traditional cytotoxic therapies in their ability to produce durable hematologic and cytogenetic responses with a more favorable toxicity profile [64]. Oral BCR-ABL TKIs are generally well tolerated and adverse events associated with their use are typically mild to moderate in intensity, can be easily controlled, and subside after the first few months of treatment [36, 64].

Toxicities can usually be managed by dose reductions, interruptions in therapy, or supportive treatment using anti-diarrheals, anti-emetics, corticosteroids, colony stimulating factors, or others [4, 50]. Currently, imatinib, dasatinib, and nilotinib are approved as first-line agents for the treatment of patients newly diagnosed with CP-CML [65]. Treatment selection should be guided by patient-specific parameters such as use of dasatinib and nilotinib should be avoided in patients who have or may develop QT interval prolongation; avoid use of nilotinib in patients with a history of pancreatitis, avoid dasatinib in patients with lung diseases [64]. From the BELA study, bosutinib did not show an improvement of CCgR [53]. However, MMR was observed; therefore it can be used as second-line agent for CML resistance or intolerance to prior therapy [65]. Follow-up data from clinical trials revealed an increase in ponatinib-related vascular occlusion events which led the FDA to require additional safety measures for marketing of the agent [64]. Consequently, indications for ponatinib use are limited for treatment of T315I positive CML, T315I positive Ph^+ ALL, and CML or ALL for whom no other TKI is indicated [65]. Although TKIs have changed the treatment landscape for CML and dramatically improved overall survival of patients diagnosed with CML, these inhibitors cannot eradicate all CML cells *in vitro* study. Achievement of BCR-ABL transcript DNA levels of $\leq$ 10% at 3 or 6 months, an early molecular response following initiation of TKI therapy, generally predicts better long-term outcomes for patients progression-free survival and overall survival [66]. However, even in patients with undetectable levels of BCR-ABL transcripts, TKI therapy must be continued indefinitely, since withdrawal of therapy can result in relapse [4, 50]. An important goal and challenge for the future will be to develop therapies with the ability to overcome drug resistance, minimize residual disease, eradicate residual stem cells, and decrease the need for long-term treatment to maintain disease remission [67].

References

[1] Fausel, CA; Kiel, PJ. Chronic Leukemias. In: DiPiro JT, Talbert RL, Yee GE, eds. *Pharmacotherapy: A Pathophysiologic Approach*, 9th ed. New York, NY: McGraw Hill, 2014, 2277-93.

[2] Chu, E; Sartorelli, AC. Cancer chemotherapy. In: Katzung BG, Trevor, AJ, Eds. *Basic & Clinical Pharmacology*. 13th ed. New York, NY: McGraw Hill, 2015, pp. 918-40.

[3] Arora, A; Scholar, EM. Role of tyrosine kinase inhibitors in cancer therapy. *J Pharmacol Exp Ther*, 2005, 315(3), 971-79.

[4] Apperley, JF. Chronic myeloid leukaemia. *Lancet*, 2015, 385(9976), 1447-59.

[5] Fausel, C. Targeted chronic myeloid leukemia therapy: seeking a cure. *Am J Health Syst Pharm*, 2007, 64(Suppl 15), S9-15.

[6] Schiffer, CA. BCR-ABL tyrosine kinase inhibitors for chronic myelogenous leukemia. *N Engl J Med*, 2007, 357(3), 258-65.

[7] Finley, RS. Overview of targeted therapies for cancer. *Am J Health Syst Pharm*, 2003, 60(24 Suppl 9), S4-10.

[8] DeVita, VT; Chu, E. A history of cancer chemotherapy. *Cancer Res*, 2008, 68(21), 8643-53.

[9] Chabner, BA; Barnes, J; Neal, J; et al. Targeted therapies: tyrosine kinase inhibitors, monoclonal antibodies, and cytokines. In: Brunton LL, Chabner BA, Knollmann BC, Eds. Goodman & Gilman's *The Pharmacological Basis of Therapeutics*, 12th ed. New York, NY: McGraw Hill, 2011, pp. 1731-34.

[10] Nishioka, Y; Aono, Y; Sone, S. Role of tyrosine kinase inhibitors in tumor immunology. *Immunotherapy*, 2011, 3(1), 1077-116.

[11] Zhang, J; Yang, PL; Gray, NS. Targeting cancer with small molecule kinase inhibitors. *Nat Rev Cancer*, 2009, 9(1), 28-39.

[12] Vlahovic, G; Crawford, J. Activation of tyrosine kinases in cancer. *Oncologist*, 2003, 8(6), 531-38.

[13] Paul, MK; Mukhopadhyay, AK. Tyrosine kinase – role and significance in cancer. *Int J Med Sci*, 2004, 1(2), 101-15.

[14] Krause, DS; Van Etten, RA. Tyrosine kinases as targets for cancer therapy. *N Engl J Med*, 2005, 353(2), 172-87.

[15] Bari, SB; Adhikari, S; Surana, SJ. Tyrosine kinase receptor inhibitors: a new target for anticancer drug development. *Journal of Pharma Sci Tech*, 2012, 1(2), 36-45.

[16] Madhusudan, S; Ganesan, TS. Tyrosine kinase inhibitors in cancer therapy. *Clin Biochem*, 2004, 37(7), 618-35.

[17] Gross, S; Rahal, R; Stransky, N; Lengauer, C; Hoeflich, KP. Targeting cancer with kinase inhibitors. *J Clin Invest*, 2015, 125(5), 1780-89.

[18] Gerber, DE. Targeted therapies: a new generation of cancer treatments. *Am Fam Physician*, 2008, 77(3), 311-19.

[19] Shord, SS; Medina, PJ. Cancer treatment and chemotherapy. In: DiPiro JT, Talbert RL, Yee GE, eds. *Pharmacotherapy: A Pathophysiologic Approach*, 9th ed. New York, NY: McGraw Hill, 2014, 2055-100.

[20] Strome, SE; Sausville, SE; Mann, D. A mechanistic perspective of monoclonal antibodies in cancer therapy beyond target-related effects. *Oncologist*, 2007, 12(9), 1084-95.

[21] Gotink, KJ; Verheul, HM. Anti-angiogenic tyrosine kinase inhibitors: what is their mechanism of action? *Angiogenesis*, 2010, 13(1), 1-14.

[22] Hojjat-Farsangi, M. Small-molecule inhibitors of the receptor tyrosine kinases: promising tools for targeted cancer therapies. *Int J Mol Sci*, 2014, 15(8), 13768-801.

[23] Gleevec [package insert]. *Novartis Pharmaceuticals Corporation*, East Hanover, NJ, August 2016. https://www.pharma.us.novartis.com/sites/www.pharma.us.novartis.com/files/gleevec_tabs.pdf. Accessed September 26, 2016.

[24] O'Brien, SG; Guilhot, F; Larson, RA; et al. Imatinib compared with interferon and low-dose cytarabine for newly diagnosed chronic-phase chronic myeloid leukemia. *N Engl J Med*, 2003, 348(11), 994-1004.

[25] Druker, BJ; Guilhot, F; O'Brien, SG; et al. Five-year follow-up of patients receiving imatinib for chronic myeloid leukemia. *N Engl J Med*, 2006, 355(23), 2408-17.

[26] Deininger, M; O'Brien, SG; Guilhot, F; et al. International Randomized Study of Interferon vs ST1571 (IRIS) 8-year follow up: sustained survival and low risk for progression or events in patients with newly diagnosed chronic myeloid leukemia in chronic phase (CML-CP) treated with imatinib. ASH 2009 Annual Meeting Abstracts. *Blood*, 2009, 114, 1126.

[27] Whirl-Carrillo, M; McDonagh, EM; Hebert, JM; et al. Pharmacogenomics Knowledge for Personalized Medicine<https://www.ncbi.nlm.nih.gov/pubmed/22992668, "*Clinical Pharmacology & Therapeutics*, (2012) 92(4), 414-417.

[28] Gorre, ME; Mohammed, M; Ellwood, K; et al. Clinical resistance to STI-571 cancer therapy caused by BCR-ABL gene mutation or amplification. *Science*, 2001, 293(5531), 876-80.

[29] Cortes, J; Jabbour, E; Kantarjian, H; et al. Dynamics of BCR-ABL kinase domain mutations in chronic myeloid leukemia after sequential treatment with multiple tyrosine kinase inhibitors. *Blood*, 2007, 110(12), 4005-11.

[30] Peng, B; Lloyd, P; Horst, S. Clinical pharmacokinetics of imatinib. *Clin Pharmacokinet*, 2005, 44(9), 879-94.

[31] Di Gion, P; Kanefendt, F; Lindauer, A; et al. Clinical Pharmacokinetics of tyrosine kinase inhibitors: focus on pyrimidines, pyridines, and pyrroles. *Clin Pharmacokinet.*, 2011, 50(9), 551-603.

[32] Sprycel [package insert]. Bristol-Myers Squibb Company, Princeton, NJ: October 2015. http://packageinserts.bms.com/pi/pi_sprycel.pdf. Accessed September 26, 2016.

[33] Tasigna [package insert]. Novartis Pharmaceuticals Corporation, East Hanover, NJ, January 2015. https://www.pharma.us.novartis.com/sites/www.pharma.us.novartis.com/files/tasigna.pdf. Accessed September 26, 2016.

[34] Bosulif [package insert]. Pfizer, Inc., New York, NY, April 2016. http: //labeling.pfizer.com/ShowLabeling.aspx?id=884#section-11.1. Accessed September 26, 2016.

[35] Iclusig [package insert]. Ariad Pharmaceuticals, Inc., Cambridge, MA, June 2016. http://www.iclusig.com/pi. Accessed September 26, 2016.

[36] Eckstein, N; Röper, L; Haas, B; et al. Clinical pharmacology of tyrosine kinase inhibitors becoming generic drugs: the regulatory perspective. *J Exp Clin Cancer Res*, 2014, 33, 15.

[37] Kantarjian, H; Shah, NP; Hochhaus, A; et al. Dasatinib versus imatinib in newly diagnosed chronic-phase chronic myeloid leukemia. *N Engl J Med*, 2010, 362(24), 2260-70.

[38] Steinberg, M. Dasatinib: a tyrosine kinase inhibitor for the treatment of chronic myelogenous leukemia and Philadelphia chromosome-positive acute lymphoblastic leukemia. *Clin Ther.*, 2007, 29(11), 2289-308.

[39] Soverini, S; Colarossi, S; Gnani, A; et al. Contribution of ABL kinase domain mutations to imatinib resistance in different subsets of Philadelphia-positive patients: by the GIMEMA Working Party on Chronic Myeloid Leukemia. *Clin Cancer Res*, 2006, 12(24), 7374-79.

[40] Kantarjian, HM; Shah, NP; Cortes, JE; et al. Dasatinib or imatinib in newly diagnosed chronic-phase myeloid leukemia: 2-year follow-up from a randomized phase 3 trial (DASISION). *Blood*, 2012, 119(5), 1123-29.

[41] Matsuoko, A; Takahashi, N; Miura, M; et al. H2-receptor antagonist influences dasatinib pharmacokinetics in a patient with Philadelphia-positive acute lymphoblastic leukemia. *Cancer Chemother Pharmacol*, 2012, 70(2), 351-52.

[42] van Leeuwen, RW; van Gelder, T; Mathijssen, RH; Jansman, FG. Drug-drug interactions with tyrosine-kinase inhibitors, a clinical perspective. *Lancet Oncol*, 2014, 15(8), e315-26.

[43] Montani, D; Bergot, E; Günther, S; et al. Pulmonary arterial hypertension in patients treated by dasatinib. *Circulation*, 2012, 125(17), 2128-37.

[44] Kantarjian, H; Giles, F; Wunderle, L; et al. Nilotinib in imatinib-resistant CML and Philadelphia chromosome – positive ALL. *N Engl J Med*, 2006, 354(24), 2542-51.

[45] le Coutre, P; Ottmann, OG; Giles, F; et al. Nilotinib (formerly AMN107), a highly selective BCR-ABL tyrosine kinase inhibitor, is active in patients with imatinib-resistant or –intolerant accelerated-phase chronic myelogenous leukemia. *Blood*, 2008, 111(4), 1834-39.

[46] Saglio, G; Kim, DW; Issaragrisil, S; et al. Nilotinib versus imatinib for newly diagnosed chronic myeloid leukemia. *N Engl J Med*, 2010, 362(24), 2251-59.

[47] Larson, RA; Hochhaus, A; Hughes, TP; et al. Nilotinib vs imatinib in patients with newly diagnosed Philadelphia chromosome-positive chronic myeloid leukemia in chronic phase: ENESTnd 3-year follow-up. *Leukemia*, 2012, 26(10), 2197-203.

[48] DeRemer, DL; Ustun, C; Natarajan, K. Nilotinib: a second-generation tyrosine kinase inhibitor for the treatment of chronic myelogenous leukemia. *Clin Ther*, 2008, 30(11), 1956-75.

[49] Tanaka, C; Yin, OQ; Sethuraman, V; et al. Clinical pharmacokinetics of the BCR-ABL tyrosine kinase inhibitor nilotinib. *Clin Pharmacol Ther*, 2010, 87(2), 197-203.

[50] Wong, SF; Mirshahidi, H. Use of tyrosine kinase inhibitors for chronic myeloid leukemia: management of patients and practical applications for pharmacy practitioners. *Ann Pharmacother*, 2011, 45(6), 787-97.

[51] Chen, MH; Kerkelä, R; Force, T. Mechanisms of cardiac dysfunction associated with tyrosine kinase inhibitor cancer therapeutics. *Circulation*, 2008, 118(1), 84-95.

[52] Engel, T; Justo, D; Amitai, M; Volchek, Y; Mayan, H. Nilotinib-associated acute pancreatitis. *Ann Pharmacother*, 2013, 47(1), e3.

[53] Cortes, JE; Kim, DW; Kantarjian, HM; et al. Bosutinib versus imatinib in newly diagnosed chronic-phase chronic myeloid leukemia: results from the BELA trial. *J Clin Oncol*, 2012, 30(28), 3486-92.

[54] Cortes, JE; Kantarjian, H; Shah, NP; et al. Ponatinib in refractory Philadelphia chromosome-positive leukemias. *N Engl J Med*, 2012, 367(22), 2075-88.

[55] Cassuto, O; Dufies, M; Jacquel, A; et al. All tyrosine kinase inhibitor-resistant chronic myelogenous cells are highly sensitive to ponatinib. *Oncotarget*, 2012, 3(12), 1557-65.

[56] Cassuto, O; Jacquel, A; Robert, GE; Augerger, P. Ponatinib circumvents all types of imatinib resistance in chronic myelogenous leukemia cell lines. *Cell Cycle*, 2013, 12(11), 1645-46.

[57] Quintás-Cardama, A; Cortes, J. Therapeutic options against BCR-ABL1 T315I-positive chronic myelogenous leukemia. *Clin Cancer Res*, 2008, 14(4), 4392-99.

[58] Mughal, A; Aslam, HM; Khan, AM; Saleem, S; Umah, R; Saleem, M. Bcr-Abl tyrosine kinase inhibitors – current status. *Infect Agent Cancer*, 2013, 8(1), 23.

[59] Cortes, JE; Kim, DW; Pinilla-Ibarz, J; et al. A phase 2 trial of ponatinib in Philadelphia chromosome-positive leukemias. *N Engl J Med*, 2013, 369(19), 1783-96.

[60] Lipton, JH; Chuah, C; Guerci-Bresler, A; et al. EPIC: a phase 3 trial of ponatinib compared with imatinib in patients with newly diagnosed chronic myeloid leukemia in chronic phase (CP-CML). *Blood*, 2014, 124(21), 519.

[61] Lipton, JH; Chuah, C; Guerci-Bresler, A; et al. Ponatinib versus imatinib for newly diagnosed chronic myeloid leukaemia: an international, randomized, open-label, phase 3 trial. *Lancet Oncol*, 2016, 17(5), 612-21.

[62] Gainor, JF; Chabner, BA. Ponatinib: accelerated disapproval [editorial]. *Oncologist*, 2015, 20(8), 847-48.

[63] Culhane, J; Li, E. Targeted therapy with tyrosine kinase inhibitors. *US Pharm*, 2008, 33(10 Oncology suppl), 3-14, 23. Available from: https://www.uspharmacist.com/article/targeted-therapy-with-tyrosine-kinase-inhibitors [cited: 26th Sep 2016].

[64] Pophali, PA; Patnaik, MA. The role of new tyrosine kinase inhibitors in chronic myeloid leukemia. *Cancer J*, 2016, 22(1), 40-50.

[65] National Comprehensive Cancer Network. NCCN Clinical Practice Guidelines in Oncology. *Chronic Myelogenous Leukemia*. V.1.2016. [cited: 26th September 2016]. Available from: https://www.nccn.org/professionals/physician_gls/pdf/cml.pdf.

[66] Hughes, TP; Saglio, G; Kantarjian, HM; et al. Early molecular response predicts outcomes in patients with chronic myeloid leukemia in chronic phase treated with frontline nilotinib or imatinib. *Blood*, 2014, 123(9), 1353-60.

[67] O'Dwyer M. First-line treatment of chronic myeloid leukemia. *Ther Adv Hematol*, 2010, 1(1), 15-22.

In: Frontiers in Leukemia Pharmacotherapy
Editor: Lunawati L. Bennett
ISBN: 978-1-53614-960-9

Chapter 6

MYELODYSPLASTIC SYNDROME

Zachery R. Halford*[*]*, PharmD
Union University, College of Pharmacy, Jackson, Tennessee, US

ABSTRACT

Myelodysplastic syndrome (MDS) is a heterogeneous group of hematological disorders characterized by dysplastic and ineffective hematopoiesis resulting in qualitative and quantitative marrow defects. A disease of the elderly, the median age for diagnosis in the United States is 76 years. With limited treatment options for this frail population, MDS tends to follow an indolent course with most patients living 5 to 10 years after diagnosis. Significant progress has been made over the past decade as researchers continue to gain understanding into the pathogenesis and genetic determinants of MDS.

This chapter provides a broad overview of the epidemiology, etiology, pathogenesis, disease classification, clinical presentation, pathologic features, diagnosis, prognosis, and general treatment options for myelodysplastic syndrome. Particular emphasis is placed on discussing specific treatment options based on risk stratification and symptomotology.

Keywords: myelodysplastic syndrome, pre-leukemia, cytopenias, chromosome 5q deletion, lenalidomide, erythropoietin-stimulating agents, azacitidine, decitabine, DNA methyltransferase inhibitors

ABBREVIATIONS

AML	acute myeloid leukemia
ATG	anti-thymocyte globulin

[*] Corresponding Author Email: zhalford@uu.edu.

DMTI	DNA methyltransferase inhibitor
EPO	erythropoietin
ESA	erythropoiesis stimulating agent
FAB	French-American-British
FDA	Food and Drug Administration
G-CSF	granulocyte-colony stimulating factor
HSCT	hematopoietic stem cell transplantation
IMiD	immunomodulatory drug
IPSS	International Prognostic Scoring System
IPSS-R	International Prognostic Scoring System - Revised
IST	immunosuppressive therapy
LDH	lactate dehydrogenase
MDS	myelodysplastic syndrome
NCCN	National Comprehensive Cancer Network
RBC	red blood cell
REMS	Risk Evaluation and Mitigation Strategy program
SEER	Surveillance, Epidemiology and End Results Program
TPO	thrombopoietin
WHO	World Health Organization

INTRODUCTION

MDS is a malignant and heterogeneous group of acquired hematopoietic stem cell disorders characterized by dysplastic and ineffective hematopoiesis [1]. Historically, MDS was referred to as oligoblastic leukemia, smoldering acute leukemia, preleukemia or refractory anemia. These syndromes may arise *de novo* or occur secondary to mutagenic therapy or exposure to environmental toxins [1]. Over time, MDS demonstrates an inherent predisposition to transform into acute myeloid leukemia (AML) [2].

Patients with MDS exhibit variable degrees of bone marrow dysfunction resulting in anemia, thrombocytopenia and neutropenia. Furthermore, cells may also contain qualitative functional defects. The combination of qualitative and quantitative abnormalities typically result in sequelae including infections, bleeding, bruising and anemic manifestations. The general course of MDS progression varies significantly from patient to patient. Some experience a chronic indolent course while others present with a highly proliferative and aggressive disease with rapid progression to AML [3].

MDS is often diagnosed incidentally following the findings of abnormal blood counts upon examination. In general, MDS is a disease of the elderly with a median age of diagnosis around 76 years and a male predominance (estimated male-to-female ratio of

1.75 to 1) [4]. Most MDS patients will die because of the consequences of bone marrow dysregulation and not leukemic transformation. Research has dramatically improved our understanding of MDS over the past decade. For instance, the World Health Organization (WHO) revised its classification system in 2008 and again in 2016 to better reflect MDS subtypes and the unique biomarkers associated with diagnostic and prognostic criteria [5]. In addition, important advances in the management of MDS can also be noted over the last decade. Iron chelation, hematopoietic growth factors, epigenetic and immunomodulatory therapy all highlight these recent improvements. The first randomized clinical trial showing survival improvement in MDS was published in 2009. Clinicians and researchers continue to build on this success with additional ongoing trials looking to unlock the complex pathways surrounding MDS evolution and pathogenesis [6].

EPIDEMIOLOGY

A disease of the elderly, MDS is often diagnosed late in life or, in many cases, never diagnosed at all. Failure to diagnosis may result from a lack of reporting, overlap with various other myeloproliferative disorders or a misconception of poor available treatment options in elderly patients with comorbidities. Onset of disease before the age of 50 is rare with the exception of treatment-related MDS. The precise incidence of *de novo* MDS is unknown. An estimated 3 to 12 cases of MDS are annually diagnosed per 100,000 persons with a conservative estimate of approximately 10,000 new cases diagnosed annually in the United States [4]. The Surveillance, Epidemiology and End Results (SEER) Program estimates nearly 20,000 new cases of MDS each year in the United States [7]. Furthermore, reimbursement analysis of medical claims estimate the incidence of MDS in the United States to be closer to 30,000 new cases each year [8]. Currently, at least 60,000 Americans with MDS are alive in the country. With an aging population and improved awareness, this number will likely only continue to climb in the future.

ETIOLOGY AND PATHOGENESIS

The etiology of MDS remains unclear in most patients and is likely multifactorial involving a stepwise acquisition of genetic abnormalities and driver mutations. MDS may present *de novo* or following mutagenic exposure. Predisposing factors are uncovered in only 20-30% of patients [9]. The development of MDS has been associated with exposure to environmental, occupational, and treatment-related chemicals and radiation [10]. For example, MDS has been linked to atomic bomb survivors in Japan and Chernobyl nuclear plant workers [11]. Individuals with a family history of hematologic malignancy have also shown a predisposition to developing MDS [10]. Certain modifiable risk factors for developing MDS have been identified and include smoking and obesity [12]. Furthermore, recent studies suggest chronic immune stimulation from infectious and/or autoimmune diseases may serve as a trigger for MDS development [13].

Therapy-related MDS accounts for 10% to 15% of all cases [14]. Increased chemotherapy utilization in conjunction with amplified chemotherapy doses may account for some of the rising MDS incidence noted over the last decade. With improved survival rates following chemotherapy and radiation, cancer survivors are now at an increased risk of acquiring MDS with rates as high as 10% to 15% at ten years following primary treatment [15]. For those with therapy-related MDS, chromosomal abnormalities are found in roughly 90% of patients, which is significantly higher than the 50% figure reported in *de novo* MDS [15-16]. Additional risk factors for therapy-related MDS include exposure to alkylating agents, topoisomerase II inhibitors, older age, and radiotherapy prior to hematopoietic stem cell transplantation (HSCT). Table 1 provides more information on chemotherapy agents implicated in therapy-related MDS. Alkylating agents, in particular, are well documented in the development of MDS; typically lagging for about 4-7 years between exposure and MDS occurrence. Topoisomerase II inhibitors such as etoposide and teniposide typically result in MDS 2 to 3 years following exposure and also present with higher rates of chromosomal abnormalities such as 11q23 and 21q22 [14].

Table 1. Causative agents in the development of hematologic neoplasms [14]

Topoisomerase Inhibitors	Anthracyclines	Alkylating Agents	Other
Etoposide	Doxorubicin	Cyclophosphamide	Vinca alkaloids
Teniposide	Daunorubicin	Melphalan	Antimetabolites
Actinomycin	Mitoxantrone	Busulfan	Taxanes
		Carboplatin	Mycophenolate
		Cisplatin	
		Thiotepa	
		CCNU/BCNU	
		Dacarbazine	

For those with MDS, the bone marrow is characteristically hypercellular and likely suffering from ineffective hematopoiesis. As a clonally-driven process, it is believed that MDS develops from a single transformed hematopoietic progenitor cell line [17]. Studies suggest cellular dysfunction and dysplasia result from the acquisition of several mutations within the cell of origin [18]. Progressive and ongoing bone marrow failure resulting in cytopenias are the hallmark characteristic of MDS. Despite our gaps in understanding MDS pathogenesis, a multistep biochemical pathway has been proposed [1]. The affected clonal population of hematopoietic cells display enhanced self-renewal and proliferative capacity in conjunction with impaired cell differentiation, evasion of immunosurveillance, and anti-apoptotic mechanisms. These acquired changes allow the clonal population to become dysplastic and avoid destruction [19].

Myelodysplasia results in cellular dysfunction with increased cytokines, impaired cellular differentiation, loss of regulatory control, and genomic instability [1]. Within the bone marrow microenvironment, cellular division occurs at a high rate; however, these cells also experience increased apoptosis leading to ineffective cell cycling. This high rate of cellular turnover within the bone marrow results in peripheral cytopenias and a lack of mature peripheral blood cells.

Genomic instability results from a multistep process when one or more transformations within the dysplastic cell confer growth advantages to the now predominate cell line. These transformative cytogenetic abnormalities require addition evaluation; current studies detect genomic additions or deletions in roughly 50% of *de novo* MDS.

Disease Classification

Two classification structures exist for evaluating MDS. The French-American-British (FAB) Cooperative Group system was developed in 1982 and utilized a morphology-based process to predict survival rates and the likelihood of transformation to AML. The FAB approach is mainly of historical interest now but is still included in the Food and Drug Administration (FDA) approved package inserts for certain MDS treatment options. In addition, the FAB system served as the foundation for developing the WHO classification system [20]. The WHO began an effort to develop a classification update in 1997. Since then there have been multiple updates with the most recent occurring in 2016 [5]. The WHO classification system is based on a combination of morphology, genetic, immunophenotype, and clinical features of MDS. Childhood MDS exists but is considered a separate entity by the WHO classification scheme. This system attempts to identify patients with various biological subtypes with the goal of future patient-specific targeted therapy based on molecular pathways. Both systems are complicated and require expert hematopathologist consultation. The 2016 WHO classification system identifies six general entities within MDS based on cell lineage, morphology, and cytogenetic abnormalities [5].

Table 2. WHO disease classification [5]

Subtype	Description	Estimated % of MDS patients
MDS-SLD	MDS with single lineage dysplasia	<5
MDS-RS	MDS with ring sideroblasts	<5
MDS-MLD	MDS with multilineage dysplasia	70
MDS-EB	MDS with excess blasts	25
MDS-5q	MDS with isolated del(5q)	5
MDS-U	MDS, unclassified	<5

MDS = myelodysplastic syndrome; WHO = World Health Organization.

Clinical Presentation

Signs and symptoms of MDS are rather non-specific at diagnosis and many patients discover they have the disease after inadvertent findings on routine blood counts. Others may report symptoms consistent with previously undiagnosed cytopenias. Anemia is the most noted cytopenia in MDS and can manifest as weakness, fatigue, exercise intolerance, dizziness, cognitive impairment, angina as well as numerous other complaints [21]. Systemic symptoms of fever and weight loss are generally uncommon but may represent late manifestations of the disease. Approximately 17% of patients over the age of 65 with anemia of unknown origin have peripheral blood counts consistent with MDS [22]. The clinical course is variable with most patients presenting with asymptomatic disease or mild anemia. These patients then progress to transfusion dependence over many years. Those with more aggressive MDS may rapidly evolve to acute leukemia over a short period.

Infectious complications remain the principle cause of death in MDS and frequently occur in patients with neutropenia and granulocyte dysfunction [23]. These infections are predominately bacterial with skin being the most commonly noted site. Fungal, viral and mycobacterial infections are all uncommon and typically only present in those taking immunosuppressive agents.

Pathologic Features

Abnormal cellular morphology and quantitative changes in one of more hematologic cell lines define MDS. Obtaining a complete blood count to evaluate for cytopenias is a routine practice when suspecting MDS. Pancytopenia at the time of diagnosis is documented in up to 50% of patients. Anemia tends to be uniformly present with a mean corpuscular volume in the normal to macro range. The red blood cell distribution width shows increased red blood cell size and variability. Furthermore, leukopenia resulting from neutropenia occurs in 50% of patients at diagnosis [24]. Nearly 25% of patients with MDS present with thrombocytopenia. Unlike anemia, isolated thrombocytopenia is an uncommon finding of early MDS.

Peripheral blood smears are useful for identifying MDS as they often demonstrate evidence of erythrodysplasia. Various erythroid abnormalities can be morphologically identified with peripheral smears, including elliptocytes, ovalomacrocytes, teardrops and Howell-Jolly bodies. Bone marrow aspirate and biopsy should also be conducted to determine the percentage of blasts within the marrow. Bone marrow evaluation also allows for an in-depth analysis and cytologic evaluation of blastic and other noteworthy cell types. A bone marrow biopsy will often show the classic paradox of marrow hypercellularity despite low peripheral blood counts.

Lastly, cytochemistry and immunochemistry studies should be conducted to identify a decrease of loss of normal myeloid maturation antigens [25]. Flow cytometry may be useful for diagnostic and prognostic purposes in patients with MDS. Furthermore, immunochemical analysis helps identify specific clonal irregularities. Although MDS is diagnosed based on bone marrow biopsy and peripheral blood smear, the detection of various chromosomal abnormalities via routine cytogenetic testing can help distinguish between MDS and leukemia. Cytogenetic testing can also help identify the classification of MDS and determine risk stratification. Genetic testing for chromosomal abnormalities is now considered routine practice [26]. If found, certain cytogenetic abnormalities help diagnose either MDS or AML [27, 28]:

Table 3. Cytogenetic abnormalities in MDS and AML

MDS	AML
del(7q)	*RUNX1-RUNX1T1*
del(5q)	inv(16)(p13.1q22)
del(13q)	t(16;16)(p13.1;q22)
del(11q)	t(15;17)(q22;q21.1)
del(12p) or t(12p)	
del(9q)	
Idic(x)(q13)	
t(17p)	
T(11;16)(q23;p13.3)	

AML = acute myeloid leukemia; MDS = myelodsysplastic syndrome.

Diagnosis and Prognosis

MDS involve a host of hematologic conditions best characterized by chronic cytopenias with abnormal cellular maturation. Therefore, those with MDS are at risk of developing symptomatic anemia, bleeding, bruising, infection and progression to AML. Those with MDS typically die from disease sequelae involving bone marrow failure rather than leukemic transformation. Unfortunately, the distinction between MDS and AML can often be blurry, as the diagnostic criteria can overlap depending on classification system.

In patients with unexplained cytopenia, the potential diagnosis of MDS should be considered. In addition to blood smears and cytogenic testing, pertinent patient history details regarding alcohol and drug use, medications, possible mutagenic exposures, and nutritional status should be obtained. An initial evaluation for suspected MDS includes a thorough evaluation of a peripheral blood smear and counts, cytogenetics, morphology as well as a comprehensive patient history [28]. A formal diagnosis of MDS can be tricky due to morphologic changes resulting from various medications and/or concomitant diseases (e.g., viral infections). To help ensure consistent diagnosing practices, the International Consensus Working Group recommends the following criteria [29]:

1) Unexplained and stable cytopenia for at least 6 months (some exceptions for specific karyotypes and bilineage abnormalities).
2) Exclusion of other potential causes of dysplasia or cytopenia
3) At least one of the following – dysplasia (≥10% in at least one of the three major marrow lineages); blast count between 5% and 19%; positive for a known specific MDS-associated karyotype (e.g., del(5q), del(7q)

The International Prognostic Scoring System (IPSS) was created in 1997 based on survival data from over 800 patients with *de novo* MDS. Fifteen years after the original IPSS tool was published, a large international coalition led by researchers at Stanford University developed an updated prognostic tool using a broader array of cytogenetic knowledge to bolster prognostic accuracy. Although cumbersome and difficult to memorize, online tools exist (https://www.mds-foundation.org/ipss-r-calculator/) to help clinicians navigate the various factors involved in the IPSS-R tool. The International Prognostic Scoring System – Revised (IPSS-R) data only supports evaluating patients with *de novo* MDS and at the time of their initial diagnosis. Another limitation involves patient co-morbidities, which can certainly affect quality and duration of life. This is especially true in elderly patients where the severity of a patient's co-morbid conditions plays a more significant role in determining life expectancy than their MDS. The IPSS-R tool incorporates several additional cytogenetic abnormalities and divides MDS patients into one of five prognostic camps (Table 5) [3].

Table 4. International prognostic scoring system-revised (IPSS-R)

Points	0	0.5	1	1.5	2	3	4
Blasts	≤2%	-	2%-4%	-	5%-10%	>10%	-
Hemoglobin (g/dL)	>10	-	8-10	<8	-	-	-
ANC (x 10^9/L)	≥0.8	<0.8	-	-	-	-	-
Platelets (x 10^9/L)	>100	50-100	<50	-	-	-	-
Cytogenetics	Very good	-	Good	-	Inter-mediate	Poor	Very poor

ANC = absolute neutrophil count.

Few patients with MDS will survive a decade after their initial diagnosis. Most patients with MDS, unfortunately, will die within a few years of diagnosis and some will have a life expectancy of only a few months. It is because of these disparate life expectancies that prognostic tools are so vital for evaluating and managing patients with MDS. Several important cytogenetic abnormalities have been identified over the last decade, which explains the overall heterogeneity of MDS and, in part, the incongruent prognosis among MDS patients. Table 6 highlights the five various risk stratifications along with their frequency and median survival. The time it takes for 25% of patients within each stratification to develop AML is also listed.

Table 5. IPSS-R cytogenetic risk groups [3]

Risk Group	Karyotypes	Points	Median Survival (years)	Time until AML evolution for 25% of patients (years)	Proportion of patients in each group
Very Good	-Y, del(11q)	0	5.4	-	4%
Good	Normal, del(5q), del(20q), del(12)	1	4.8	9.4	72%
Intermediate	del(7q), +8, +19, i(17q), any other single or double clones not listed	2	2.7	2.5	13%
Poor	-7, abnormal 3q, double including 7/del(7q), complex with 3 abnormalities	3	1.5	1.7	4%
Very Poor	Complex with >3 abnormalities	4	0.7	0.7	7%

AML = acute myeloid leukemia; IPSS-R = International Prognostic Scoring System – Revised.

Table 6. IPSS-R classification [3]

Risk group	Total Points	% of patients in study (n=7,012)	Median survival (years)	Time until AML evolution for 25% of patients (years)
Very low	0 – 1.5	19%	8.8	-
Low	2.0 – 3.0	38%	5.3	10.8
Intermediate	3.5 – 4.5	20%	3	3.2
High	5.0 – 6.0	13%	1.5	1.4
Very high	>6.0	10%	0.8	0.7

AML = acute myeloid leukemia; IPSS-R = Internation Prognostic Scoring System – Revised.

TREATMENT OVERVIEW

Treating MDS is complex and dependent on a number of patient- and disease-specific factors. Furthermore, not all patients with MDS even require immediate treatment. General treatment strategies may include supportive care, suppression of clonal abnormalities, identification of leukemic transformation, chemotherapy or immunotherapy to improve bone marrow function, and potentially curative allogeneic HSCT. The disparities in treatment approaches arise, in part, because of the following factors:

1) MDS is a heterogeneous disease with varying rates of disease progression [1].
2) Most cases of MDS cannot be cured with conventional chemotherapy alone [10].
3) Due to the increased age of most MDS patients, the goal of therapy often revolves around symptom management and improved quality of life rather than curing the patient [28].
4) Asymptomatic patients may not benefit from MDS treatment [30].

The IPSS-R assessment tool provides a way to evaluate risk and is often used in the initial stages of treatment planning. In addition to the IPSS-R tool, clinicians should also evaluate patient age, the presence of co-morbidities, patient performance status and patient-specific treatment desires when identifying appropriate treatment options. All patients with MDS should receive guideline-based supportive care. The National Comprehensive Cancer Network (NCCN) then arranges patients into one of two groups [28]:

1) Lower-risk patients – IPSS-R very low, low, and intermediate risk
2) Higher-risk patients – IPSS-R intermediate, high, and very high risk

Patients who fall under the IPSS-R intermediate risk may be treated as either low or high risk, depending on other prognostic factors such as age, performance status, and laboratory markers (serum ferritin and LDH levels). Regardless of risk stratification, all MDS patients should be offered best supportive care and, when available, counseled on enrollment into a clinical trial [28].

Supportive Care

Standard care for all MDS patients involves supportive care measures [28]. This should include observation, psychosocial support, routine quality of life assessments, and thorough clinical monitoring. Every effort should be undertaken to ensure the highest quality of life possible and should incorporate all life domains (spiritual, physical, emotional, functional, and social). Cytopenias are the single most important culprit of disease-related mortality in MDS patients.

Thrombocytopenia is a common supportive care issue resulting from both a hypoproliferative bone marrow with reduced endogenous thrombopoietin (TPO) production and an increased rate of megakaryocyte destruction. Several studies have evaluated TPO receptor agonists for the treatment of thrombocytopenia in lower-risk MDS patients [31, 32]. These small phase I/II studies have found an improved platelet response for both romiplostim and eltombopag; however, these agents are not FDA approved for the treatment of MDS and concerns that TPO mimetics could lead to proliferation and transformation of leukemic cells remain. Larger, prospective clinical trials are needed to fully elucidate their role in the management of thrombocytopenia secondary to MDS. Profound thrombocytopenia is associated with an increased bleeding risk requiring platelet transfusion [28].

Patients with MDS often present with varying degrees of normocytic or macrocytic anemia. Over 80% of patients initially diagnosed with MDS present with an underlying anemia and nearly 50% with a hemoglobin < 10g/dL [33]. At diagnosis, the degree of anemia is a prognostic indicator in patients with MDS. These patients can often present with fatigue, altered cognition, angina, weakness, headache, and exercise intolerance. Red blood cell transfusions are a vital component of MDS supportive care and are often required chronically to maintain quality of life [28]. Transfusion thresholds vary from institution to institution and from patient to patient, but most asymptomatic patients will require a packed RBC transfusion when the hemoglobin falls below 8 g/dL [28]. To minimize complications of leukocyte-containing RBC products (viral infections, transfusion reactions, immunosuppression), the standard of care is to provide leukoreduced RBC transfusions for patients with MDS. Some high-risk patients may also require irradiated RBC transfusions. Fortunately, RBC transfusions provide a rapid increase in hemoglobin and help MDS patients feel an improved energy level and overall quality of life [30].

Frequent RBC transfusions are a poor prognostic factor in patients with MDS. Chronic transfusions can lead to hemochromatosis and subsequent long-term hepatic, endocrine and cardiac complications. To help avoid these concerns, iron chelation therapy has been evaluated in MDS patients and multiple options exist to reduce the total body iron burden. The NCCN guidelines currently recommend treating iron overload patients with chelation therapy [28]. A meta-analysis evaluating iron-chelation therapy in eight observation studies found that those receiving chelation had a significant improvement in overall survival (61.2 months) compared to MDS patients who did not receive iron-chelation therapy [34]. A paucity of data remains and additional clinical trials looking specifically at iron-chelation therapy are needed to substantiate the findings from these observational studies. Several ongoing prospective clinical trials are attempting to evaluate deferasirox, an oral iron-chelating agent, in patients with MDS. One completed clinical trial evaluated 173 MDS patients receiving deferasirox and found that it reduced serum ferritin and labile plasma iron in transfusion-dependent patients [35]. Over the 3-year study, 138 of the 173 (80%) patients discontinued deferasirox; 43 of these patients discontinued therapy because of adverse side effects or disease progression. The most common toxicities were gastrointestinal disturbances and increased serum creatinine. The FDA assigned black box warnings to deferasirox in 2010 for case reports of acute renal or hepatic failure. Therefore, patients receiving deferasirox should receive serum creatinine and liver function test monitoring prior to initiating therapy and routinely thereafter. According to the FDA label, deferasirox should not be given to patients with a creatinine clearance less than 40 mL/min [36].

Patients with low-risk MDS and symptomatic anemia may receive erythropoiesis-stimulating agents (ESAs) such as epoetin alfa and darbepoetin alfa with or without the addition of granulocyte-colony stimulating agents (G-CSFs) [28]. Due to their synergistic erythropoietin effects and enhance RBC survival, adding a G-CSF to ESAs may be beneficial and should be considered. Individuals with a low serum erythropoietin (EPO) level and low transfusion requirement are more likely receive benefit from ESAs. Studies evaluating filgrastim in MDS have shown an increase in neutrophil production; however, this has not led to reduced infections or an improvement in overall survival [37]. Clinical trials have found both epoetin alfa and darbepoetin alfa to be effective at raising hemoglobin levels and minimizing transfusion requirements in selected patients with low-risk MDS [38]. Both agents appear to be similar in efficacy and safety and neither agent has demonstrated a survival benefit in this patient population. The desired hemoglobin concentration ranges from 10 to 12 g/dL. Nearly 40% of patients treated with ESAs respond to therapy, which typically takes 6-8 weeks to occur, and the median duration of response is 24 months [39]. As highlighted in Table 7, multiple dosing strategies are available.

Table 7. Dosing strategies for ESAs and G-CSF [40-42]

Medication	Dosing
Epoetin alfa	150-300 units/kg subcutaneous daily
	450-1000 units/kg subcutaneous per week in divided doses
	60,000 units once weekly
Darbepoetin alfa	150-300 mcg subcutaneous once weekly
	500 mcg subcutaneous every 2-3 weeks
G-CSF	Filgrastim 1-2 mcg/kg subcutaneous daily

ESA = erythropoietin-stimulating agent; G-CSF = granulocyte-colony stimulating factor.

In 2007, the FDA issued "black box warnings" on ESA safety concerns in patients with non-MDS cancer. These alerts significantly altered treatment paradigm within oncology practice; however, the use of ESAs in patients with MDS remains unchanged. These ESA agents have been used safely in adult patients with MDS and play an important role in their quality of care and overall transfusion requirement [37]. The NCCN panel along with the American Society of Hematology, and the American Society of Clinical Oncology recommend ESAs in MDS patients with symptomatic anemia [43, 44].

As a result of neutropenia and granulocyte impairment, MDS has a high propensity to develop infectious complications, which remains the primary cause of death in these patients [45]. Although most infections are bacterial, other infectious pathogens such as viral, mycobacterial and fungal infections can occur in patients receiving immunosuppressant therapy for MDS management. Preventative therapy is important and several strategies have been studied, including vaccination, prophylactic antibiotics, and myeloid growth factors. According to the NCCN guidelines, at this time, only routine vaccination is a recommended strategy [28]. Recommended vaccines include influenza and pneumococcal with pertussis and haemophilus influenza B likely being beneficial as well. Live vaccines should not be given to patients with MDS.

Treating Asymptomatic MDS

Patient with asymptomatic MDS should be routinely monitored with laboratory studies and examinations to determine rate and depth of disease progression. While patients are in this asymptomatic phase, every effort should be made to ensure they are properly vaccinated and to thoughtfully encourage smoking cessation, if applicable. Treatment should be re-evaluated once the patient develops a transfusion requirement or recurrent infections. Table 8 summarizes the treatment options available to help treat and manage patients with symptomatic MDS.

Table 8. MDS treatment strategies [28]

Treatment Aim	Treatment Options
Supportive Care	Blood transfusion
	Iron-chelation
	Antimicrobials
	Growth factors (EPO, G-CSF)
IPSS-R Very Low Risk, Low Risk, Intermediate Risk	Supportive care alone
	DNA hypomethylating agent
	Immunosuppressive therapy
	Lenalidomide (5q deletion)
IPSS-R Intermediate Risk, High Risk, Very High Risk	Bone marrow transplantation
	Intensive chemotherapy
	DNA hypomethylating agent

EPO = erythropoietin; G-CSF = granulocyte-colony stimulating factor; IPSS-R = International Prognostic Scoring System – Revised.

TREATING SYMPTOMATIC MDS

Low Intensity Therapy

Patients with an IPSS-R score of ≤3 (very low, low) should primarily receive supportive care, as detailed above, with or without the addition of DNA hypomethylating agents or lenalidomide [28]. IPSS-R intermediate patients may also fall into the low-intensity treatment group. There is no standard of care for treating symptomatic patients with MDS and each patient should be counselled on enrolling in a clinical trial whenever possible. The patient's performance status, treatment desires, IPSS-R risk stratification score, and co-morbidities must all be considered when selecting individualized treatment plans [28]. Low intensity therapy may consists of supportive care measures, DNA hypomethylating agents (azacitidine or decitabine), immunosuppressive therapy, or lenalidomide. Most of these strategies have minimal treatment-related complications and can be administered in the outpatient setting for patient convenience. It is important to remember that these strategies may provide symptom relief and improve quality of life, but they are not curative and should be viewed as a palliative measure. The primary goal for treating MDS patients with pharmacotherapy is to alter the natural progression of the disease and avoid recurrent and/or refractory MDS.

DNA Hypomethylating Agents

The DNA methyltransferase inhibitor (DMTI) hypomethylating agents consists of azacitidine and decitabine. These agents have been shown in randomized phase III clinical trials to reduce the likelihood of leukemic transformation and possibly improve overall survival [46, 47]. Approximately 50% of patients in these trials experienced a hematologic response and both agents have FDA-approved indications for MDS. A meta-analysis evaluating over 950 patients receiving a hypomethylating agent for MDS found a significant improvement in overall survival (hazard ratio 0.72, 95% CI 0.60-0.85) and time to AML transformation or death (hazard ratio 0.69, 95% CI 0.58-0.82) [48].

Azacitidine (Vidaza®) is a pyrimidine nucleoside analog that elicits direct cytotoxicity of abnormal bone marrow cells via DNA hypomethylation. Results from one phase III clinical trial involving 191 low or intermediate risk MDS patients showed a superior complete or partial response with azacitidine compared to supportive care (23% versus 0%) [46]. Furthermore, the 75mg/m^2 subcutaneous dose of azacitidine given daily for 7 days every 28 days showed a longer median time to leukemic transformation (21 versus 13 months) and improved median survival (18 versus 11 months). Alternative azacitidine dosing strategies have been studied and may be beneficial; however, survival benefit has only been demonstrated with the 7-day schedule [49, 50]. Hematological responses to azacitidine therapy may take several months to materialize and most patients will experience at least one episode of neutropenic fever requiring hospitalization during treatment. A 2006 study showed completed remissions occurred in 10% to 17% of azacitidine-treated patients and the median number of cycles to first response was three, with 90% of responses occurring by cycle 6 [51]. A quality-of-life analysis reported azacitidine, when compared to supportive care alone, improved several issues including physical functioning, dyspnea, mood, psychosocial distress, and fatigue [52]. Common side effects noted with azacitidine therapy include significant cytopenias (nadir: 10-17 days), injection site reactions, fever, fatigue, skin rash, dizziness, peripheral edema, nausea, vomiting, constipation, weakness, and cough [53].

A large open-label, randomized, phase III clinical trial evaluated 358 higher risk MDS patients who were randomized to azacitidine or conventional care that could include supportive care alone, low-dose cytarabine, or AML-type induction [54]. Overall, 175 patients received azacitidine, 145 received best supportive care, 45 received low-dose cytarabine, and 17 received AML-type induction. A median overall survival benefit was seen, with azacitidine patients living 9 months longer than those with conventional care (24.5 versus 15 months) and 51% of azacitidine patients surviving 24 months compared to just 26% of conventional care patients. This was the first prospective, randomized controlled trial in MDS demonstrating an improvement in overall survival. In addition to improved overall survival, azacitidine also exhibited less toxicity and fewer hospitalizations compared to conventional care.

Decitabine (Dacogen®) is another pyrimidine nucleoside analog of cytidine that is incorporated into DNA and inhibits methyltransferase causing hypomethylation and cell death. Various clinical trials have proven decitabine's clinical worth in de novo MDS, relapsed disease, and in patients previously treated with azacitidine [47, 55]. One trial evaluated 170 randomized patient with MDS assigned to decitabine 15mg/m^2 IV over three hours every 8 hours for three consecutive days and repeated every 6 weeks or best supportive care [47]. Decitabine was found to be clinically effective in the management of MDS with a significantly higher overall response rate (17% versus 0%) and longer median time to AML progression or death. Similar to azacitidine, toxicity concerns are real and worthy of consideration. The most common toxicity complaints identified in the trial were cytopenias, fever, sepsis, infection, and nausea/vomiting [47]. Another phase III clinical trial in higher risk MDS patients who were at least 60 years of age compared decitabine to best supportive care [56]. These patients were ineligible for intensive therapy, but decitabine significantly improved progression free survival (6.6 versus 3 months) and reduced the risk of AML progression at one year (22% versus 33%). Despite improvements in progression free survival and AML progression, decitabine showed no statistically significant benefit in the primary outcome of overall survival (10 versus 8.5 months). Patients receiving decitabine did report improved quality of life, which is an important dimension of care to consider in this patient population.

DNA hypomethylating agents in combination with other therapeutic options do not improve response rates and should therefore be avoided. Azacitidine was studied in combination with either lenalidomide or vorinostat but neither group displayed a clinically significant benefit compared to the azacitidine monotherapy [57].

Immunosuppressant Therapy

Aplastic anemia has historically been treated with various immunosuppressant agents with moderate success. Bone marrow failure is a common feature of both aplastic anemia and myelodysplastic syndrome. There is mounting evidence that the underlying cytopenias of MDS arise from a dysregulated autoimmune system, at least in certain patient populations [58]. Patients with MDS are also more likely to suffer from other autoimmune disorders such as rheumatoid arthritis, polymyalgia, thyroid disease, glomerulonephritis, polyneuropathy, and idiopathic thrombocytopenic purpura [59].

Immunosuppressant therapy (IST) with agents such as antithymocyte globulin (ATG), alemtuzumab (Campath®), tacrolimus (Prograf®) or cyclosporine (Gengraf®, SandIMMUNE®) has produced hematologic responses in certain MDS patients [3]. Treating MDS with IST remains controversial and exploratory. Finding the correct subset of patients who will respond to immunosuppressant therapy has been the primary challenge surrounding IST implementation [28]. Some recent studies indicate that IST is most effective in patients with low risk disease, marrow hypoplasia, normal cytogenetics, and certain clonal features. The National Institutes of Health created a scoring system based on past studies to determine who might benefit the most from IST [60, 61].

Antithymocyte globulin is produced from either equine (Atgam®) or rabbit (Thymoglobulin®) sources and both appear to be active in MDS. One randomized, phase III clinical trial compared ATG in combination with cyclosporine to best supportive care and found the combination resulted in significantly higher rates of hematologic response (29% versus 9%) [62]. The study, however, did not show a survival benefit. Toxicity concerns with ATG are significant, requiring hospital admission and close monitoring. Continued research with IST in various MDS patient subsets is required to further elucidate this potential treatment option.

Lenalidomide

Lenalidomide (Revlimid®) is an oral immunomodulatory drug (IMiD) that also displays antiangiogenic and antineoplastic characteristics through selective inhibition of cytokine secretion and anti-CD3 stimulation [28]. Lenalidomide received FDA approval in 2005 for the treatment of low to intermediate risk MDS in patients with deletion 5q chromosomal abnormality and transfusion-dependent anemia. A deletion involving the 5q chromosome, also known as del(5q), may occur in up to 30% of patients with MDS. The WHO created a new term for MDS patients with isolated 5q chromosomal deletion called "5q- Syndrome" [63].

A landmark multicenter, phase II clinical trial evaluated oral lenalidomide 10 mg per day for 21 days every 4 weeks or just 10 mg daily [64]. Out of 148 patients, 112 (76%) had reduced transfusion requirements and 99 patients (67%) no longer required transfusions. Researchers found that patients rapidly responded to lenalidomide therapy with a median time to response of 4.6 weeks. In addition to reducing transfusion requirements, lenalidomide was also shown to reverse cytologic and cytogenetic abnormalities in 38 out of 106 and 62 out of 85 evaluable patients with 5q deletion, respectively. A confirmatory phase III trial compared lenalidomide with best supportive care in lower risk MDS patients exhibiting del(5q) [65]. With over 200 randomized patients, lenalidomide 5 mg or 10 mg daily resulted in lower transfusion rates and higher cytogenetic responses. Lenalidomide was well tolerated with a manageable side effect profile. Unfortunately, nearly 50% of patients will experience a clinical and cytogenetic relapse 2 to 3 years after treatment with lenalidomide [65].

In transfusion-dependent MDS patients with del(5q) with or without other cytogenetic abnormalities, lenalidomide is the treatment of choice [28]. Lenalidomide should be started at 10 mg daily for 21 days each month with dose adjustments based on efficacy and tolerability. A reduction in transfusion requirements is typically observed within 4 months and may last a year or longer. Lenalidomide can also be considered in symptomatic MDS patients without the del(5q) abnormality who failed to respond to initial therapy.

Lenalidomide has black box warnings for hematologic toxicity, embryo-fetal toxicity, and venous thromboembolism. In the United States, lenalidomide use requires registration and adherence to the risk evaluation and mitigation strategy (REMS) program (RevAssist – www.revlimid.com) to help avoid the potential for pregnancy among patients taking lenalidomide. Other potential concerning side effects include peripheral neuropathy, constipation, cytopenias, and edema. Rash, hypothyroidism, pruritus and dizziness can also occur with lenalidomide, however, these rarely lead to discontinuation. Despite these toxicities, lenalidomide is the standard of care in patients with lower risk MDS, anemia, and del(5q) [28].

High Intensity Therapy

As noted in previous sections, not all patients with MDS require treatment; however, with high-risk disease (IPSS-R >4.5), immediate treatment is often required [28]. Similar to patients with IPSS-R very low, low, and intermediate risk disease, there is no standard of care for treating this disease. High intensity treatment is generally reserved for high-risk patients with a poor overall prognosis. High intensity therapy includes supportive care measures, intensive combination chemotherapy, and allogeneic HSCT. Unlike low intensity regimens, patients receiving these high intensity therapies typically require hospital admission due to the significant treatment-related complications.

Patients requiring high intensity therapy have an estimated median survival of 8-18 months with supportive care alone [3]. In patients with good performance status and minimal comorbidities, intensive chemotherapy and/or allogeneic HCT may be indicated. Most patients with higher risk disease should receive more intensive therapy, but DNA hypomethylating agents may provide benefit in select patients based on their preferences. Although both agents (azacitidine and decitabine) can be used in this setting, some prefer azacitidine because it can be administered on an outpatient basis. The NCCN guidelines recommend azacitidine over decitabine in high risk patients, even though both appear to be therapeutically similar. Additional prospective studies are required to determine if azacitidine truly is superior to decitabine from an efficacy standpoint. Oral formulation for both azacitidine and decitabine are currently being studied in patients with MDS. This would be a welcomed advancement as MDS patients receiving these agents spend a great deal of time receiving treatment in a healthcare setting.

Hematopoietic Stem Cell Transplant

Allogeneic HSCT is the only curative option for patients with MDS [28]. Preferred transplant patients include those who are young, have HLA identical siblings, and are relatively healthy. The median age of MDS at diagnosis is 75 years of age, which means most patients are ineligible for transplantation referral [7]. In fact, fewer than 5% of patients are even considered because of their age at the time of diagnosis [66]. Up to 50% of patients who receive allogeneic HSCT for MDS will experience prolonged disease-free survival. Unfortunately, treatment-related morbidity and mortality is common amongst HSCT recipients and finding matched marrow donors can be difficult. Recent advances in supportive care management and HLA matching allows more transplant-eligible patients. The common age cutoff for transplantation consideration is 70 years of age [67]. Numerous factors such as HLA matching, type of transplant, FAB subtype, patient comorbidities, and time from diagnosis to transplantation help determine HSCT outcomes. Rates of long-term disease-free survival in high risk MDS undergoing HSCT varies from 20% to 60% dependening on the patient's match and overall health [67]. Deciding what patients should be transplanted and the optimal timing of HSCT has been a controversial topic with most institutions opting to only consider HSCT in high risk patients or those with low risk disease who have a new cytogenetic abnormality, advanced cytopenia, or progression to high risk disease [68]. Moreover, MDS patients with very low, low, and intermediate disease should be closely observed and transplanted once disease progression occurs. Prospective, randomized, controlled trials are needed to compare outcomes and determine best practice for HSCT therapy in MDS patients.

Reduced intensity HSCT using nonmyeloablative chemotherapy has become more common as clinicians attempt to improve the safety of HSCT therapy. A reduced-intensity regimen relies on a graft-versus-tumor effect to help eradicate the myelodysplastic clone. Retrospective studies evaluating nonmyeloablative and myeloablative chemotherapy regimens failed to conclusively find a superior method. It appears, however, that patients receiving nonmyeloablative therapy experience lower treatment-related mortality at the expense of increased rates of disease relapse [69]. The clinical dilemma surrounding HSCT is balancing treatment-related complications with disease recurrence and long-term immunosuppression. The comparison of reduced-intensity with myeloablative transplantation remains hotly contested with additional prospective studies needed to determine the optimal approach to transplantation.

High Intensity Chemotherapy

Intensive AML-like induction therapy or HSCT make up high intensity options for treating MDS and both carry significant treatment-related morbidity and mortality.

However, unlike the low intensity options, both AML-like induction therapy and HSCT have the potential to alter the natural progression of MDS and can even be curative. Intensive chemotherapy should be considered in high risk patients lacking a HSCT donor or for those patients with a high marrow blast count (>10%). Due to the toxic nature of intensive chemotherapy, these patients should also be relatively younger (<60 years old) with a good performance status and few co-morbidities. Various chemotherapy regimens exist but a paucity of data exists to effectively determine a preferred regimen [33]. Specific chemotherapy agents may include idarubicin, cytarabine, fludarabine, mitoxantrone, etoposide, and/or topotecan. One prospective multicenter study evaluated 184 patients with either MDS or secondary AML [1]. These patients received AML-like induction chemotherapy followed by auto- or allogeneic HSCT. The 4-year overall survival rate was 26% with a median survival of 13 months. Similar to AML, chemotherapy-resistance leading to diminished response rates and remission duration is a common concern when treating high risk MDS. In the original IPSS trial, high risk MDS patients were treated with either best supportive care or non-intensive chemotherapy which resulted in a four-year overall survival rate of 0% [3].

Recurrent or Refractory MDS

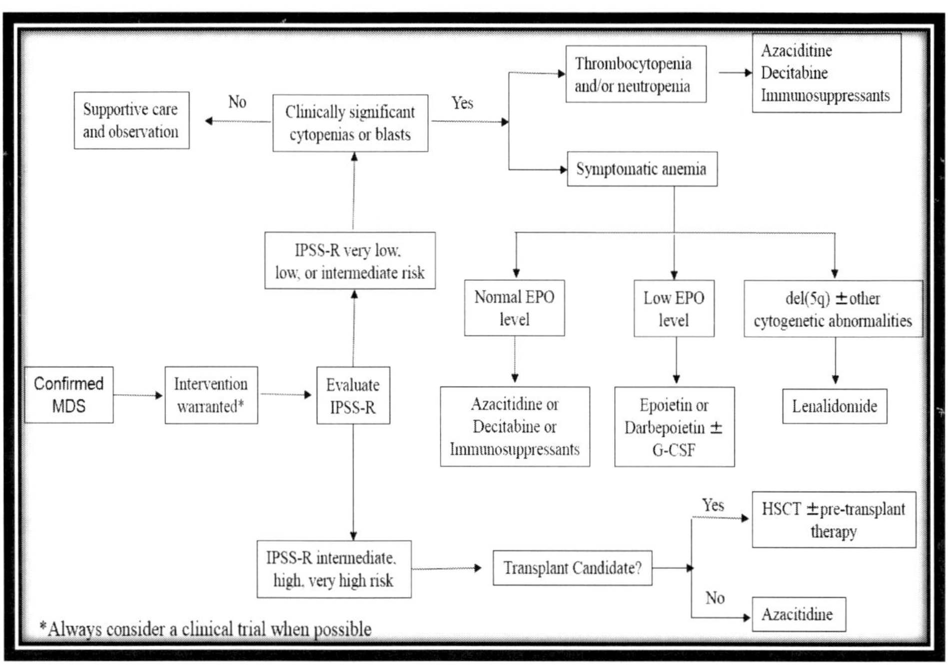

EPO = erythropoietin; G-CSF = granulocyte-colony stimulating factor; HSCT = hematopoietic stem cell transplant; IPSS-R = International Prognostic Scoring System – Revised; MDS = myelodysplastic syndrome.

Figure 1. Risk-Adjusted Treatment Schema for MDS Management.

If possible, patients with recurrent MDS or those who are refractory to standard therapy should be encouraged to enroll in a clinical trial. Aside from clinical trials, treating this patient population is largely dependent on their previous therapy as well as preferences. In recurrent or refractory patients who have not attempted DNA hypomethylation therapy (azacitidine or decitabine), this should be considered first. If the patient has failed one DNA hypomethylating agent, there is a paucity of data surrounding the use of another agent within the same class. For most patients with disease progression despite treatment, best supportive care will often be the treatment of choice unless they qualify for either lenalidomide or HSCT [28].

CONCLUSION

MDS are a group of clonal irregularities originating from an erroneous hematopoietic progenitor cell. Nearly 30% of all MDS cases progress to a fatal form of acute leukemia called AML [70]. Genetic mutations are common with MDS development and nearly half of all MDS patients display some form of pertinent genetic mutation. The most important risk factor for developing MDS is aging with a significant risk-spike after the age of 65 years old. Therapy-related MDS accounts for 10% to 15% of all cases and are associated with exposure to radiation, chemotherapy or a combination of the two [14]. Several prognostic tools exist for aiding in risk stratification and therapy selection. Overall, older patients with identifiable cytogenetic abnormalities and severe cytopenias tend to have the worst disease course and long-term outlook. Based on IPSS-R scoring, patients are divided into very low, low, intermediate, high, and very high-risk categories. In low risk disease, supportive care alone may suffice. Treatment, in addition to best supportive care, becomes necessary once the patient is symptomatic. Various treatment options exist for those qualifying. DNA hypomethylating agents (decitabine or azacitidine) are useful as first line therapy in low risk patients and azacitidine showed improved survival compared to supportive care in high risk patients [54]. Lenalidomide is preferred in MDS with del(5q) [65]. The only potential cure for MDS is allogeneic HSCT, which is the preferred treatment modality for relatively young and healthy high risk patients with a matched related donor.

REFERENCES

[1] Tefferi A and Vardiman JW: Myelodysplastic syndromes. *N Engl J Med* 2009;361(19):1872–1885.

[2] Vardiman JW, Harris NL, Brunning RD. The World Health Organization (WHO) classification of the myeloid neoplasms. *Blood* 2002;100:2292–2302.

[3] Greenberg PL, Tuechler H, Schanz J, et al. Revised International Prognostic Scoring System (IPSS-R) for myelodysplastic syndromes. *Blood* 2012;120:2454-2465.

[4] Ma X. Epidemiology of myelodysplastic syndromes. *Am J Med* 2012;125:S2–S5.

[5] Arber DA, Orazi A, Hasserjian R, et al. The 2016 revision to the World Health Organization classification of myeloid neoplasms and acute leukemia. *Blood* 2016;127(20):2391-2405.

[6] Stein EM, DiNardo C, Altman JK, et al. Safety and efficacy of AG-221, a potent inhibitor of mutant IDH2 that promotes differentiation of myeloid cells in patients with advanced hematologic malignancies: results of a phase 1/2 trial. *Blood* 2015;126:323.

[7] Howlader N, Noone AM, Krapcho M, et al. *SEER Cancer Statistics Review*, 1975–2010, National Cancer Institute. Bethesda, MD.

[8] Cogle CR, Craig BM, Rollison DE, List AF. Incidence of the myelodysplastic syndromes using a novel claims-based algorithm: high number of uncaptured cases by cancer registries. *Blood* 2011;117(26):7121.

[9] Nagata C, Shimizu H, Hirashima K, et al.: Hair dye use and occupational exposure to organic solvents as risk factors for myelodysplastic syndrome. *Leuk Res* 1999; 23: 57–62.

[10] Jadersten M, Hellstrom-Lindberg E. Myelodysplastic syndromes: Biology and treatment. *J Intern Med* 2009;265:307–328.

[11] Iwanaga M, Hsu WL, Soda M, et al. Risk of myelodysplastic syndromes in people exposed to ionizing radiation: A retrospective cohort study of Nagasaki atomic bomb survivors. *J Clin Oncol* 2011;29:428–434.

[12] Ma X, Lim U, Park Y, et al. Obesity, lifestyle factors, and risk of myelodysplastic syndromes in a large US cohort. *Am J Epidemiol* 2009;169:1492–1499.

[13] Kristinsson SY, Bjorkholm M, Hultcrantz M, et al. Chronic immune stimulation might act as a trigger for the development of acute myeloid leukemia or myelodysplastic syndromes. *J Clin Oncol* 2011;29:2897–2903.

[14] Czader M, Orazi A. Therapy-related myeloid neoplasms. *Am J Clin Pathol* 2009;132:410–425.

[15] Armitage JO, Carbone PP, Connors JM, et al. Treatment trelated myelodysplasia and acute leukemia in nonHodgkin's lymphoma patients. *J Clin Oncol* 2003;21:897–906.

[16] Haase D, Germing U, Schanz J, et al. New insights into the prognostic impact of the karyotype in MDS and correlation with subtypes: Evidence from a core dataset of 2124 patients. *Blood* 2007;110:4385–4395.

[17] Woll PS, Kjällquist U, Chowdhury O, et al. Myelodysplastic syndromes are propagated by rare and distinct human cancer stem cells in vivo. *Cancer Cell* 2014;25(6):794-808.

[18] Pang WW, Pluvinage JV, Price EA, et al. Hematopoietic stem cell and progenitor cell mechanisms in myelodysplastic syndromes. *Proc Natl Acad Sci U S A.* 2013;110(8):3011.

[19] Bejar R, Levine R, Ebert BL. Unraveling the molecular pathophysiology of myelodysplastic syndromes. *J Clin Oncol* 2011;29:504–515.

[20] Vardiman JW, Thiele J, Arber DA, et al. The 2008 revision of the World Health Organization (WHO) classification of myeloid neoplasms and acute leukemia: Rationale and important changes. *Blood* 2009;114:937–951.

[21] Foucar K, Langdon RM 2nd, Armitage JO, et al. Myelodysplastic syndromes. A clinical and pathologic analysis of 109 cases. *Cancer* 1985;56(3):553.

[22] Guralnik JM, Eisenstaedt RS, Ferrucci L, et al. Prevalence of anemia in persons 65 years and older in the United States: evidence for a high rate of unexplained anemia. *Blood* 2004; 104: 2263–2268.

[23] Pomeroy C, Oken MM, Rydell RE, et al. Infection in the myelodysplastic syndromes. *Am J Med* 1991;90(3):338.

[24] French registry of acute leukemia and myelodysplastic syndromes. Age distribution and hemogram analysis of the 4496 cases recorded during 1982-1983 and classified according to FAB criteria. Groupe Francais de Morphologie Hematologique. *Cancer* 1987;60(6):1385.

[25] Hokland P, Kerndrup G, Griffin JD, et al. Analysis of leukocyte differentiation antigens in blood and bone marrow from preleukemia (refractory anemia) patients using monoclonal antibodies. *Blood* 1986;67(4):898.

[26] Greenberg PL, Tuechler H, Schanz, et al. Revised international prognostic scoring system for myelodysplastic syndromes. *Blood* 2012;120(12):2454.

[27] Swerdlow SH, Campo E, Harris NL, et al. *World Health Organization classification of tumours of haematopoietic and lymphoid tissues*, IARC Press, Lyon 2008.

[28] *The NCCN Clinical Practice Guidelines in Oncology™ Myelodysplastic Syndromes* (Version 2.2018). National Comprehensive Cancer Network, Inc. Available at: www.NCCN.org. Accessed May 12, 2018.

[29] Valent P, Horny HP, Bennett JM, et al. Definitions and standards in the diagnosis and treatment of the myelodysplastic syndromes: consensus statements and report from a working conference. *Leuk Res* 2007;31:727-736.

[30] Malcovati L, Hellstrom-Lindberg E, Bowen D, et al. Diagnosis and treatment of primary myelodysplastic syndromes in adults: recommendations from the European Leukemia Net. *Blood* 2013;122:2943–2964.

[31] Brierley CK, Steensma DP. Thrombopoiesis-stimulating agents and myelodysplastic syndromes. *Br J Haematol* 2015;169:309–323.

[32] Kantarjian H, Fenaux P, Sekeres MA, et al. Safety and efficacy of romiplostim in patients with lower-risk myelodysplastic syndromeand thrombocytopenia. *J Clin Oncol* 2010;28:437-444.

[33] Steensma DP, Bennett JM. The myelodysplastic syndromes: diagnosis and treatment. *Mayo Clin Proc* 2006;81(1):104.

[34] Mainous AG 3rd, Tanner RJ, Hulihan MM, et al. The impact of chelation therapy on survival in transfusional iron overload: a meta-analysis of myelodysplastic syndrome. *Br J Haematol* 2014;167(5):720-3.

[35] List AF, Baer MR, Steensma DP, et al. Deferasirox reduces serum ferritin and labile plasma iron in RBC transfusion-dependent patients with myelodysplastic syndrome. *J Clin Oncol* 2012;30(17):2134.

[36] *Food and Drug Administration.* Prescribing information. Exjade (deferasirox) tablets for oral suspension. 2013. Available at http://www.accessdata.fda.gov/ drugsatfda_docs/label/2013/021882s019lbl.pdf. Accesses May 23, 2018.

[37] Greenberg P, Taylor K, Larson RA. Phase III randomized multicenter trial of G-CSF vs observation for myelodysplastic syndromes (MDS). *Blood* 1993;82:196a.

[38] Ross SD, Allen IE, Probst CA, et al. Efficacy and safety of erythropoiesis-stimulating proteins in myelodysplastic syndrome: a systematic review and meta-analysis. *Oncologist* 2007;12:1264–1273.

[39] Jadersten M, Malcovati L, Dybedal I, et al. Erythropoietin and grnulocyte-colony stimulating factor treatment associated with improved survival in myelodysplastic syndrome. *J Clin Oncol* 2008;26:3607-3613.

[40] Epoetin alfa. Lexi-Drugs. *Lexicomp.* Wolters Kluwer Health, Inc. Riverwoods, IL. Available at: http://online.lexi.com. Accessed May 24, 2018.

[41] Darbepoetin alfa. Lexi-Drugs. *Lexicomp.* Wolters Kluwer Health, Inc. Riverwoods, IL. Available at: http://online.lexi.com. Accessed May 24, 2018.

[42] Filgrastim. Lexi-Drugs. *Lexicomp.* Wolters Kluwer Health, Inc. Riverwoods, IL. Available at: http://online.lexi.com. Accessed May 24, 2018.

[43] Rizzo JD, Brouwers M, Hurley P, et al. American Society of Hematology/American Society of Clinical Oncology clinical practice guideline update on the use of epoetin and darbepoetin in adult patients with cancer. *Blood* 2010;116(20):4045.

[44] Rizzo JD, Brouwers M, Hurley P, et al. American Society of Clinical Oncology/American Society of Hematology clinical practice guideline update on the use of epoetin and darbepoetin in adult patients with cancer. *J Clin Oncol* 2010;28(33):4996.

[45] Pomeroy C, Oken MM, Rydell RE, et al. Infection in the myelodysplastic syndrome. *Am J Med* 1991;90(3):338.

[46] Silverman LR, Demakos EP, Peterson BL, et al. Randomized controlled trial of azacitidine in patients with the myelodysplastic syndrome: a study of the cancer and leukemia group B. *J Clin Oncol* 2002;20(10):2429.
[47] Kantarjian H, Issa JP, Rosenfeld CS, et al. Decitabine improves patient outcomes in myelodysplastic syndromes: results of a phase III randomized study. *Cancer* 2006;106:1794–1803.
[48] Gurion R, Vidal L, Gafter-Gvili A, Belnik Y, et al. 5-azacitidine prolongs overall survival in patients with myelodysplastic syndrome--a systematic review and meta-analysis. *Haematologica* 2010;95(2):303.
[49] Lyons RM, Cogriff TM, Modi SS, et al. Hematologic response to three alternative dosing schedules of azacitidine in patients with myelodysplastic syndromes. *J Clin Oncol* 2009;27:1850-1856.
[50] Martin MG, Walgren RA, Procknow E, et al. A phase II study of 5-day intravenous azacitidine in patients with myelodysplastic syndromes. *Am J Hematol* 2009;84:560-564.
[51] Silverman LR, McKenzie DR, Peterson BL, et al. Further analysis of trials with azacitidine in patients with myelodysplastic syndrome: studies 8421, 8921, and 9221 by the Cancer and Leukemia Group B. *Clin Oncol* 2006;24(24):3895.
[52] Kornblith AB, Herndon JE, Silverman LR, et al. Impact of azacytidine on the quality of life of patients with myelodysplastic syndrome treated in a randomized phase III trial: a Cancer and Leukemia Group B study. *J Clin Oncol* 2002;20:2441–2452.
[53] Azacitidine. Lexi-Drugs. *Lexicomp*. Wolters Kluwer Health, Inc. Riverwoods, IL. Available at: http://online.lexi.com. Accessed May 24, 2018.
[54] Fenaux P, Mufti GJ, Hellstrom-Lindberg E, et al. Efficacy of azacitidine compared with that of conventional care regimens in the treatment of higher-risk myelodysplastic syndromes: a randomised, open-label, phase III study. *Lancet Oncol* 2009;10:223–232.
[55] Wijermans P, Lübbert M, Verhoef G, et al. Low-dose 5-aza-2'-deoxycytidine, a DNA hypomethylating agent, for the treatment of high-risk myelodysplastic syndrome: a multicenter phase II study in elderly patients. *J Clin Oncol* 2000;18(5):956.
[56] Lübbert M, Suciu S, Baila L, et al. Low-dose decitabine versus best supportive care in elderly patients with intermediate- or high-risk myelodysplastic syndrome (MDS) ineligible for intensive chemotherapy: final results of the randomized phase III study of the European Organisation for Research and Treatment of Cancer Leukemia Group and the German MDS Study Group. *J Clin Oncol* 2011;29(15):1987-96.
[57] Sekeres MA, Othus M, List AF, et al. Randomized Phase II Study of Azacitidine Alone or in Combination With Lenalidomide or With Vorinostat in Higher-Risk

Myelodysplastic Syndromes and Chronic Myelomonocytic Leukemia: North American Intergroup Study SWOG S1117. *J Clin Oncol* 2017;35(24):2745.
[58] Olnes MJ, Sloand EM. Targeting immune dysregulation in myelodysplastic syndromes. *JAMA* 2011 Feb 23; 305(8):814-9.
[59] Giannouli S, Kanellopoulou T, Voulgarelis M. Myelodysplasia and autoimmunity. *Curr Opin Rheumatol* 2012;24(1):97-102.
[60] Sloand EM, Wu CO, Greenberg P, et al. Factors affecting response and survival in patients with myelodysplasia treated with immunosuppressive therapy. *J Clin Oncol* 2008;26(15):2505.
[61] Saunthararajah Y,Nakamura R, Wesley R, et al. A simple method to predict response to immunosuppressive therapy in patients with myelodysplastic syndrome. *Blood* 2003;102(8):3025.
[62] Passweg JR, Giagounidis AA, Simcock M, et al. Immunosuppressive therapy for patients with myelodysplastic syndrome: a prospective randomized multicenter phase III trial comparing antithymocyte globulin plus cyclosporine with best supportive care--SAKK 33/99. *J Clin Oncol* 2011;29(3):303.
[63] Vardiman JW, Harris NL, Brunning RD, et al. The World Health Organization (WHO) classification of the myeloid neoplasms. *Blood* 2002;100(7):2292-2302.
[64] List A[1], Dewald G, Bennett J, et al. Lenalidomide in the myelodysplastic syndrome with chromosome 5q deletion. *N Engl J Med* 2006 Oct 5;355(14):1456-65.
[65] Fenaux P, Giagounidis A, Selleslag D, et al. A randomized phase 3 study of lenalidomide versus placebo in RBC transfusion-dependent patients with Low-/Intermediate-1-risk myelodysplastic syndromes with del5q. *Blood* 2011;118(14):3765-76.
[66] Sekeres MA, Schoonen WM, Kantarjian H, et al. Characteristics of US patients with myelodysplastic syndromes: results of six cross-sectional physician surveys. *J Natl Cancer Inst* 2008;100:1542–1551.
[67] Lim Z, Brand R, Martino R, et al. Allogeneic hematopoietic stem-cell transplantation for patients 50 years or older with myelodysplastic syndromes or secondary acute myeloid leukemia. *J Clin Oncol* 2010;28:405–411.
[68] Cutler CS, Lee SJ, Greenberg P, et al. A decision analysis of allogeneic bone marrow transplantation for the myelodysplastic syndromes: delayed transplantation for low-risk myelodysplasia is associated with improved outcome. *Blood* 2004;104(2):579.
[69] Martino R, Iacobelli S, Brand R, et al. Retrospective comparison of reduced-intensity conditioning and conventional high-dose conditioning for allogeneic hematopoietic stem cell transplantation using HLA-identical sibling donors in myelodysplastic syndromes. *Blood* 2006;108:836–846.
[70] Walter MJ, Shen D, Ding L, et al. Clonal architecture of secondary acute myeloid leukemia. *N Engl J Med* 2012;366(12):1090-1098.

In: Frontiers in Leukemia Pharmacotherapy
Editor: Lunawati L. Bennett
ISBN: 978-1-53614-960-9

Chapter 7

ACUTE MYELOID LEUKEMIA

Zachery R. Halford*, PharmD and Heath McLean
Union University, College of Pharmacy,
Jackson, Tennessee, US

ABSTRACT

Acute myeloid leukemia (AML) is a heterogeneous group of hematologic diseases characterized by aberrant precursor cells and abnormal cellular proliferation resulting from one or more genetic mutations. AML is the second most common leukemia in adults and frequently presents with non-specific signs and symptoms. Historically, acute leukemia survival rates were abysmal with few patients living longer than one year post-diagnosis. Despite AML being the leading cause of leukemia-related mortality in the U.S., long-term survival rates can exceed 50% in certain AML cohorts following intensive chemotherapy and allogeneic hematopoietic stem cell transplantation (HSCT). Unfortunately, most patients with AML will die from their disease regardless of treatment intensity or duration.

This chapter aims to highlight the epidemiology, etiology, pathogenesis, diagnosis, disease classification, prognostic factors, and general treatment approach for adult patients with acute myeloid leukemia. Novel treatment options will also be discussed for patients with relapsed and/or refractory disease.

Keywords: acute myeloid leukemia, acute promyelocytic leukemia, cytopenias, induction, consolidation, hematopoietic stem cell transplantation, FLT3

---

* Corresponding Author Email: zhalford@uu.edu.

Abbreviations

ALL	acute lymphocytic leukemia
AML	acute myeloid leukemia
APL	acute promyelocytic leukemia
ATO	arsenic trioxide
ATRA	all-trans retinoic acid
CNS	central nervous system
CR	complete remission
DIC	disseminated intravascular coagulopathy
ECOG	Eastern Cooperative Oncology Group
FDA	Food and Drug Administration
FISH	fluorescence in situ hydribization
FLAG	fludarabine, cytarabine, filgrastim regimen
FLT3	FMS-like tyrosine kinase 3 ligand
HiDAC	high-dose cytarabine
HSCT	hematopoietic stem cell transplantation
IDH	isocitrate dehydrogenase
MDS	myelodysplastic syndrome
MLL	mixed lineage leukemia
MRD	minimal residual disease
NCCN	National Comprehensive Cancer Network
PCR	polymerase chain reaction
SEER	Surveillance, Epidemiology, and End Results Program
TMD	transient myeloproliferative disorder
WBC	white blood cell
WHO	World Health Organization

Introduction

Acute myeloid leukemia describes a heterogeneous group of leukemias, each arising from an immature blast cell of the myeloid lineage [1]. Myeloid blast cells include the precursors of neutrophils, monocytes, macrophages, basophils, mast cells, eosinophils, erythrocytes, and platelets, among others. In 2018, AML is projected to be the deadliest leukemia and the second most commonly diagnosed leukemia in the United States [2]. The myeloblast was first characterized in 1900, allowing practitioners to differentiate between myeloid and lymphoid leukemia [3]. Over the last 100 years, AML has been further divided into 8 classic subtypes. In recent years, our understanding of the role genetic mutations play in AML has greatly increased, with it being the first neoplasm for which a whole cancer genome was successfully sequenced [3, 4]. There are now over 40 known AML-associated mutations with several showing promise for molecular targeting.

EPIDEMIOLOGY

With an estimated 19,520 new cases projected for 2018, AML is the second most commonly diagnosed leukemia in the United States, coming in just 1,400 new cases behind chronic lymphocytic leukemia. AML accounts for approximately 1.1% of all new cancer cases in the United States, and is projected to be the most deadly leukemia of 2018, with an estimated 10,670 deaths. This accounts for roughly 44% of total deaths from all leukemias, and 1.8% of all cancer deaths. While the estimated number of new cases decreased slightly from 21,380 in 2017 to 19,520 in 2018, the estimated number of deaths has remained relatively constant [2, 5]. The average lifetime risk for developing AML is around 0.5% for both sexes; however, AML seems to be slightly more common in men than in women [6]. Approximately 4.3 new cases are diagnosed per 100,000 persons, and 2.8 deaths occur per 100,000 men and women per year.

Both the average age of a patient with AML and the median age at diagnosis are estimated to be about 68 years old, with 63.8% of new cases occurring in those aged 55 to 84 years, and 83.8% of new cases occurring in those aged at least 45 years. Only 4.9% of new cases occur in those under the age of 20. The median age at death for patients with AML is 72, with 71.8% of deaths occurring in those aged 55 to 84 years, and 92.7% of deaths occurring in those aged at least 45 years. Only 1.8% of deaths occurred in those less than 20 years old [7].

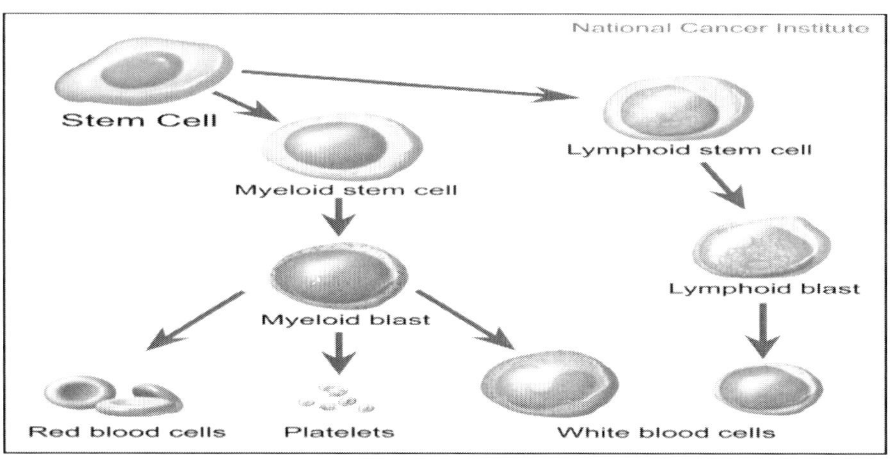

Figure 1. Hematopoietic stem cell maturing into either myeloid or lymphoid blast. Acute myeloid leukemia results from aberrant hematopoiesis following various genetic and epigenetic alterations. Illustration courtesy of National Cancer Institute.

AML appears to be slightly more common in the Caucasian population than in any other ethnic group, with 9.1 cases per 100,000 persons. Black and Hispanic populations have 7.8 and 7.2 cases per 100,000, respectively. Asian and Pacific Islander populations have 7 cases per 100,000. AML is least common in Native Americans and Alaskan Natives, with 4.9 cases per 100,000. The number of deaths per 100,000 appears to be roughly proportional to the number of cases for most ethnic groups, with the exception of Native Americans and Alaskan Natives. This group showed a death rate of 3.9 per 100,000, despite only having 4.9 cases per 100,000. The 5-year survival rate was 6.3% in 1975, and has been steadily increasing since then, with an estimated 5-year survival of 29.4% in 2010 [7].

ETIOLOGY

AML occurs when there is a mutation in an immature blast cell of the myeloid lineage. Since AML typically presents later in life, most of these mutations seem to be acquired throughout life, as opposed to being inherited at birth. Many environmental risk factors have been linked to higher risk of AML. In recent years, specific mutations have been identified that are associated with and can be used to characterize AML [3].

Several important risk factors for the development of AML exist, many of which are found in other cancers, like smoking, older age, family history of the disease, and exposure to radiation or carcinogenic chemicals, like benzene. Some genetic syndromes have shown a direct association with the development of AML, including Li-Fraumeni syndrome, Down syndrome, trisomy of chromosome 8, severe congenital neutropenia, Fanconi anemia, Bloom syndrome, and neurofibromatosis type 1, among others. Some myeloproliferative disorders also increase the risk of AML, including polycythemia vera, essential thrombocythemia, and idiopathic myelofibrosis [3]. Chemotherapeutic agents with an increased risk of developing AML include alkylating agents, platinum agents, and topoisomerase II inhibitors. Risk for developing AML seems to peak around 8 years after exposure to these agents [6].

In 2009, AML was the first neoplasm for which an entire cancer genome was successfully sequenced. Since then, more than 40 mutations associated with AML have been identified [3]. Several age-related mutations in hematopoietic stem progenitor cells accumulate before an initiating event occurs, leading to clonal expansion. Examples of mutations that have been identified as initiating mutations in AML are mutations such as NPM1, DNMT3A, IDH1, TET2, and PML-RARA fusion. Initiating events vary among subtypes of AML [4].

After the initiating event, a progression event often occurs, giving rise to the founding clone of malignant cells. This founding clone will give rise to all subsequent malignant cells. It is estimated that 1 to 5 progression events occur in most cases of

AML. A mutation of FMS-like tyrosine kinase 3 ligand (FLT3) has been identified as one example of a progression event. It is unknown how much time may pass between initiating events and progression events. Small additional mutations in the founding clone may lead to the development of multiple subclones [4].

FLT3, the most commonly identified mutation associated with a progression event, has recently become a target for drug therapy [4]. FLT3 is a receptor tyrosine kinase involved in signaling cascades that mediates cell growth and differentiation, and is mutated in 30% of adults newly diagnosed with AML [8]. Midostaurin, a tyrosine kinase inhibitor, inhibits the activity of FLT3, leading to downstream dysregulation, inhibiting proliferation, and inducing apoptosis in cells expressing mutant FLT3 [9]. Midostaurin is currently recommended by the National Comprehensive Cancer Network (NCCN) for the treatment of newly diagnosed, FLT3 positive AML, in combination with daunorubicin and cytarabine for induction and consolidation therapy [10].

Classification

Since AML is typically present in the bone marrow and blood, and sometimes various other tissues, a staging system is neither practical nor useful as a prognostic indicator. Instead, treatment decisions and prognosis are often based on the patient's age, laboratory markers, and subtype of AML present. Two systems exist to classify AML into subclasses. The French-American-British (FAB) classification system divides AML into subtypes based on the cell type of the founding clone of malignant cells. The World Health Organization (WHO) classification system also uses the presence of chromosome translocations and genetic abnormalities to characterize subtypes of AML [11].

The FAB classification system was devised in the 1970s by a collection of French, American, and British experts, and divided AML into subclasses based on the morphology of malignant cells observed under a microscope. Although the use of the FAB system alone is no longer common for classifying AML, it can be useful for understanding how various leukemias arise. There are eight classic FAB subtypes of AML, M0-M7, which are based on the cell type from which the leukemia arose and overall cell maturity [11].

The WHO system of classification, in addition to the origin of the neoplasm, takes into account the presence of various chromosome translocations and cytogenetic abnormalities when dividing AML into subtypes [11]. Many genetic abnormalities have been identified that can help guide prognosis and treatment in AML. Some of these include mutations of CEBPA, RUNX1, FLT3, BCR-ABL1 rearrangement, and numerous chromosome translocations [12]. The WHO system also differentiates between AML with and without myelodysplasia-related changes, and AML associated with prior chemotherapy or radiation. AML not otherwise specified includes leukemias that do not fit into any of the other defined categories, and uses a system of classification similar to the FAB system [11]. Many of these cytogenetic and molecular abnormalities are now used to assess risk status in AML, and have been incorporated into the 2018 NCCN AML guidelines [10].

Table 1. AML subtypes based on FAB and WHO [11-13]

AML Subtype	Cell of Origin	Incidence (per 1 million person-years)	Percent of AML Patients
AML not otherwise specified	-	16.8	43.9
AML with minimal differentiations (M0)	Myeloblast	1.5	3.9
AML without maturation (M1)	Myeloblast	2.1	5.5
AML with maturation (M2)	Myeloblast	2.4	6.4
AML with t(8;21) (M2)	Myeloblast	0.6	1.6
APL with t(15;17) (M3)	Promyelocyte	2.7	7.4
Acute myelomonocytic leukemia (M4)	Myelomonocyte	3.4	9.1
AML with inv(16) or t(16;16) (M4)	Myelomonocyte	0.4	1.0
Acute monoblastic and monocytic leukemia (M5)	Monocyte	2.8	7.5
Acute erythroid leukemia (M6)	Reticulocyte	0.7	1.8
Acute megakaryoblastic leukemia (M7)	Megakaryoblast	0.4	1.1
Acute panmyelosis with myelofibrosis	-	0.3	0.7
Myeloid sarcoma	-	0.3	0.9
AML with 11q23 abnormalities	-	0.3	0.7
AML with myelodysplasia-related changes	-	2.4	6.1
Therapy-related myeloid neoplasms	-	0.9	2.3

AML = Acute myeloid leukemia; APL = acute promyelocytic leukemia; FAB = French-American-British; WHO = World Health Organization.

PRESENTATION

Patients with AML generally have non-specific symptoms, including unexplained weight loss, fatigue, loss of appetite, bone or joint pain, and night sweats; however, many other pathologies also elicit these symptoms. Most patients present with signs and symptoms of leukemia resulting from secondary pancytopenia. This occurs because the malignant cells proliferate at a much faster rate than normal cells, taking over the bone marrow, and preventing normal hematopoiesis. AML symptoms associated with pancytopenia are due to anemia, thrombocytopenia, and neutropenia [6].

Anemic patients often complain of fatigue, weakness, cold extremities, feeling dizzy or lightheaded, and shortness of breath in more severe cases. These symptoms can all be attributed to the decreased oxygen transport capacity of an anemic patient's blood. Patients with thrombocytopenia often experience excessive bleeding and bruising [6].

Neutropenic patients will often experience frequent or recurrent infections due to a decreased number of functional WBC. Infections are normally associated with fever, and require antibiotics in these patients. Patients may have a low, normal, or high WBC count in AML. Normal or elevated levels of WBCs can occur in patients with FAB subtypes M0-5 AML, since these occur due to malignancies and abnormal proliferation of immature lymphocytes. Even though the WBC count may be elevated, these patients are still functionally neutropenic due to the inherent dysfunction of malignancy cells [6].

Other symptoms of AML include hepatosplenomegaly and lymphadenopathy due to collection of leukemia cells in the spleen and lymph nodes. Leukemia cells may also spread to other organs, including the skin or gums. If AML spreads to the gums, it may cause pain, swelling, or bleeding. If it spreads to the skin, the patient may present with chloromas, which are tumor-like collections of leukemia cells under the skin [6]. Early recognition of AML symptoms, and prompt diagnosis is crucial to patient survival, since AML is often very aggressive.

Diagnosis and Prognosis

Patients who present with symptoms consistent with AML should have a complete blood count with differential drawn. A detailed history and physical exam should also be conducted, in addition to a complete metabolic panel, platelet count, uric acid level, and lactate dehydrogenase level. A bone marrow core biopsy and aspirate analysis may be completed if there is a high level of clinical suspicion that leukemia is present. A diagnosis of AML is typically made if the blood contains at least 20% blasts of the myeloid lineage, although this is not required for diagnosis if certain genetic abnormalities are detected [12].

Other potentially beneficial labs include prothrombin time, partial thromboplastin time, and computed tomography scan of the brain to assess for hemorrhaging. Human leukocyte antigen typing should be performed if the patient is a potential candidate for HSCT in the future. An magnetic resonance imaging scan of the brain with contrast may be performed to exclude leukemic meningitis in patients with major neurologic symptoms at diagnosis. A lumbar puncture should also be performed in patients who present with major neurologic symptoms [10].

Cytogenetic analyses and characterization of cytogenetic abnormalities have been areas of prominent investigation in recent years. Fluorescence in situ hybridization (FISH) is a test that can detect genetic abnormalities in human cells, some of which can now be used to diagnose AML and help guide treatment. A diagnosis of AML may be made in patients with less than 20% blasts present if t(15;17), t(8,21), t(16;16), or inv(16) are detected. There are also a number of cytogenetic abnormalities that can be used to karyotype AML [10].

Numerous prognostic factors have been identified for adult patients with AML, including age, duration of CR, comorbidities, extramedullary involvement, underlying myelodysplastic syndrome (MDS), multi-drug resistance gene expression, elevated initial WBC (>100,000/mm3), and therapy-related AML [14]. While cytogenetic information is unknown at the time of diagnosis, karyotype remains the most important prognostic factor for determing remission rates and long-term syrvival [10].

Table 2. Risk stratification considerations for AML [10, 14]

Risk Category	Risk Factors
Favorable	Age < 50 Karnofsky score >60% MRD negative No antecedent hematologic disorder No previous chemotherapy NPM1 and/or CEBPA mutation t(8;21), inv(16)/t(16;16), t(15;17)
Intermediate	Normal karyotype
High	Age > 60 Karnofsky score <60% Complex karyotype FLT3-ITD mutation Therapy-related AML MRD positive IDH mutation

AML = acute myeloid leukemia; IDH = isocitrate dehydrogenase; FLT3 = FMS-like tyrosine kinase 3 ligand; MRD = minimal residual disease.

A population-based retrospective trial out of the United Kingdom included over 11,000 AML patients. This analysis showed an overall survival rate of only 15%, up from 10% in the 1970s, with a wide range of outcomes based on age at diagnosis [15]. The following overall survival rates were recorded based on patient age:

1) 15 to 24 years old – 53% (n=289)
2) 25 to 39 years old – 49% (n=702)

3) 40 to 59 years old – 33% (n=2170)
4) 60 to 69 years old – 13% (n=2208)
5) 70 to 79 years old – 3% (n=3258)
6) 80 years and older – 0% (n=2676)

Similar findings for overall survival based on age at diagnosis are reported in the SEER database (Figure 2) [7].

Performance status is also highly associated with both age and overall survival. The Karnofsky performance status and Eastern Cooperative Oncology Group (ECOG) performance tools are commonly used to help estimate a patient's ability to tolerate chemotherapy based on comorbidities and functional status. The Karnofsky scale (Table 3) ranges from 0 to 100 whereas the ECOG tool ranges from 0 to 5 (Table 4). As an example of performance status affecting overall survival, Estey et al. conducted a trial at the M.D. Anderson Cancer Center evaluating mortality during induction therapy in AML. Estey found that an ECOG performance status of ≥3 resulted in higher rates of death within the first month across all age groups [16].

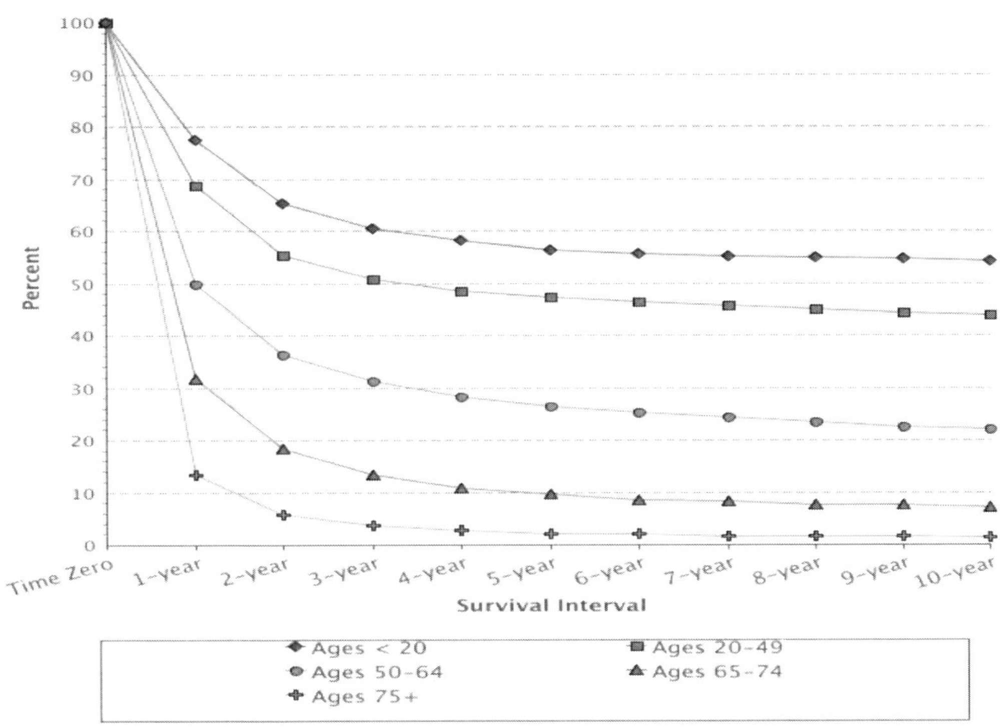

Courtesy of National Cancer Institute.
Source: https://seer.cancer.gov/faststats/selections.php?series=age.

Figure 2. Relative Survival by Age at Diagnosis from 1988-2014 [7].

Table 3. Karnofsky performance status [17]

Score (%)	State of Health
100	Normal; no complaints; no evidence of disease
90	Able to carry on normal activities; minor signs of disease
80	Normal activity with effort; some signs of disease
70	Cares for self; unable to carry on normal activities or work
60	Requires occasional assistance but is able to care for most needs
50	Requires considerable assistance and care
40	Disabled and requires special care
30	Severly disabled; hospitalization is indicated
20	Very sick; hospitalization required; active support treatment needed
10	Moribund; fatal process
0	Dead

Table 4. ECOG performance status [18]

ECOG Value	Description
0	Fully active, able to carry on all pre-disease performance without restriction
1	Restricted in physically strenuous activity but ambulatory and able to carry out light work
2	Ambulatory and capable of selfcare but unable to carry out work activities. Up and about more than 50% of waking hours
3	Capable of only limited selfcare. Confined to bed or chair more than 50% of waking hours
4	Completely disabled and incapable of carrying out selfcare.
5	Dead

TREATMENT FOR ADULT DE NOVO AML

At diagnosis, an AML patient may have 10^{12}/L leukemic cells. Induction therapy should kill 99.9% of these cells leaving roughly 10^{9}/L leukemic cells. Additional chemotherapy eradicates the remaining billion cells in order to avoid disease relapse and provide long-term survival. In light of this, treatment goals are multipronged and multi-dimensional. Ultimately, clinicians seek to obtain a CR and long-term disease-free survival in healthy AML patients. Current treatment strategies yield mixed results, with approximately 70% of patients obtaining a complete remission but only 20% to 40% becoming long-term survivors [19]. Before initiating AML treatment, clinicians must first evaluate the patient's performance status, age, previous cancer treatment, and disease progression. Molecular markers are powerful tools for long-term AML prognosis; however, they are not frequently incorporated into initial treatment planning at this time.

Treatment for relatively healthy adults with AML is typically divided into two sequential phases – induction chemotherapy followed by post-remission consolidation. Obtaining a complete remission from induction chemotherapy is a vital first step in reducing the leukemia burden, restoring normal hematopoiesis, and improving the life-altering symptoms common to AML. The short-term goal of obtaining a CR following induction chemotherapy is defined as restoration of normal hematopoiesis, no clinically detectable disease, and a bone marrow blast count less than 5% [20]. Following a CR, the goal of consolidation therapy is to maintain a continuous remission without disease recurrence.

Post-remission consolidation is intense and requires a good performance status to pursue. AML is a disease of the elderly, therefore certain patients will be unable to tolerate intense chemotherapy. The best option for these older patients may be low-intensity chemotherapy with the goal of improving quality of life and prolonging survival. All patients with AML should be counseled and encouraged to enroll into a clinical trial whenever possible. In addition, all patients should receive best supportive care to prevent and manage common complications arising from AML and the adverse events of chemotherapy. For all transplant candidates, human leukocyte antigen testing should be performed as soon as possible to help find a matched sibling or unrelated donor [10].

Induction

Age is an important determinant of long-term survival in patients with AML. Current guidelines use 60 years of age as a line of therapeutic demarcation [10]. Patients under 60 years of age are considered "young" and are often given induction chemotherapy. For those patients over 60 years of age, they are deemed "old" and frequently receive less intensive chemotherapy depending on their performance status. These older patients cannot routinely tolerate intensive chemotherapy required to obtain a CR. Furthermore, they tend to have unfavorable cytogenetics as well as an underlying myelodysplasia that prevents hematopoietic restoration following myelosuppressive chemotherapy. The goal for these older, frail AML patients is to improve quality of life, minimize treatment complications, and prolong life. Some older patients with significant comorbidities cannot tolerate even low-intensity chemotherapy and will require best supportive care in lieu of other treatment options. Recently, age cutoffs for intensive treatment have been questioned and evaluated. One clinical trial studied 3,365 AML patients using a multicomponent stratification looking at not only age but performance status, platelet count, de novo disease or secondary disease, and various other factors [21]. This trial found that age alone might not be predictive and treatment decisions should also include performance status and co-morbidities.

Unfortunately, little has changed over the past half century for AML induction therapy. The backbone of induction remains a combination of an anthracycline with standard or high dose cytarabine (Table 5). In patients with impaired cardiac function, non-anthracycline regimens need to be considered. Most patients only require one induction cycle to obtain a complete remission. Anthracyclines such as daunorubicin and idarubicin are commonly employed in AML induction with similar safety and efficacy profiles. A meta-analysis of 29 randomized clinical trials evaluating these two anthracyclines showed idarubicin had fewer remission failures compared to daunorubicin, but this did not translate to any appreciable survival benefit [22]. This study also found that high dose daunorubicin or idarubicin produced overall survival rates of 50% to 60%. Dose intensity for daunorubicin has also been studied in several prospective clinical trials [23-25]. A phase III clinical trial evaluating daunorubicin 45 mg/m^2 versus 90 mg/m^2 in younger (15-60 year old) AML patients found that those assigned to 90 mg/m^2 had higher remission rates (71% versus 57%), longer survival (24 months versus 16 months), and similar rates of severe toxicities. Another large, prospective, randomized clinical trial evaluated daunorubicin 60 mg/m^2 versus 90 mg/m^2 in high risk AML and MDS patients under the age of 60 years. Findings with this clinical trial included no overall difference in remission rates (73% versus 75%) and an increase in 60-day mortality (10% versus 5%) in patients receiving 90 mg/m^2 of daunorubicin. Overall survival was similar between the two dosing schemes. Based on these various trials, the NCCN guidelines currently list both 60 mg/m^2 and 90 mg/m^2 dosing options as category 1 recommendations [10].

Another induction option is the high-dose cytarabine (HiDAC) regimen that utilizes 1000 to 3000 mg/m^2 of cytarabine IV every 12 hours for 8 to 12 doses in addition to an anthracycline. High doses of cytarabine provide excellent anti-leukemic activity with high intracellular drug concentrations that can help overcome residual disease and drug resistance. The use of HiDAC in adult AML patients remains controversial due to questionable survival benefit in the face of increased treatment-related complications. One trial evaluated 860 "younger" adults (≤60 years) who were randomized to either standard dose cytarabine or HiDAC [26].

Patients receiving HiDAC therapy showed similar rates of CR (82% versus 80%), event free survival (35% versus 34%), and overall survival (42% and 40%) at 5 years compared to standard cytarabine doses. Those in the HiDAC arm did experience significantly higher rates of severe toxicity (61% versus 51%) including delayed neutrophil and platelet recovery, skin reactions, gastrointestinal and ocular toxicities. A meta-analysis including 22 trials and nearly 5,600 "younger" AML patients found that HiDAC therapy improved relapse-free survival but with increased toxicity [27]. Future studies are required to better identify what patient cohort can tolerate the toxicities while maintaining a survival advantage.

Table 5. Common adult AML induction regimens

Regimen	Dosing	Comments
Cytarabine with Daunorubicin	Cytarabine – 100 to 200 mg/m^2 IV daily as a continuous infusion x 7 days Daunorubicin – 60 to 90 mg/m^2 IV on days 1 through 3	Known as the "7 + 3" induction regimen Complete remission in 60% to 88% of patients "7 + 3" with idarubicin may have better remission rates but overall survival appears to be similar
Cytarabine with Idarubicin	Cytarabine – 100 to 200 mg/m^2 IV daily as a continuous infusion x 7 days Idarubicin – 12 mg/m^2 IV on days 1 through 3	
High-dose Cytarabine with Daunorubicin	Cytarabine – 1 to 3 g/m^2 twice daily for 12 doses Daunorubicin – 45 mg/m^2 IV daily for 3 days	Higher remission rate than "7 + 3" induction (90% vs 70%) Significantly higher rates of toxicity

AML = Acute myeloid leukemia.

Some centers use a double induction chemotherapy course that incorporates the re-administration of induction chemotherapy with "7+3" or HiDAC [28]. One phase III randomized clinical trial evaluated 860 patients between the ages of 18 and 60 with newly diagnosed AML. Event-free and overall survival were similar in patients receiving double induction and those randomized to either timed-sequential or control "7+3" induction. NCCN guidelines currently recommend standard dose cytarabine regimens as a category 1 recommendation for all patients. HiDAC regimens are also considered a category 1 recommendation but only for patients who are 45 years or younger [10]. High doses of cytarabine require frequent administration of saline or steroid eye drops due to chemical conjunctivitis resulting from appreciable concentrations in tear production. HiDAC also can lead to significant cytopenias and cerebellar toxicities including somnolence, confusion, cognitive dysfunction, and seizures.

Consolidation Overview

Standard induction therapy will result in a CR in roughly 70% of AML patients. Nearly 5% of patients undergoing induction will die from treatment-related complications such as bleeding or infection. Once induction therapy has finished, a bone marrow aspirate and biopsy ensuring a CR are required prior to initiating post-remission consolidation therapy. In patients who failed to obtain a CR, re-induction therapy is required and may include additional chemotherapy agents and/or dose intensification. If a patient fails to obtain a CR, they are considered to have a poor prognosis with refractory disease requiring salvage therapy.

Consolidation therapy is required following induction because remissions are fleeting and will inevitably relapse within a few months due to the clinically undetectable MRD still present following induction chemotherapy. The goals of post-remission consolidation are to eliminate residual leukemic disease and achieve long-term disease-free survival using one or more high-intensity chemotherapy courses. For older AML patients who cannot tolerate the rigors of high-intensity consolidation therapy, lower intensity therapies may be an option.

Three consolidation options are currently available for AML patients in a CR: intensive chemotherapy, autologous HSCT, or allogeneic HSCT. The preferred pathway depends on risk stratification, age, cytogenetic and molecular abnormalities.

Consolidation for Favorable-Risk AML

Following induction therapy, consolidation may be initiated once a CR has been confirmed and the patient recovers from any significant treatment-related complications. For AML patients with good cytogenetics and favorable disease, consolidation therapy may consist of high-dose chemotherapy with or without allogeneic HSCT. The benefit and timing of HSCT remains controversial and requires additional studies. Currently, NCCN guidelines list high dose chemotherapy with HiDAC as their only category 1 recommendation for this patient population. Several meta-analyses were conducted to evaluate allogeneic HSCT. The most recent study evaluated over 6,000 patients and found that allogeneic HSCT in favorable-risk patients did not provide a relapse-free survival benefit compared to autologous HSCT [29]. Furthermore, favorable-risk AML patients have significantly better survival rates than those with intermediate- or unfavorable-risk cytogenetics (55% versus 24% versus 5%) [30]. Evidence suggests favorable-risk AML patients do not benefit from more-intensive therapy and may experience significant treatment-related morbidity and mortality. Therefore, these patients should receive chemotherapy for post-remission consolidation without transplantation.

The primary intensive chemotherapy regimen for post-remission consolidation remains HiDAC in favorable-risk patients. Various trials have been conducted to improve remission rates and reduce toxicities; however, HiDAC continues to be the preferred option. Cytarabine doses can vary from 1,000 mg/m^2 twice daily up to 3,000 mg/m^2 twice daily. High dose cytarabine is superior to low dose regimens in consolidation. One clinical trial evaluated 100 mg/m^2/day, 400 mg/m^2/day, and 3,000 mg/m^2/dose every 12 hours in younger AML patients undergoing post-remission chemotherapy [31]. This study found higher rates of disease-free survival in the 3,000 mg/m^2 arm compared to the 100 mg/m^2 and 400 mg/m^2 arms (44% versus 29% and 24%, respectively). In addition, overall survival rates were superior (52% versus 40% and 35%, respectively).

Unfortunately, the high dose arm did confer additional treatment-related toxicities. The exact number of HiDAC cycles in favorable-risk AML is unknown. The NCCN guidelines recommend 3 to 4 cycles in consolidation [10]. Following each course, at least 28 days is required to make a hematologic recovery before beginning the next cycle. Typical parameters include an absolute neutrophil count of at least 1,000 x 10^6/L and platelets $\geq$ 100 x 10^9/L.

Consolidation for Intermediate-Risk AML

Similar to favorable-risk AML, consolidation and eradication of MRD can be achieved through intensive chemotherapy. In addition, this patient cohort should also be assessed for autologous or allogeneic HSCT. All three modalities are options in these patients. Koreth conducted a meta-analysis evaluating relapse-free survival and overall survival benefit of allogeneic HSCT following CR [29]. Twenty four clinical trials were assessed with over 6,000 total AML patients, 2,499 having intermediate-risk disease. Unlike favorable-risk patients, those with intermediate- and unfavorable-risk AML showed a significant survival benefit when given allogeneic HSCT compared to autologous HSCT. Selection of intensive chemotherapy versus HSCT is dependent on comorbidities, age, preference, and donor availability. In younger patients with few comorbidities, strong consideration should be given to allogeneic HSCT due to the improved survival benefit despite the risk of treatment-related morbidity and mortality inherent in transplantation. Pfirrmann developed a prediction calculator for post-remission survival in AML [32]. This tool utilizes age, CD-34 count, FLT-ITD ratio, cytogenetic risks, and de novo or secondary AML status to help identify optimal treatment strategies for the various AML cohorts. This multicenter trial found that patients with intermediate-risk AML displayed superior survival rates with autologous HSCT compared to chemotherapy or allogeneic HSCT (66% versus 41% and 44%, respectively). The NCCN guidelines recommend either allogeneic HSCT or 3 to 4 cycles of HiDAC are preferred consolidation options in intermediate-risk AML. Generally, they recommend 2,000 mg/m^2 to 3,000 mg/m^2 of cytarabine in otherwise healthy individuals with the option of reducing the dose to 1,000 mg/m^2 in less fit patients.

Consolidation for Unfavorable-Risk AML

Patients with unfavorable-risk AML in a CR following induction therapy should be strongly encouraged to enroll in a clinical trial whenever possible. These high-risk patients should undergo allogeneic HSCT as soon as possible, preferably with a matched sibling donor. Unfortunately, only 25% to 30% of potential transplant candidates have a matched sibling donor. For those patients without a matched sibling donor, matched unrelated donors are appropriate and encouraged. A myeloablative regimen is preferred over reduced-intensity or nonmyeloablative. Consolidation therapy with HiDAC may be required to maintain a CR while a bone marrow donor is being located. Unfavorable-risk AML confers a poor overall prognosis with high-dose chemotherapy alone. Five year overall survival rates range from 15% to 30% and the incorporation of allogeneic HSCT can increase survival rates to 40%, which is still unacceptably low. Allogeneic HSCT is significantly better at eradicating residual leukemic disease because it provides a graft-versus-leukemia effect that persists long after treatment cessation. Unfortunately, graft-versus-host-disease is also closely linked with this graft-versus-leukemia effect and is a noteworthy concern in transplant patients.

Post-Consolidation Management

Unlike ALL, maintenance therapy with relatively low doses of chemotherapy was not shown to provide any survival benefit in AML (aside from patients with M3 AML). Upon completion of induction and consolidation therapy, patients are required to undergo monitoring at periodic intervals to evaluate remission status and potential late-effects from chemotherapy. Patients are most likely to relapse following post-remission consolidation within one to two years; therefore, frequent surveillance is required during this time frame to catch recurrence as early as possible. A unilateral bone marrow aspirate is required to identify a bone marrow relapse. Cytogenetic testing, even if already completed, should be evaluated as well to help determine prognosis and potentially identify targetable mutations.

Treatment of Relapse/Refractory AML

Nearly 50% of older adult AML patients will never achieve a CR following induction chemotherapy. These patients are determined to have refractory disease and have a poor prognosis. Relapse is considered once a patient has obtained a CR but experience disease recurrence in the bone marrow, central nervous system, peripheral blood, or some other extramedullary site. Once relapse has been confirmed, several assessments are required including patient performance status, age, transplant eligibility, a viral panel, comorbidities, and patient preference. Transplant eligibility varies across institutions with a common age cutoff around 65 years. This cutoff, however, is changing as recent advancements in transplantation and supportive care have reduced infections, organ toxicity, and graft-versus-host-disease following allogeneic HSCT.

Allogeneic HSCT following myeloablative chemotherapy remains the best treatment option for curing relapsed/refractory AML. Patients will typically fare better if entering transplantation in a CR; however, transplantation can still be undertaken in those with MRD. Obtaining a second complete remission using re-induction chemotherapy is ideal but not always feasible and needs to be considered on a patient-by-patient basis. Duval developed a scoring system to help clinicians determine what patients should receive re-induction chemotherapy prior to transplantation [33]. They identified five key variables that significantly affect survival:

1) First CR lasting less than 6 months.
2) Circulating blast cells at the time of disease recurrence.
3) Non-sibling HSCT donor
4) Performance status - Karnofsky or Lansky score less than 90 (no longer able to carry on normal activities).
5) Poor-risk cytogenetics.

Each variable was given a 1-point value. This study evaluated 1,673 relapsed/refractory AML patients and found that rates of overall survival correlated with the total number of points a patient had prior to transplantation. Overall survival rates for those with 0, 1, 2, and 3 points were 42%, 28%, 15%, and 6%, respectively. Based on these findings, some institutions will proceed to HSCT without re-induction chemotherapy if a patient's score is ≤ 2. For those individuals with a score of 3 or greater, HSCT does not appear to be beneficial in patients who are not in a complete remission. Therefore, those with a score of 3 or greater should undergo re-induction chemotherapy to obtain a second CR before undergoing HSCT. Unfavorable-risk patients who do not qualify for HSCT are unlikely to respond to conventional chemotherapy and investigational agents should be considered.

Re-induction chemotherapy typically involves aggressive, cytotoxic chemotherapy (Table 3). Older frail patients cannot tolerate re-induction chemotherapy. Few novel therapies exist for relapsed or refractory AML, however, in August of 2017, the FDA approved enasidenib (Idhifa) based on findings from phase I/II clinical trials for the treatment of relapsed or refractory AML in patients with the isocitrate dehydrogenase (IDH) gene [34]. Enasidenib was found to produce a complete remission in 19.3% of patients with IDH-2 positive relapsed/refractory AML. Median duration of remission was 8.2 months. Nearly 10% of patients with relapsed/refractory AML are positive for the IDH mutation. A phase III clinical trial is currently enrolling participants and will compare enasidenib to standard therapy in older AML patients.. In 2018, the FDA approved the first isocitrate dehydrogenase-1 (IDH-1) inhibitor for patients with relapsed/refractory AML. Ivosidenib (Tibsovo®), a small-molecule inhibitor of mutant IDH-1 protein, was studied in 174 adult patients harboring the IDH-1 mutation [35]. The rate of CR following treatment with ivosidenib was 24.7%. The overall median duration of remission was 8.2 months. Common adverse events included fatigue, leukocytosis, diarrhea, QT prolongation, rash, edema, dyspnea, and differentiation syndrome. The FDA gave ivosidenib a black box warning for differentiation syndrome, which can be fatal if left untreated. Other IDH-targeting agents are also in the therapeutic pipeline [36].

Several viable intensive chemotherapy regimens exist for re-induction therapy following AML relapse or in refractory disease. The preferred regimen depends on patient- and treatment-specific factors such as previous exposure, comorbidities, clinical experience, leukemic mutations, etc. Moreover, no one regimen stands out over the others. One large international randomized phase III clinical trial evaluating regimens based on clinician preference versus an investigation drug, elacytarabine, found that no one regimen provided benefit in terms of long-term survival, response rate or relapse-free survival [37]. This trial confirmed that the only patients receiving a long-term survival benefit were those who achieved a complete remission and proceeded to allogeneic HSCT. Several intensive regimens exist for the treatment of relapsed/refractory AML.

Table 6. Common re-induction regimens for relapsed/refractory AML

Regimen	Components	CR Rate
HiDAC [38, 39]	Cytarabine 3,000 mg/m^2 every 12 hours on days 1 through 6	32% - 47%
FLAG [40, 41]	Fludarabine 30 mg/m^2 days 1-5 Cytarabine 2,000 mg/m^2 days 1-5 Filgrastim 5 mcg/kg daily	48% - 55%
FLAG-IDA [42]	Fludarabine 30 mg/m^2 days 1-5 Cytarabine 2,000 mg/m^2 days 1-5 Filgrastim 300 mcg daily Idarubicin 10 mg/m^2 days 1-3	63%
MEC [43, 44]	Mitoxantrone 6 mg/m^2 days 1-6 Etoposide 80 mg/m^2 days 1-6 Cytarabine 1,000 mg/m^2 days 1-6	59% - 66%
Gemtuzumab ozogamicin [45]	Gemtuzumab ozogamicin 3 mg/m^2 (max = 4.5 mg/dose) on days 1, 4, and 7	42%
Clofarabine + Cytarabine [46]	Clofarabine 40 mg/m^2 days 2-6 Cytarabine 1,000 mg/m^2 days 1-5	28% - 51%
FLAD [47]	Fludarabine 30 mg/m^2 days 1-3 Cytarabine 2,000 mg/m^2 days 1-3 Liposomal daunorubicin 100 mg/m^2 days 1-3	53%

AML = Acute myeloid leukemia; FLAD = fludarabine, cytarabine, liposomal daunorubicin; FLAG = fludarabine, cytarabine, filgrastim; HiDAC = high dose cytarabine; IDA = idarubicin; MEC = mitoxantrone, etoposide, cytarabine.

Once re-induction chemotherapy has finished, eligible patients will move forward with allogeneic HSCT as soon as possible (Figure 3). For patients who are ineligible for intensive therapy or HSCT, other treatment options exist to help improve symptoms and prolong survival without the life-threatening complications of intensive chemotherapy. Low dose cytarabine, single-agent clofarabine, azacitidine, and decitabine are all chemotherapy options with significantly fewer complications compared to the intensive chemotherapy. Several investigational agents are also worth consideration in patients with relapsed/refractory AML. These include targeted agents for FLT3 and C-KIT mutations. FLT3 is identified in 10% to 30% of AML patients. This mutation leads to an extremely poor prognosis with overall survival of only 20% [48]. A number of FLT3-specific tyrosine kinase inhibitors are FDA approved including midostaurin, lestaurtinib, sorafenib, and sunitinib. The overall benefit of these tyrosine kinase inhibitors in FLT3-positive AML is not fully understood and requires additional evaluation.

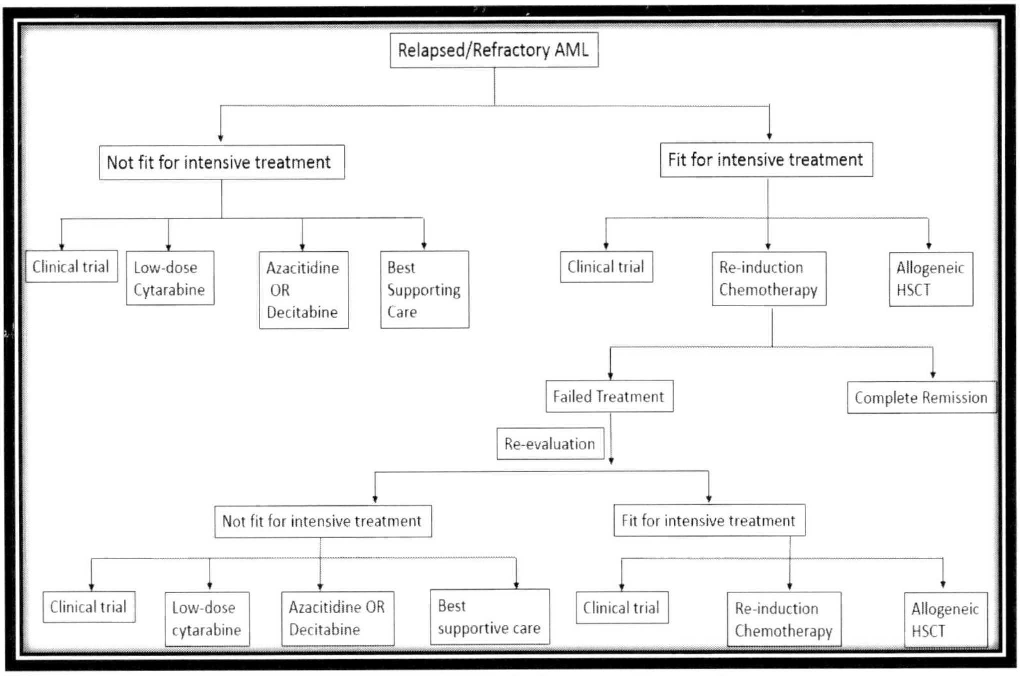

AML = acute myeloid leukemia; HSCT = hematopoietic stem cell transplant.

Figure 3. Treatment Schema for Relapsed/Refractory AML.

SUPPORTIVE CARE

AML patients require frequent hospitalizations for treatment and symptom management and experience a variety of long-term sequelae. These patients are often extremely ill, requiring comprehensive management including bone marrow support with red blood cell and platelet transfusions, infectious prophylaxis, nutritional support, correction of coagulopathies, tumor lysis syndrome prevention, and growth factor support. Following allogeneic HSCT, clinicians must continuously monitor for signs and symptoms of graft-versus-host-disease and navigate the tumultuous terrain of therapeutic immunosuppression. Furthermore, hypervigilant surveillance is required to identify and diagnose disease recurrence at the earliest possible opportunity.

Conclusion

AML is a heterogeneous disease of the myeloid cell line with eight morphological subtypes. Historically, AML survival rates were abysmal with few patients living longer than one year post-diagnosis. Despite AML being the leading cause of leukemia-related mortality in the U.S., long-term survival rates exceed 50% in certain AML cohorts following intensive chemotherapy and allogeneic HSCT. AML has a number of important prognostic indicators including age, WBC count at diagnosis, MRD following induction, cytogenetic abnormalities, patient performance status, and prior hematologic disorders. Treatment for traditional AML consists of intensive chemotherapy with or without HSCT for otherwise healthy individuals. Transplantation eligibility is an important component and guide for managing AML. Standard therapy consists of remission induction with combination chemotherapy followed by post-induction consolidation. Allogeneic HSCT plays an important role in sustaining remission and preventing disease recurrence; however, most patients cannot tolerate the acute and chronic complications resulting from myeloablative treatment and transplantation. Despite substantial improvements in managing AML complications, newer treatment paradigms are needed to increase long-term survival.

References

[1] Dohner H, Weisdorf D, Bloomfield C. Acute Myeloid Leukemia. *New England Journal of Medicine* 2015; 373: 1136-52.

[2] Siegel RL, Miller KD, Jemal A. Cancer Statistics, 2018. *CA: A Cancer Journal for Clinicians* 2018; 68: 7–30.

[3] Freireich EJ, Wiernik PH, Steensma DP. The Leukemia: A Half-Century of Discovery. *Journal of Clinical Oncology* 2014;32:3463-3469.

[4] Welch JS, Ley TJ, Link DC, et al. The Origin and Evolution of Mutations in Acute Myeloid Leukemia. *Cell* 2012; 150: 264-78.

[5] Siegel RL, Miller KD, Jemal A. Cancer Statistics, 2017. *CA: A Cancer Journal for Clinicians* 2017; 67: 7–30.

[6] American Cancer Society. *Acute Myeloid Leukemia: Early Detection, Diagnosis, and Types* [Internet]. Last revised 02/22/2016; cited 06/29/2018. Available from https://www.cancer.org/cancer/acute-myeloid-leukemia/detection-diagnosis-staging/how-classified.html.

[7] Noone AM, Howlader N, Krapcho M, et al. *SEER Cancer Statistics Review*, 1975-2015, National Cancer Institute. Bethesda, MD, https://seer.cancer.gov/csr/1975_2015/, based on November 2017 SEER data submission, posted to the SEER web site, April 2018.

[8] Stone R, Mandrakar S, Sanford B, et al. Midostaurin plus Chemotherapy in Acute Myeloid Leukemia with a FLT3 Mutation. *New England Journal of Medicine* 2017; 377:454-64.

[9] National Cancer Institute. *Midostaurin* [Internet]. Version 18.05d; released 05/29/2018; cited 06/21/2018. Available from https://ncit.nci.nih.gov/ncitbrowser/ConceptReport.jsp?dictionary=NCI_Thesaurus&ns=NCI_Thesaurus&code=C1872.

[10] *NCCN Clinical Practice Guidelines in Oncology. Acute Myeloid Leukemia*. Version 1:2018. cited 06/21/2018. Available from https://www.nccn.org/professionals/physician_gls/pdf/aml.pdf.

[11] American Cancer Society. *How is Acute Myeloid Leukemia Classified?* Revised 02/22/2016; cited 06/21/2018. Available from https://www.cancer.org/cancer/acute-myeloid-leukemia/detection-diagnosis-staging/how-classified.html.

[12] Arber D, Orazi A, Hasserjian R. The 2016 revision to the World Health Organization classification of myeloid neoplasms and acute leukemia. *Blood* 2016. 127(20):2391-405.

[13] G Dores, S Devesa, R Curtis, et al. Acute leukemia incidence and survival among children and adults in the United States, 2001-2007. *Blood* 2012; 119:34-43.

[14] Estey EH. Acute myeloid leukemia: 2013 update on risk-stratification and management. *Am J Hematol* 2013;88:318-327.

[15] Shah A, Andersson TM, Rachet B, et al. Survival and cure of acute myeloid leukaemia in England, 1971-2006: a population-based study. *Br J Haematol* 2013;162(4):509-516.

[16] Estey EH. Therapeutic options for acute myelogenous leukemia. *Cancer* 2001;92(5):1059.

[17] Karnofsky DA, Burchenal JH. The clinical evaluation of chemotherapeutic agents in cancer. In: *Evaluation of chemotherapeutic agents*. MacLeod CM, editor. New York: Columbia University Press; 1949. pp. 191–205.

[18] Oken MM, Creech RH, Tormey DC, et al. Toxicity and response criteria of the Eastern Cooperative Oncology Group. *Am J Clin Oncol* 1982; 5:649.

[19] Dohner H, Weisdorf DJ, Bloomfield CD. Acute myeloid leukemia. *N Eng J Med* 2015;373:1136-1152.

[20] Cheson BD, Bennett JM, Kopecky KJ, et al. Revised recommendations of the International Working Group for Diagnosis, Standardization of Response Criteria, Treatment Outcomes, and Reporting Standards for Therapeutic Trials in Acute Myeloid Leukemia. *J Clin Oncol* 2003;21:4642–4649.

[21] Walter RB, Othus M, Borthakur G, et al.: Prediction of early death after induction therapy for newly diagnosed acute myeloid leukemia with pretreatment risk scores: a novel paradigm for treatment assignment. *J Clin Oncol* 2011;29:4417-4423.

[22] Teuffel O, Leibundgut K, Lehrnbecher T, et al. Anthracyclines during induction therapy in acute myeloid leukemia: a systematic review and meta-analysis. *Br J Haematol* 2013;161:192-203.

[23] Ohtake S, Miyawaki S, Fujita H, et al. Randomized study of induction therapy comparing standard-dose idarubicin with high-dose daunorubicin in adult patients with previously untreated acute myeloid leukemia: the JALSG AML201 Study. *Blood* 2011;117(8):2358.

[24] Fernandez HF, Sun Z, Yao X, et al. Anthracycline dose intensification in acute myeloid leukemia. *N Engl J Med* 2009;361(13):1249.

[25] Burnett AK, Russell NH, Hills RK, et al. A randomized comparison of daunorubicin 90 mg/m2 vs 60 mg/m2 in AML induction: results from the UK NCRI AML17 trial in 1206 patients. *Blood* 2015;125(25):3878-3885.

[26] Löwenberg B, Pabst T, Vellenga E, et al. Cytarabine dose for acute myeloid leukemia. *N Engl J Med* 2011;364(11):1027.

[27] Li W, Gon x, Sun M, et al. High-dose cytarabine in acute myeloid leukemia treatment: a systemic review and meta-analysis. *PLoS One* 2014;9:e110153.

[28] Castaigne S, Chevret S, Archimbaud E, et al. Randomized comparison of double induction and timed-sequential induction to a "3 + 7" induction in adults with AML: long-term analysis of the Acute Leukemia French Association (ALFA) 9000 study. *Blood* 2004;104(8):2467.

[29] Koreth J, Shclenk R, Kopecky KJ, et al. Allogeneic stem cell transplantation for acute myeloid leukemia in first complete remission: systematic review and meta-analysis of prospective clinical trials. *JAMA* 2009;301(22):2349.

[30] Byrd JC, Mrozek K, Dodge RK, et al. Pretreatment cytogenetic abnormalities are predictive of induction success, cumulative incidence of relapse, and overall survival in adult patients with de novo acute myeloid leukemia: results from Cancer and Leukemia Group B (CALGB 8461). *Blood* 2002:100:4325-4336.

[31] Mayer RJ, Davis RB, Schiffer CA, et al. Intensive postremussion chemotherapy in adults with acute myeloid leukemia. Cancer and Leukemia Group B. *N Engl J Med* 1994;331(14):896.

[32] Pfirrmann M, Ehninger G, Thiede C, et al. Prediction of post-remission survival in acute myeloid leukaemia: a post-hoc analysis of the AML96 trial. *Lancet Oncol* 2012;13(2):207-214.

[33] Duval M, Klein JP, He W, et al. Hematopoietic stem-cell transplantation for acute leukemia in relapse or primary induction failure. *J Clin Oncol* 2010;28(23):3730.

[34] *Food and Drug Administration.* Prescribing information Idhifa (enasidenib) tablets for oral suspension. 2017. Available at https://www.fda.gov/drugs/informationon drugs/approveddrugs/ucm569482.htm (Accessed on June 09, 2018).

[35] DiNardo CD, De Bottom S, Stein EM, et al. Ivosidenib (AG-120) in mutant IDH1 AML and advanced hematologic malignancies: results of a phase 1 dose escalation and expansion study. *Blood* 2017;130;725.

[36] DiNardo CD, Stein EM, de Botton S, et al. Durable remissions with Ivosidenib in IDH1-mutated relapsed or refractory AML. *N Engl J Med* 2018 [Epub ahead of print].

[37] Roboz GJ, Rosenblat T, Arellano M, et al. International randomized phase III study of elacytarabine versus investigator choice in patietns with relapsed/refractory acute myeloid leukemia. *J Clin Oncol* 2014;32:1919.

[38] Karanes C, Kopecky K.J., Head D, et al. A phase III comparison of high dose ARA-C (HIDAC) versus HIDAC plus mitoxantrone in the treatment of first relapsed or refractory acute myeloid leukemia Southwest Oncology Group Study. *Leuk Res* 1999;23:787–794.

[39] Herzig R.H, Lazarus H.M, Wolff, S.N., et al. High-dose cytosine arabinoside therapy with and without anthracycline antibiotics for remission reinduction of acute nonlymphoblastic leukemia. *J Clin Oncol* 1985;3:992–997.

[40] Lee SR, Yang DH, Ahn, JS, et al. The clinical outcome of flag chemotherapy without idarubicin in patients with relapsed or refractory acute myeloid leukemia. *J Korean Med Sci* 2009;24:498–503.

[41] Montillo M, Mirto S, Petti MC, et al. Fludarabine, cytarabine, and G-CSF (FLAG) for the treatment of poor risk acute myeloid leukemia. Am. *J Hematol* 1998;58:105–109.

[42] Virchis A, Koh M, Rankin P, et al. Fludarabine, cytosine arabinoside, granulocyte-colony stimulating factor with or without idarubicin in the treatment of high risk acute leukaemia or myelodysplastic syndromes. Br. *J Haematol* 2004;124:26–32.

[43] Amadori S, Arcese W, Isacchi G, et al. Mitoxantrone, etoposide, and intermediate-dose cytarabine: An effective and tolerable regimen for the treatment of refractory acute myeloid leukemia. *J Clin Oncol* 1991;9:1210–1214.

[44] Trifilio SM, Rademaker AW, Newman D, et al. Mitoxantrone and etoposide with or without intermediate dose cytarabine for the treatment of primary induction failure or relapsed acute myeloid leukemia. *Leuk Res* 2012;6:394–396.

[45] Walter RB, Medeiros BC, Gardner KM, et al. Gemtuzumab ozogamicin in combination with vorinostat and azacitidine in older patients with relapsed or refractory acute myeloid leukemia: A phase I/II study. *Haematologica* 2014;99:54–59.

[46] Faderl S, Gandhi V, O'Brien S, et al. Results of a phase 1-2 study of clofarabine in combination with cytarabine (ARA-C) in relapsed and refractory acute leukemias. *Blood* 2005;105:940–947.

[47] De Astis E, Clavio M, Raiola AM, et al. Liposomal daunorubicin, fludarabine, and cytarabine (FLAD) as bridge therapy to stem cell transplant in relapsed and refractory acute leukemia. *Ann. Hematol* 2014;93:2011–2018.

[48] Marcucci G, Maharry K, Whitman SP, et al. High expression levels of the ETS-related gene, ERG, predict adverse outcome and improve molecular risk-based classification of cytogenetically normal acute myeloid leukemia: a Cancer and Leukemia Group B Study. *J Clin Oncol* 2007;25(22):3337.

In: Frontiers in Leukemia Pharmacotherapy
Editor: Lunawati L. Bennett
ISBN: 978-1-53614-960-9

Chapter 8

ACUTE LYMPHOBLASTIC LEUKEMIA

Zachery R. Halford*, PharmD
Union University, College of Pharmacy, Jackson, Tennessee, US

ABSTRACT

Acute lymphoblastic leukemia (ALL) is a heterogeneous disease resulting from a series of mutational events occurring primarily in precursor lymphoblasts. These mutations thwart lymphoid maturation and normal hematopoiesis, manifesting with signs and symptoms of anemia, thrombocytopenia, and neutropenia. Significant progress has been made over the past 50 years in the identification, diagnosis, risk stratification, treatment, and overall management of acute leukemia. Cure rates for pediatric ALL is 80% to 90%; however, adult patients fare significantly worse with an overall survival rate of 30% to 40% despite similar treatment strategies.

This chapter aims to highlight the epidemiology, etiology, pathogenesis, diagnosis, disease classification, prognostic factors, and general treatment approach for adult patients with acute lymphoblastic leukemia. Novel treatment options will also be discussed for patients with relapsed and/or refractory disease.

Keywords: acute lymphoblastic leukemia, pre-leukemia, cytopenias, induction, consolidation, maintenance, bone marrow transplantation, philadelphia chromosome, tyrosine kinase inhibitor

---

* Corresponding Author Email: zhalford@uu.edu

ABBREVIATIONS

6-MP	6-mercaptopurine
ALL	acute lymphocytic leukemia
AML	acute myeloid leukemia
ANC	absolute neutrophil count
AYA	adolescents and young adults
BiTE	bispecific T-cell-engager
CD	cluster of differentiation
CNS	central nervous system
CR	complete remission
DIC	disseminated intravascular coagulopathy
FAB	French-American-British
FDA	Food and Drug Administration
FISH	fluorescence in situ hybridization
HSCT	hematopoietic stem cell transplantation
LBL	lymphoblastic lymphomas
MRD	minimal residual disease
MLL	mixed lineage leukemia
MPAL	mixed phenotype acute leukemia
NCCN	National Comprehensive Cancer Network
PCR	polymerase chain reaction
Ph^+	Philadelphia chromosome
SEER	Surveillance, Epidemiology, and End Results Program
TDT	terminal deoxytransferase
TKI	tyrosine kinase inhibitor
TPMT	thiopurine S-methyltransferase
WHO	World Health Organization

INTRODUCTION

Acute Lymphoblastic Leukemia (ALL) is a heterogeneous hematologic disorder of immature (blast) lymphoid cells characterized by excessive progenitor proliferation [1]. These blastic cells eventually overtake the bone marrow and inhibit normal cellular maturation thereby resulting in anemia, neutropenia, and thrombocytopenia. In addition to these pancytopenic complications, ALL patients will also experience blastic infiltration of various tissue such as skin, liver, central nervous system, spleen, and lymph nodes. ALL is an aggressive form of leukemia requiring urgent treatment when diagnosed. ALL can occur in both children and adults, however, children fare significantly better than adults with nearly 90% of pediatric ALL patients surviving long-term compared to only 35% of adults with ALL.

Lymphoid progenitor cells can become one of three cell types: B lymphocytes, T lymphocytes, or natural killer cells. Multiple ALL subtypes exist and are characterized by morphologic, immunophenotypic, cytogenetic, and molecular determinants. The World Health Organization (WHO) divides ALL into two primary categories based on cell lineage: precursor B cell ALL and precursor T cell ALL [2]. Treatment and prognosis for these two classifications differ significantly. Furthermore, additional delineation is made to distinguish ALL from acute lymphoblastic lymphomas (LBL). Despite important clinical and laboratory similarities, lymphoblastic leukemias are diagnosed when blasts counts exceed 20% within the bone marrow regardless of the presence or absence of lesions. LBLs are slightly different, requiring the presence of lesions and < 25% blasts in the bone marrow for diagnosis. It is important to remember that both ALL and LBL are considered the same disease with different manifestations.

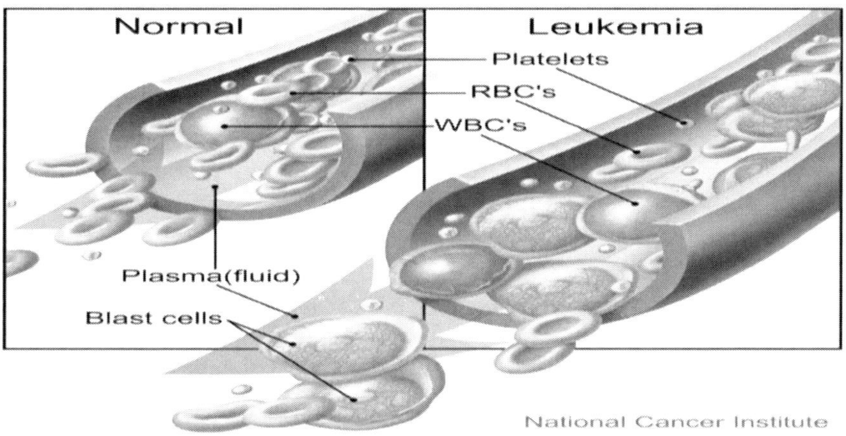

Figure 1. Normal blood compared with blood cells in leukemia. Courtesy of the National Institutes of Health.

EPIDEMIOLOGY

In 2018, the SEER estimates 5,960 new cases of ALL will occur in the United States with a resulting 1,470 deaths [3]. Acute leukemia is more common in males than females (~3400 males and 2600 females annually) and whites than blacks in the United States [3]. The age-adjusted incidence of ALL is 1.48 per 100,000 people per year [4]. The median age at diagnosis for ALL is 15 years with 55.4% of these patients being diagnosed under the age of 20 years [3]. The lifetime risk for an individual of acquiring ALL and dying from the disease is 0.04%. ALL comprises nearly 20% of all newly diagnosed acute leukemias in adults with most cases occurring *de novo* [1]. Therapy-related ALL can occur with certain chemotherapy agents including topoisomerase II inhibitors and DNA alkylators. The 5-year survival rate for adult and pediatric ALL is 68.7%. In children, ALL is the most common malignancy and remains the leading cause of cancer-related mortality in patients under 20 years of age. The peak age for ALL diagnosis is 1 to 4 years [3].

Etiology and Pathogenesis

Similar to other cancers, ALL likely arises from various interactions between exogenous and endogenous exposures, inherited genes, and simple chance. An exact mechanism detailing the pathogenesis of leukemia is unknown at this time and further studies are required to fully elucidate this disease process. Researchers do know, however, that ALL development is a multifactorial process involving several potential factors such as genetic mutations, environmental, socioeconomic, viral exposure, immunologic abnormalities, and toxins. Infections include Epstein-Barr virus and Human T-lymphocyte virus along with genetic disorders have the strongest causation correlation with ALL development [5]. Less than 5% of ALL cases are associated with inherited genetic syndromes such as Down's syndrome, Bloom's syndrome, Li Fraumeni syndrome, and Nijmegen breakage syndrome.

Pathologic Features

Normal hematopoiesis occurs with several tightly-regulated and synchronous steps involving pluripotent stem cells differentiating into either myeloid or lymphoid stem cells. These lymphoid stem cells further differentiate into T lymphocytes, B lymphocytes or natural killer cells. ALL can result at any stage of development and within any of these cell lines. Various genetic mutations may induce the advancement of leukemia. Noteworthy mutations leading to the initial development of ALL include proto-oncogenes, tumor suppressor gene deletion, and loss of apoptotic signaling pathways. A transformed cell may expand and acquire additional mutations, eventually resulting in a highly proliferative monoclonal population of leukemic cells. These leukemic cells expand to the point of bone marrow suffocation, stifling other cell lines from dividing and maturing.

Cytogenetic and molecular analysis including fluorescence in situ hybridization (FISH) commonly reveal chromosomal abnormalities in roughly 80% of ALL patients [6]. These abnormalities include chromosomal additions or deletions as well as translocations and inversions. Chromosomal translocations can occur in ALL and frequently identify specific disease subtypes. For instance, nearly 25% of precursor B cell ALL involves the TEL-AML1 (ETV6-RUNX1) fusion gene generated by the reciprocal translocation of t(12;21)(p13;q22) [7]. In adult ALL patients, the most common chromosomal translocation occurring in 25% of patients is the Philadelphia chromosome, otherwise known as t(9;22). This *BCR-ABL1* fusion gene results in constitutive tyrosine kinase activity and is associated with a poor prognosis. Overall, leukemias are steeped in genetic alterations and researchers are only beginning to scratch the molecular surface. Further genetic analysis will hopefully yield additional abnormalities that can be exploited with targeted therapy.

DISEASE CLASSIFICATION

ALL is divided into subtypes and classified based on the specific lymphocyte clone identified through lymphoblast analysis and immunophenotyping. Flow cytometry analyzes specific cell surface antigens commonly called clusters of differentiation (CD) and helps to distinguish between lymphoid and myeloid leukemias. Leukemia is also characterized by the presence or absence of important cytogenetic abnormalities. Historically, the French-American-British (FAB) system was used to classify ALL based on morphological assessment [2]. Prior to the 2008 World Health Organization (WHO) classification, clinicians frequently utilized the FAB scheme to determine prognosis and treatment options. FAB classification is antiquated and no longer relied upon.

Table 1. French-American-British classification [2]

FAB Subtype	Leukemia Cell	Description
L1	Pre-B or T cell	Small and homogenous
L2	Pre-B or T cell	Large and heterogeneous
L3	B cell	Large, mature cells

Table 2. WHO classification of acute leukemia [2]

<table>
<tr><td rowspan="2">Acute leukemias of ambiguous lineage</td><td>Acute undifferentiated leukemia</td></tr>
<tr><td>Mixed phenotype acute leukemia (MPAL)</td></tr>
<tr><td rowspan="8">B cell lymphoblastic leukemia/lymphoma (B-ALL)</td><td>B-lymphoblastic leukemia/lymphoma</td></tr>
<tr><td>B-lymphoblastic leukemia/lymphoma with t(9;22)</td></tr>
<tr><td>B-lymphoblastic leukemia/lymphoma with TEL-AML1</td></tr>
<tr><td>B-lymphoblastic leukemia/lymphoma with hyperdiploidy</td></tr>
<tr><td>B-lymphoblastic leukemia/lymphoma with hypodiploidy</td></tr>
<tr><td>B-lymphoblastic leukemia/lymphoma with t(5;14)</td></tr>
<tr><td>B-lymphoblastic leukemia/lymphoma with t(1;19)</td></tr>
<tr><td>B-lymphoblastic leukemia/lymphoma with recurrent genetic abnormalities</td></tr>
<tr><td>T cell lymphoblastic leukemia/lymphoma (T-ALL)</td><td>T cell lymphoblastic leukemia/lymphoma</td></tr>
</table>

ALL = acute lymphoblastic leukemia; WHO = World Health Organization.

In 2008 the WHO released their leukemia classification system which incorporated addition factors such as chromosomal abnormalities, immunophyenotyping, molecular and morphological features into their classification of acute leukemia.

Clinical Presentation

Patients who develop ALL typically present after weeks to months of non-specific complications that include fatigue, lethargy, dizziness, recurrent infections, easy bruising, fever, night sweats, weight loss, and bone or joint pain [1]. These patients will often complain of feeling unwell but will not typically appear in immediate distress. Hepatomegaly, splenomegaly, and/or lymphadenopathy can also arise secondary to leukemia infiltration in up to 50% of adult patients. ALL frequently leads to pancytopenic complications resulting from malignant clonal cells overtaking and suppressing normal hematopoiesis. The majority of early complications occur because of these resulting cytopenias. Bruising, bleeding, ecchymoses, and epistaxis can occur from thrombocytopenia. Anemic patients may complain of pallor, dyspnea on exertion, fatigue, palpitations and malaise. Neutropenia can result in fever and infectious complications.

Clinical signs and symptoms of leukemia are often accompanied by laboratory derangements and pathology irregularities. A complete blood count is often the first laboratory test clinicians use to initially evaluate leukemia. Other laboratory findings may include hyperuricemia, hyperkalemia, hyperphosphatemia, and hypocalcemia secondary to rapid cellular turnover indicative of tumor lysis syndrome. Prothrombin time, D-dimer, and partial thromboplastin time may all be elevated as well.

Diagnosis

A comprehensive leukemia workup is required to properly diagnose, classify, and treat ALL. In patients with suspected leukemia, a bone marrow aspirate and biopsy is required to facilitate morphological review, comprehensive flow cytometry, and identification of the leukemic clone. A formal diagnosis of ALL occurs with demonstration of ≥ 20% bone marrow lymphoblasts [3]. Additional tests include a history and physical, laboratory analysis, urinalysis, echocardiogram, pregnancy test, viral testing, CT/MRI scans, and a lumbar puncture. Assessment of cardiac function is particularly important due to the frequent use of anthracycline-based therapy. Patients presenting with ALL are also at a high risk for tumor lysis syndrome, requiring careful evaluation of baseline laboratory values and renal function.

Table 3. Common immunophenotyping panels for diagnostic workup

ALL Subtype	Immunophenotype
Precursor B-cell	CD10, CD19, CD20, CD22, CD79a, IgM, Pax5, terminal deoxytransferase
T-cell	CD1a, CD2, CD3, CD4, CD5, CD7, CD8
Other	CD34, CD38

CD = cluster of differentiation; IgM = Immunoglobulin M.

Table 4. ALL workup requirements and considerations

Evaluation	Comments
History and physical	
Laboratory	CBC, CMP, LFTs, DIC panel, TLS panel
Urinalysis	
Viral testing	Hepatitis B/C, HIV, CMV
Pregnancy	Counsel on fertility preservation
CT Scan	Neck, chest, abdomen, pelvis CT/MRI of head if neurological signs present
Lumbar puncture	First dose of IT chemotherapy given concomitantly
Testicular exam	Sanctuary site
Echocardiogram	Baseline needed prior to Anthracycline use
Infectious concerns	Opportunistic infections

CBC = complete blood count; CMP = complete metabolic panel; CMV = cytomegalovirus; CT = computed tomography; DIC = disseminated intravascular coagulopathy; HIV = human immunodeficiency virus; MRI = magnetic resonance imaging; TLS = tumor lysis syndrome.

Hematopathology assessment includes morphological evaluation, immune-phenotyping, and clonal characterization. Identifying genetic abnormalities in ALL patients is also critical for proper classification and treatment. On peripheral blood smears, morphological evaluation will identify lymphoblast size, the presence of Auer rods, and cytoplasmic features, among other things. Immunophenotyping involves flow cytometry and helps determine the presence of lymphoblast surface antigens. Three main cellular distinctions arise following flow cytometry: 1) precursor B cell leukemia, 2) mature B cell leukemia, and 3) T cell leukemia. Precursor B cell leukemia is the most common, making up nearly 90% of pediatric ALL cases and 70% of adult cases [7]. Common B cell markers include CD19, CD22, CD20 and CD79a, and CD10 [1]. Precursor B cell leukemia is positive for terminal deoxytransferase (TdT) which helps distinguish it from mature B cell leukemia which is negative for TdT. T cell leukemias make up nearly 25% of adult ALL cases and commonly express CD3 and CD1a, CD2, CD5, CD7, and TdT [1].

Cytogenetic testing is an important component of a comprehensive ALL workup and the results have prognostic and treatment implications. The frequency of genetic alterations also differs between adults and children with ALL. For instance, the Philadelphia chromosome (*BCR-ABL1*) is present in 25% of adult ALL cases but only 2-4% of pediatric cases. The presence of *BCR-ABL1* has a significant effect on overall survival and treatment decisions. Conversely, TEL-AML1 is much more common in children (22%) than adults (2%) and confers a positive survival benefit. These discrepancies are widespread and help explain why survival rates in pediatric ALL differ from their adult counterparts.

Another common genetic subtype found in B-cell ALL is the BCR-ABL1-like genes. This subgroup of patients is negative for the Philadelphia translocation but their molecular profile signature has other similarities to the BCR-ABL1 population, including poor overall survival. The Ikaros gene mutation (*IKZF1*) is associated with a poor prognosis and increased disease recurrence. A high co-occurrence rate exists between *IKZF1* and *BCR-ABL1* or BCR-ABL1-like gene mutations. Furthermore, patients with *BCR-ABL1* and BCR-ABL1-like ALL show heightened kinase activity, which helps explain their positive response to TKIs such as imatinib. A plethora of genetic mutations have been discovered in ALL, however, further research is required to continue identifying independent genetic risk factors, such as the Philadelphia chromosome, and fully elucidate their effects and determine appropriate risk stratification strategies and treatment requirements.

Acute lymphoblastic Lymphoma (LBL) was historically categorized as a non-Hodgkin's lymphoma until the 2008 WHO classification list designated LBL as a leukemia, distinguishable only by the primary location of disease occurrence. The WHO made this change because ALL and LBL contain indistinguishable morphologic, genetic, and immunophenotypic features. Furthermore, as we will discuss later, both ALL and LBL require similar treatment regimens.

Prognosis and Risk Stratification

ALL is increasingly recognized as a genetically heterogeneous cancer with an assortment of genetic defects. Complete remission rates, duration of remissions, and long-term survival are all associated with various clinical and biological features evaluated at diagnosis. Proper evaluation of these risk factors is a vital component of risk stratification and treatment selection in ALL patients. As discussed previously, ALL is a disease with many subtypes and varying degrees of treatment success. Identifying which patients require more intensive and longer periods of treatment is key to providing optimal care. Conversely, certain low risk patients may require less intensive therapy, thus sparing them from treatment-related complications.

Table 5. Common cytogenetic abnormalities in ALL [8-10]

Gene	Mutation	Frequency in Adults	Frequency in Children
BCR-ABL1	t(9:22) Philadelphia chromosome	25%	2-4%
TEL-AML1 ETV6-RUNX1	t(12:21)	22%	2%
BCR-ABL1-like	Multiple	10% - 30%	15%
IKZF1	Ikaros	25% - 35%	12% - 17%

Important prognostic factors in ALL include both tumor and patient-specific characteristics. Historically, age at diagnosis and initial white count were vital determinants of overall risk stratification. Patients over the age of 35 or those with an initial white count above 30 $x10^9/L$ for B cell ALL or 100 x $10^9/L$ for T cell ALL were at significant greater risk of disease recurrence. One of the largest ALL studies to date determined that both older age and/or higher initial white count were both independent prognostic factors for decreased survival in non-*BCR-ABL1* patients [11]. More recently, genetic mutations and flow cytometry findings have also been incorporated into survival estimates. Patient response to initial therapy is another emerging indicator of treatment success. Coupled together, patient characteristics, leukemic features, and response to initial therapy are the most significant determinants of long-term survival in ALL patients.

Substantial debate surrounding ALL risk assessment in adults persists, however, the National Comprehensive Cancer Network (NCCN) guidelines recommend classifying patients between the ages of 15 and 39 as Adolescents and Young Adults (AYA) who may benefit from pediatric-like treatment protocols [12]. This AYA population is generally separated from the adult population (aged 40 and over) who tend to have a worse prognosis and in whom intensive pediatric protocols are not feasible.

Adult ALL patients over the age of 65 are again separated and placed into a different stratification. In addition to age, the Philadelphia chromosome can play an important prognostic role in ALL patients and is therefore evaluated at diagnosis. The presence of the Philadelphia chromosome (Ph^+) automatically places the patient at high risk. For those patients who are less than 65 and in otherwise good health, they can fall into either standard risk or high-risk cohorts. Commonly, adult ALL patients without the Philadelphia chromosome will be considered high risk if they have an elevated white count as described above. Additional high-risk features include various cytogenetic mutations, which, although not always tied to treatment outcomes, appear to be indispensable for prognostication and stratification. Examples of high risk cytogenetic features include hypodiploidy (< 44 chromosomes), Philadelphia chromosome, and t(4;11) with MLL-AF4 fusion [7]. Overall prognosis is dependent on these various factors. For instance, adult ALL patients with the Philadelphia chromosome have a 5-year overall survival of only 25% compared to 41% in ALL patients without the translocation. Furthermore, high-risk ALL has a 5-year overall survival of 25% compared to 54% for standard risk patients [11].

TREATMENT OVERVIEW FOR BCR-ABL1 (-) ALL

Once diagnosis has been confirmed, ALL therapy should be initiated quickly with curative intent. Current ALL treatment is one of the most complex and intensive programs found in oncology practice. Treatment options vary depending on risk and subtype, but the general treatment pathway remains similar. The initial goal for ALL treatment involves rapid achievement of a complete remission (CR) defined as marrow blast cells < 5% with no signs of extramedullary disease and restoration of normal hematopoiesis. The long-term treatment goal is to maintain a CR without disease remission. Once the patient maintains a CR status for 5 years, they are considered cured.

Historically, ALL treatment resulted in abysmal survival outcomes with cure rates of less than 10% in the 1960s prior to Sydney Farber's pivotal chemotherapy trials using aminopterin and other primitive chemotherapy regimens. With the discovery of several leukemocidal agents over the last three decades, cure rates in children rose to nearly 90% [13]. Treatment outcomes for adults with ALL is worse than that for children; however, modern intensive chemotherapy regimens has increased complete remission rates following induction to 60% to 85% with cure rates of 30% to 40% [14, 15].

Table 6. Poor prognostic factors in adult ALL

Prognostic Factor	Comments
Age	≥ 35 years
White count at diagnosis: (a) B-cell ALL (b) T-cell ALL	 $\geq 30 \times 10^9$/L $\geq 100 \times 10^9$/L
Morphological response	Not achieving a complete remission within 4 weeks of induction
Cytogenetics	Philadelphia chromosome (BCR-ABL1) t(4;11) Hypodiploidy BCR-ABL1-like ALL *IKZF1*
MRD	MRD positivity any time after induction therapy
CNS Involvement	Positive CNS disease at diagnosis

ALL = acute lymphoblastic leukemia; CNS = central nervous system; MRD = minimal residual disease;

ALL treatment is extremely complex with most regimens following a general treatment strategy involving three distinct phases known as induction, consolidation, and maintenance. Central Nervous System prophylaxis is also required and is administered longitudinally throughout treatment.

Induction

The intent of induction therapy is to reduce the initial leukemic burden from approximately one trillion cells (10^{12}) to one billion cells (10^9) with a marrow blast count < 5%. This eradication of more than 99.9% of leukemic cells allows for restoration of normal hematopoiesis and clinical stability. The remaining leukemia cells make up the minimal residual disease (MRD) which has important prognostic and monitoring implications. MRD evaluation using cytometry allows for detection of one leukemia cell in 10,000 normal cells, which is far more sensitive and reliable than conventional morphological evaluation. Bone marrow MRD levels < 0.01% is a positive predictor of treatment success and is an important component of treatment evaluation [16].

Multi-agent chemotherapy remains the primary treatment modality for adult patients with ALL. Surgery and radiation have no role in induction therapy. Pediatric chemotherapy regimens have the best long-term efficacy data in ALL treatment; however, these can often be too intense for adult patients and therefore require refinement and dose reductions. Numerous induction regimens exist but head-to-head clinical trials are sparse and there is currently no identifiable induction regimen with proven superiority to other regimens. Patients are highly encouraged to enroll in clinical trials whenever possible.

Since the advent of VAMP (vincristine, aminopterin, 6-mercaptopurine, and prednisone) by Emil Frei and Emil Freireich at the National Cancer Institute in 1961, ALL treatment with multiple chemotherapy classes has been routine and the standard of care. This bold and maligned approach by Frei and Freireich forever changed the course and trajectory of ALL treatment. The specific doses, schedules, and drugs have evolved over time, but the general concept of reducing leukemic burden and obtaining a complete remission through combination chemotherapy remains the same. Exact survival benefits for each agent are unknown due to the heterogeneous studies conducted through the decades. The majority of adult ALL induction regimens include an anthracycline (e.g., doxorubicin, daunorubicin), corticosteroid (e.g., prednisone, dexamethasone) and vincristine with various other agents such as cyclophosphamide, methotrexate, etoposide, L-asparaginase, cytarabine and 6-mercaptopurine (6-MP) added to augment these core agents [17]. Cyclophosphamide and L-asparaginase are especially beneficial in adult ALL patients with T cell disease [18]. In the presence of *BCR-ABL1* translocation, small molecule tyrosine kinase inhibitors (imatinib, dasatinib, nilotinib) are added to induction regimens.

Dexamethasone likely exhibits superior efficacy to prednisone in treating ALL due to improved CNS penetration. Of consequence, multiple studies have associated dexamethasone with significantly higher risk of adverse events including death, myopathy, infections, bone deterioration and neuropsychiatric complications [19]. Which corticosteroid a patient receives will depend on various patient-specific factors as well as the treatment protocol used to guide their therapy. L-asparaginase products are frequently used in pediatric ALL protocols and in some adult regimens. All asparaginase products are bacterially derived from either *Escherichia coli* (*E. coli*) or *Erwinia chrysanthemi*. Asparaginase is an enzyme responsible for catalyzing the hydrolysis of asparagine into aspartic acid and ammonia. Asparagine is a non-essential amino acid found in normal cells; however, in leukemia cells it is essential for survival and proliferation due to a dependence on exogenous sources for protein, RNA, and DNA synthesis. By depleting asparagine stores, leukemia blast cells are deprived of a vital amino acid and proliferation is arrested. Asparaginase therapy is considered an important component of therapy in certain ALL cohorts. Unfortunately, several dose-limiting toxicities exist requiring careful evaluation. All asparaginase products have the propensity to cause hypersensitivity reactions resulting from foreign protein immunogenicity [20]. Other noteworthy complications of asparaginase therapy include coagulopathies, pancreatitis, hyperglycemia, hyperbilirubinemia, and liver dysfunction. In the United States, pegylated asparaginase (Oncaspar®) is the most common asparaginase product used in ALL. For patients who have a severe hypersensitivity reaction to this *E. coli*-based product, Erwinia asparaginase (Erwinaze®) substitution provides asparagine depletion, thus maintaining optimal therapy.

Although numerous induction regimens exist, relatively common induction regimen in adult ALL patients is hyper-CVAD, which contains 8 alternative treatment cycles with regimens "A" and "B" each administered at 21-day intervals. Regimen "A" utilizes hyperfractionated cyclophosphamide, vincristine, doxorubicin, and dexamethasone and regimen "B" contains high-dose methotrexate and cytarabine. CNS-directed prophylaxis using small doses of intrathecal methotrexate and cytarabine are also incorporated into each cycle of hyper-CVAD therapy [21]. The dose-intensive treatment lasts six to seven months with a subsequent maintenance schedule lasting 24 to 30 months. Complete remissions were noted in 92% of patients with a five year overall survival rate of 38%. Death during induction therapy occurred in only 5% of patients and was significantly more likely in patients older than 60 years. Philadelphia chromosome negative patients did slightly better with an overall survival rate of 42%.

Other induction regimens include the GRAALL, CALGB 8811, and CALGB 9111 protocols [22-24]. These regimens contain similar drugs at differing doses and schedules and are considered to be more complex. The CALGB 9111 regimen does include asparaginase. All induction regimens require hospital admission due to their complexity and intensity. A multicenter, randomized, phase III clinical trial evaluated the GRAALL regimen with or without the addition of rituximab in patients with untreated CD20-positive ALL. Rituximab was shown to lower relapse rates, improve event-free survival and achieve similar response rates to the comparator regimen [24].

Consolidation

Following induction therapy and achievement of a CR, patients will proceed down one of three paths: nonmyeloablative chemotherapy, autologous transplantation, or allogeneic transplantation. One of these pathways will be selected based on risk stratification, physician comfort, clinical features, patient performance status, and donor availability. The goal of post-induction consolidation therapy is to further eradicate remnant leukemic cells. Similar to induction therapy, consolidation relies on combination chemotherapy with similar drugs and doses. The consolidation phase of therapy involves “consolidation”, “delayed intensification” and “interim maintenance” and typically lasts seven months. A variety of chemotherapy agents with differing mechanisms of action are employed in consolidation therapy with cyclophosphamide, 6-MP, cytarabine, vincristine, and anthracyclines being common agents in most protocols. CNS-directed prophylactic intrathecal therapy is continued and given throughout consolidation therapy.

Table 7. Hyper-CVAD regimen for adult ALL patients [21]

Drug	Dose	Days
Regimen “A”		
Cyclophosphamide **Mesna**	300 mg/m^2 IV over 3 hours every 12 hours x 6 doses 600 mg/m^2 IV daily over 24 hours	Days 1 to 3 Days 1 to 3
Doxorubicin	50 mg/m^2 IV over one hour	Day 4
Vincristine	2 mg IV over 10 minutes daily	Days 4 and 11
Dexamethasone	40 mg IV or PO daily	Days 1 to 4 Days 11 to 14
Regimen “B”		
Methotrexate **Leucovorin**	1000 mg/m^2 IV over 24 hours 25 mg/m^2 IV every 6 hours until methotrexate has cleared	Day 1 Day 2
Cytarabine	3000 mg/m^2 IV over 2 hours every 12 hours x 4 doses	Days 2 and 3

IV = intravenous; PO = by mouth.

Maintenance

Extended maintenance therapy is employed to prevent disease recurrence following post-consolidation therapy. The rationale behind prolonged maintenance therapy lasting two to three years is to eradicate slow-growing malignant cells and bolster the immune system's ability to thwart leukemic proliferation. Optimal duration and sequencing of maintenance chemotherapy is unknown and requires further evaluation. The rare case of mature B-cell ALL does not require maintenance therapy. For those requiring maintenance therapy, combination chemotherapy is required. Similar to induction and consolidation, multiple maintenance regimens exist with no clear-cut gold standard. Most maintenance plans contain pulse therapy with vincristine and corticosteroids, daily 6-MP, and weekly methotrexate. Oral methotrexate and 6-MP play vital roles in maintenance therapy; however, interpatient variability in their pharmacokinetic profile can lead to subtherapeutic or supratherapeutic levels and therefore affect their overall safety and efficacy. Polymorphisms in thiopurine S-methyltransferase (TPMT) can result in significantly diminished enzyme activity and an increased risk of treatment-related cytopenias. Approximately 10% of patients have heterozygous TPMT with intermediate activity and 0.3% of patients display no TPMT activity at all [25]. In these patients with homozygous TPMT-deficiency, dose reductions of 90% can be incorporated with frequent monitoring thereafter [26]. Furthermore, dose reductions may be required in patients with a persistent ANC of <1500 while on therapy. Additional considerations of pharmacokinetic variability for 6-MP includes co-administration with milk or other dairy products which contain xanthine oxidase, an enzyme that prevents the breakdown of purine metabolites. Daily oral 6-MP therapy is an important component of maintenance therapy in ALL and medication adherence can significantly alter safety and efficacy. A randomized, multi-center Children's Oncology Group clinical trial evaluated medication adherence and found that children who reported taking <95% of their 6-mercaptopurine doses exhibited a 2.7 fold increase in disease relapse [27]. Pharmacists and other healthcare professionals should provide in-depth medication education for these patients emphasizing the importance of continued medication adherence. If the ANC does not respond to increasing 6-MP doses, consider medication non-adherence. Obtaining 6-thioguanine and 6-methylmercaptopurine levels can help distinguish medication non-adherence from other culprits such as TPMT inactivity, liver dysfunction, or polymorphisms.

CNS Prophylaxis and Treatment

The original Medical Director for St. Jude's Research Hospital, Donald Pinkel, used mouse models to develop the concept of CNS leukemia, and CNS-directed therapy was soon established [28]. St. Jude's Study V conducted in the late 1960s was pivotal in proving the efficacy of CNS-directed radiation and chemotherapy in patients with ALL [28]. This 35 patient study obtained 31 complete remissions and a 50% cure rate – both were historic. At diagnosis, leukemia is rarely discovered in the CNS. One childhood study showed an incidence of CNS leukemia at diagnosis around 3%, however, CNS leukemia is a major concern for several reasons [29]. First, without prophylactic measures, most patients with ALL relapse with CNS disease following bone marrow remission. Also, most chemotherapy agents do not readily penetrate the blood-brain-barrier and therefore are ineffective at reducing leukemia in this sanctuary site.

Initial protocols incorporated brain irradiation as the primary means of preventing and/or treating CNS leukemia. Unfortunately, radiation to the brain can be extremely toxic, especially in young children. Because of the myriad acute and delayed complications resulting from craniospinal radiation, only 5% to 20% of patients with high risk disease receive irradiation [30]. Modern ALL protocols all incorporate CNS prophylactic chemotherapy throughout all phases of ALL treatment. The goal of CNS prophylaxis with intrathecal chemotherapy is to eradicate undetectable leukemia cells in the CNS while preventing untoward neurotoxic and systemic complications. Common intrathecal agents include methotrexate, cytarabine, and hydrocortisone. These can be given separately or in combination depending on the treatment protocol.

Allogeneic Hematopoietic Stem Cell Transplantation

Allogeneic Hematopoietic Stem Cell Transplantation (HSCT) remains the most intense treatment for high risk ALL patients. In young adults with high risk ALL, allogeneic HSCT results in a 10-year overall survival of 45% compared to 10% in those who receive only conventional chemotherapy. Allogeneic HSCT was recently evaluated in a large, multicenter, international trial evaluating 1,913 patients between the ages of 15 and 59 years [31]. High-risk patients were eligible for allogeneic HSCT or were randomized to autologous HSCT or chemotherapy if a matched donor could not be found. Patients fared better in the chemotherapy arm than autologous HSCT with a 5-year overall survival rate of 46% versus 37%. Furthermore, allogeneic HSCT showed a 5-year overall survival rate of 53%. This study helped confirm that allogeneic HSCT in patients experiencing their first CR was beneficial in both standard-risk and high-risk patients with a known related donor.

Matched sibling HSCT is an important treatment consideration in high-risk ALL patients. For patients without a sibling donor, unrelated donor URD transplants may become a more standardized approach with increasing evidence that they are viable and efficacious. A meta-analysis evaluating 13 randomized trials with over 3,560 patients found a significantly lower all-cause mortality in allogeneic HSCT versus autologous

HCT or chemotherapy (RR = 0.88, 95% CI 0.8 to 0.97) [32]. Furthermore, this analysis found that standard-risk ALL patients in their first CR had a lower all-cause mortality compared to autologous HSCT and chemotherapy. Chemotherapy and autologous HSCT displayed similar outcomes. The authors' concluded that allogeneic HSCT was superior in patients with ALL in first CR. The meta-analysis did have some limitations and future trials should continue to evaluate the role of transplantation in adults with ALL.

Relapsed/Refractory Disease

Despite achieving a CR in over 80% of adult ALL patients using induction and post-induction chemotherapy, most patients will ultimately relapse. The 20% of adult patients who never attain CR are defined as having primary resistant ALL. Following induction therapy, patients are routinely evaluated for relapse and disease progression by standard history and physical exams, blood work, periodic bone marrow biopsies, and lumbar punctures. Relapses can occur soon after treatment or several years down the road [33].

The most common site of relapse occurs in the bone marrow with other potential locations involving the brain or testes. The longer a patient remains in CR following treatment, the more likely they are to obtain another remission after relapsing. For instance, pediatric patients with early bone marrow relapse, defined as relapse within the first 36 months of diagnosis, did significantly worse than those with late bone marrow relapse (overall survival of 35% versus 58%) [34].

Two major clinical trials evaluating adult ALL patients showed a median overall survival of 4.5 to 6 months following disease relapse. The 5-year overall survival rate was less than 10% [35, 36]. In these studies, approximately 25% of patients experienced a second CR following intensive induction chemotherapy.

Following identification of relapse or refractory disease, remission induction using chemotherapy and/or biologic therapy should be undertaken or an allogeneic HSCT considered. In patients who are not candidates for HSCT, induction chemotherapy may help prolong survival and improve symptom management. Several novel agents are indicated for salvage therapy in relapsed or refractory ALL including blinatumomab (Blincyto®), inotuzumab ozogamicin (Besponsa®), nelarabine (Arranon®), clofarabine (Clolar®), liposomal vincristine (Marqibo), and chimeric antigen receptor T cell therapy.

Blinatumomab is a novel bispecific T-cell-engager (BiTE) targeting CD19 found universally on the cell surface of precursor and mature B-cell leukemic blasts. This first-in-class agent redirects host T cells to engage and destroy CD19-expressing cancer cells. An open-label, single-arm, phase II clinical trial was conducted at 46 centers across multiple countries evaluating blinatumomab in adult patients with persistent or recurrent MRD following a minimum of 3 blocks of intensive chemotherapy [37]. With a median follow-up of 29 months, researchers found a median overall survival of 37 months and a relapse-free survival of 19 months. Based on these results, the FDA approved blinatumomab in March of 2018 for the treatment of adults and children with MRD positive ALL. The initial FDA approval for blinatumomab was granted in 2014 for the treatment of Philadelphia chromosome-negative relapsed or refractory B-cell precursor ALL. This was later expanded in 2017 to include Philadelphia chromosome-positive ALL. A phase III clinical trial was conducted in patients with relapsed or refractory Philadelphia chromosome-negative disease [38]. Patients were randomized in a 2:1 fashion, with 271 in the blinatumomab arm and 134 in the standard of care arm. The response rates were 44% and 25%, respectively, with blinatumomab also displaying significantly improved molecular remission rates (76% versus 48%) compared to standard chemotherapy. Blinatumomab prolonged survival by 3.7 months (7.7 versus 4.0).

Tisagenlecleucel (Kymriah®), a CD19-directed genetically modified autologous T-cell immunotherapy agent, received FDA approval for the treatment of patients up to 25 years of age with relapsed or refractory B-cell precursor ALL. Please see the Pediatric ALL chapter for more information.

Treatment Overview for BCR-ABL (+) ALL

Ph^+ ALL is a clinically and biologically distinct subtype of ALL according to the WHO [2]. Nearly 25% of adult ALL patients are positive for the t(9;22) translocation and have a demonstrably worse prognosis than those without the Philadelphia chromosome. Treatment with conventional chemotherapy alone yields few survivors, but with the addition of tyrosine kinase inhibitors (TKIs) and allogeneic HSCT, up to 60% of healthy adult Ph^+ ALL patients can be cured [39]. Optimal treatment involves combination chemotherapy with the addition of a TKI (e.g., imatinib, dasatinib, nilotinib) with or without allogeneic HSCT. Patients should be enrolled in a clinical trial whenever possible. Treatment duration mirrors standard ALL therapy with most patients requiring several years of chemotherapy involving induction, post-remission consolidation, and maintenance phases to fully eradicate leukemia clones. Following induction therapy, consolidation should be initiated in patients who achieved a complete remission. If the patient is healthy and has a matched donor, allogeneic HSCT should be pursued following a CR and MRD evaluation. In older patients unable to undergo HSCT, TKI therapy should be included with low-intensity chemotherapy in order to obtain a CR.

Several TKIs targeting the *BCR-ABL1* gene exist. Currently, imatinib, dasatinib, and nilotinib are the most frequently used and have shown a significant improvement in rates of CR, overall survival, and molecular response compared to traditional chemotherapy alone [40-47].

Table 8. Tyrosine kinase studies in Philadelphia positive ALL [40-47]

Study	Number of Patients	Molecular Remission Rates	Overall Survival Rates
Imatinib			
Lee et al. 2005	N = 87	66%	33% at 5 years
Yanada et al. 2006	N = 80	50%	76% at 1 year
Daver et al. 2015	N = 54	45%	43% at 5 years
Dasatinib			
Foa et al. 2011	N = 53	15%	31% at 20 months
Ravandi et al. 2015	N = 74	65%	46% at 5 years
Rousselot et al. 2016	N = 71	24%	36% at 5 years
Nilotinib			
Ottmann et al. 2014	N = 47	42%	Not yet reported
Kim et al. 2015	N = 90	77%	72% at 2 years

Additional TKIs such as bosutinib and ponatinib have also been approved for treating Ph^+ ALL in the United States. These second- and third-generation TKIs may be used in refractory or relapsed BCR-ABL positive ALL.

Relapsed/Refractory Disease

Up to 90% of Ph^+ ALL patients with relapsed or refractory disease will have BCR-ABL mutations. One common mutation is the T315I gatekeeper which can be resistant to high concentrations of first- and second-generation TKIs. Ponatinib, a third-generation TKI, is the only current option with activity against the T315I mutation. Testing for the various BCR-ABL mutations is encouraged. After failing initial therapy, patients with relapsed/refractory disease should receive a different TKI. If possible, these patients should also be enrolled in a clinical trial. Common treatment options for these relapsed/refractory Ph^+ patients include a different TKI alone or in combination with multi-agent chemotherapy. Additional prospective clinical trials are required to further evaluate optimal TKI sequencing. In eligible patients, allogeneic HSCT is still considered the treatment of choice. Other salvage therapies include blinatumomab (Blincyto®), inotuzumab ozogamicin (Besponsa®), nelarabine (Arranon®), clofarabine (Clolar®), liposomal vincristine (Marqibo), and chimeric antigen receptor T cell therapy.

Supportive Care of the ALL Patient

ALL patients are at an increased risk for several potentially life-threatening complications resulting from their disease and intensive chemotherapy. Patients with

ALL are considered at intermediate-to-high risk for developing tumor lysis syndrome, which is a common oncologic emergency requiring early identification and management [48]. Aggressive hydration should be initiated in most patients followed by prophylactic measures such as allopurinol and, in some cases, rasburicase administration. Common metabolic derangements resulting from tumor lysis include hyperuricemia, hyperkalemia, hyperphosphatemia, and hypocalcemia. Frequent laboratory monitoring is required. ALL patients also frequently require blood product support such as packed red blood cells and platelet transfusions. Neutropenic fever remains a significant cause of morbidity and mortality in patients with acute leukemias. Early identification and appropriate empiric antibiotic coverage are essential.

Conclusion

ALL is a heterogeneous hematologic disease with several distinct subtypes. Modern treatment strategies for adults with ALL increasingly reflect those used to treat pediatric patients, integrating induction, consolidation, and maintenance therapy with or without allogeneic HSCT to achieve optimal outcomes. Historically, ALL diagnosis was a death sentence but significant progress has been made over the last several decades, including the incorporation of multi-agent chemotherapy, CNS-directed prophylactic therapy, MDS evaluation, bone marrow transplantation, BCR-ABL TKIs, and risk-based stratification. Despite substantial improvements in treatment strategies and long-term survival rates in patients with ALL, only 25% of adult patients between the ages of 40 and 59 will survive 5 years after diagnosis [49].

References

[1] Jabbour, EJ; Faderl, S; Kantarjian, HM. Adult Acute Lymphobastic Leukemia. *Mayo Clin Proc*, 2005, 80(11), 1517-1527.

[2] Arber, DA; Orazi, A; Hasserjian, R; et al. The 2016 revision to the World Health Organization classification of myeloid neoplasms and acute leukemia. *Blood*, 2016, 127(20), 2391.

[3] Noone, AM; Howlader, N; Krapcho, M; et al. *SEER Cancer Statistics Review*, 1975-2015, National Cancer Institute. Bethesda, MD, https://seer.cancer.gov/csr/1975_2015/, based on November 2017 SEER data submission, posted to the SEER web site, April 2018.

[4] Siegel, RL; Miller, KD; Jemal, A. Cancer Statistics, 2017. *CA Cancer J Clin*, 2017, 67(1), 7-30.

[5] Pui, CH; Robison, LL; Look, AT. Acute lymphoblastic leukaemia. *Lancet*, 2008, 371, 1030–1043.

[6] Moorman, AV; Chilton, L; Wilkinson, J; et al. A population-based cytogenetic study of adults with acute lymphoblastic leukemia. *Blood*, 2010, 115(2), 206.

[7] Pui, CH; Relling, MV; Downing, JR. Acute lymphoblastic leukemia. *N Engl J Med*, 2004, 350, 1535-1548.

[8] Moorman, AV; Chilton, L; Wilkinson, J; et al. A population-based cytogenetic study of adults with acute lymphoblastic leukemia. *Blood*, 2010, 115, 206-214.

[9] Roberts, KG; GU, Z; Payne-Turner, D; et al. High frequency and poor outcome of Philadelphia chromosome-like acute lymphoblastic leukemia in adults. *J Clin Oncol*, 2017, 35, 394-401.

[10] Mullighan, CG; Su, X; Zhang, J; et al. Deletion of IKZF1 and prognosis in acute lymphoblastic leukemia. *N Eng J Med*, 2009, 360, 470-480.

[11] Rowe, Jm; Buck, G; Burnett, AK; et al. Induction therapy for adults with acute lymphoblastic leukemia: results of more than 1500 patients from the international ALL trial: MRC UKALL XII/ECOG E2993. *Blood*, 2005, 106, 3760-3767.

[12] *The NCCN Clinical Practice Guidelines in Oncology™ Acute Lymphoblastic Leukemia* (Version 1.2018). National Comprehensive Cancer Network, Inc. Available at: www.NCCN.org. Accessed May 18, 2018.

[13] Hunger, SP; Mullighan, CG. Acute Lymphoblastic Leukemia in Children. *N Engl J Med*, 2015, 373, 1541–1552.

[14] Annino, L; Vegna, ML; Camera, A; et al. Treatment of adult lymphoblastic leukemia (ALL): long-term follow-up of the GIMEME ALL 0288 randomizes study. *Blood*, 2002, 99(3), 863-871.

[15] Jabbour, E; O'Brien, S; Konopleva, M; et al. New insights into the pathophysiology and therapy of adult acute lymphoblastic leukemia. *Cancer*, 2015, 121, 2517–2528.

[16] Borowitz, MJ; Devidas, M; Hunger, SP; et al. Clinical significance of minimal residual disease in childhood acute lymphoblastic leukemia and its relationship to other prognostic factors: A Children's Oncology Group Study. *Blood*, 2008, 111, 5477–5485.

[17] Rowe, JM; Buck, G; Burnett, AK; et al. Induction therapy for adults with acute lymphoblastic leukemia: results of more than 1500 patients from the international ALL trial: MRC UKALL XII/ECOG E2993. *Blood*, 2005, 106(12), 3760-3767.

[18] Landau, H; Lamanna, N. Clinical manifestations and treatment of newly diagnosed acute lymphoblastic leukemia in adults. *Curr Hematol Malig Rep*, 2006, 1, 171–79.

[19] Teuffel, O; Kuster, SP; Hunger, SP; et al. Dexamethasone versus prednisone for induction therapy in childhood acute lymphoblastic leukemia; a systemic review and meta-analysis. *Leukemia*, 2011, 25, 1232-1238.

[20] van der Sluis, IM; Vrooman, LM; Pieters, R; et al. Consensus expert recommendations for identification and management of asparaginase hypersensitivity and silent inactivation. *Haematologica*, 2016, 101(3), 279-285.

[21] Kantarjian, HM; O'Brien, S; Smith, TL; et al. Results of treatment with hyper-CVAD, a dose-intensive regimen, in adult acute lymphocytic leukemia. *J Clin Oncol*, 2000, 18, 547-561.

[22] Larson, RA; Dodge, RK; Burns, CP; et al. A five-drug remission induction regimen with intensive consolidation for adults with acute lymphoblastic leukemia: cancer and leukemia group B study 8811. *Blood*, 1995, 85(8), 2025-2037.

[23] Larson, RA; Dodge, RK; Linker, CA; et al. A randomized controlled trial of filgrastim during remission induction and consolidation chemotherapy for adults with acute lymphoblastic leukemia: CALGB study 9111. *Blood*, 1998, 92(5), 1556.

[24] Maury, S; Chevret, S; Thomas, X; et al. Rituximab in B-lineage adult acute lymphoblastic leukemia. *N Engl J Med*, 2016, 375(11), 1044.

[25] Evans, WE; Hon, YY; Bomgaars, L; et al. Preponderance of thiopurine S-methyltransferase deficiency and heterozygosity among patients intolerant to mercaptopurine or azathipprine. *J Clin Oncol*, 2001, 19(8), 2293-2301.

[26] Andersen, JB; Szumlanski, C; Weinshilboum, RM; et al. Pharmacokinetics, dose adjustments, and 6-mercaptopurine/methotrexate drug interactions in two patients with thiopurine methyltransferase deficiency. *Acta Paediatr*, 1998, 87(1), 108-111.

[27] Bhatia, S; Landier, W; Shangguan, M; et al. Nonadherence to oral mercaptopurine and risk of relapse in Hispanic and non-Hispanic white children with acute lymphoblastic leukemia: a report from the children's oncology group. *J Clin Oncol*, 2012, 30, 2094-2101.

[28] Aur, RJ; Simone, J; Hustu, HO; et al. Central nervous system therapy and combination chemotherapy of childhood lymphocytic leukemia. *Blood*, 1971, 37, 272–281.

[29] Cooper, SL; Brown, PA. Treatment of pediatric acute lymphoblastic leukemia. *Ped Clin North Am*, 2015, 62, 61–73.

[30] Pui, CH. Central nervous system disease in acute lymphoblastic leukemia: prophylaxis and treatment. *Hematology Am Soc Hematol Educ Program*, 2006, 142–146.

[31] Goldstone, AH; Richards, SM; Lazarus, HM; et al. In adults with standard-risk acute lymphoblastic leukemia, the greatest benefit is achieved from a matched sibling allogeneic transplantation in first complete remission, and an autologous transplantation is less effective than conventional consolidation/maintenance chemotherapy in all patients: final results of the International ALL Trial (MRC UKALL XII/ECOG E2993). *Blood*, 2008, 111(4), 1827-1833.

[32] Ram, R; Gafter-Gvili, A; Vidal, L; et al. Management of adult patients with acute lymphoblastic leukemia in first complete remission: systematic review and meta-analysis. *Cancer*, 2010, 116(14), 3447-3457.

[33] Brincker, H; Christensen, BE. Long-term survival and late relapses in acute leukaemia in adults. *Br J Haematol*, 1990, 74(2), 156-160.

[34] Malempati, S; Gaynon, PS; Sather, H; et al. Outcome after relapse among children with standard-risk acute lymphoblastic leukemia: Children's Oncology Group study CCG-1952. *J Clin Oncol*, 2007, 25(36), 5800-5807.

[35] Fielding, AK; Richards, SM; Chopra, R; et al. Outcome of 609 adults after relapse of acute lymphoblastic leukemia (ALL); an MRC UKALL 12/ECOG 2993 study. *Blood*, 2007, 109, 944-950.

[36] Oriol, A; Vives, S; Hernandez-Rivas, JM; et al. Outcome after relapse of acute lymphoblastic leukemia in adult patients included in four consecutive risk-adapted trials by the PETHEMA Study Group. *Haematologica*, 2010, 95, 589-596.

[37] Gokbuget, N; Dombret, H; Bonifacio, M; et al. Blinatumomab for minimal residual disease in adults with B-cell precursor acute lymphoblastic leukemia. *Blood*, 2018, 131, 1522-1531.

[38] Kantarjian, H; Stein, A; Gokbuget, N; et al. Blinatumomab versus chemotherapy for advanced acute lymphoblastic leukemia. *N Eng J Med*, 2017, 376, 836-847.

[39] Snyder, DS; Nademanee, AP; O'Donnell, MR; et al. Long-term follow-up of 23 patients with Philadelphia chromosome-positive acute lymphoblastic leukemia treated with allogeneic bone marrow transplant in first complete remission. *Leukemia*, 1999, 13(12), 2053.

[40] Yanada, M; Takeuchi, J; Sugiura, I; et al. High complete remission rate and promising outcome by combination of imatinib and chemotherapy for newly diagnosed BCR-ABL-positive acute lymphoblastic leukemia: a phase II study by the Japan Adult Leukemia Study Group. *J Clin Oncol*, 2006, 24, 460-469.

[41] Rousselot, P; Coudé, MM; Gokbuget, N; et al. Dasatinib and low-intensity chemotherapy in elderly patients with Philadelphia chromosome-positive ALL. *Blood*, 2016, 128, 774.

[42] Kim, DY; Joo, YD; Lim, SN; et al. Nilotinib combined with multiagent chemotherapy for newly diagnosed Philadelphia-positive acute lymphoblastic leukemia. *Blood*, 2015, 126, 746.

[43] Lee, KH; Lee, JH; Choi, SJ; et al. Clinical effect of imatinib added to intensive combination chemotherapy for newly diagnosed Philadelphia chromosome-positive acute lymphoblastic leukemia. *Leukemia*, 2005, 19, 1509e16.

[44] Daver, N; Thomas, D; Ravandi, F; et al. Final report of a phase II study of imatinib mesylate with hyper-CVAD for the frontline treatment of adult patients with Philadelphia chromosome-positive acute lymphoblastic leukemia. *Haematologica*, 2015, 100, 653e61.

[45] Foa, R; Vitale, A; Vignetti, M; et al. Dasatinib as first-line treatment for adult patients with Philadelphia chromosome-positive acute lymphoblastic leukemia. *Blood*, 2011, 118, 6521e8.

[46] Ravandi, F; O'Brien, S; Thomas, D; et al. First report of phase 2 study of dasatinib with hyper-CVAD for the frontline treatment of patients with Philadelphia chromosome-positive acute lymphoblastic leukemia. *Blood*, 2010, 116, 2070.

[47] Ottmann, OG; Pfeifer, H; Cayuela, JM; et al. Nilotinib (Tasigna®) and chemotherapy for first-line treatment in elderly patients with *De Novo* Philadelphia chromosome/BCR-ABL1 positive acute lymphoblastic leukemia (ALL): a trial of the European working group for adult ALL (EWALL-PH-02). *Blood*, 2014, 124, 798.

[48] Cairo, MS; Coiffier, B; Reiter, A; et al. Recommendations for the evaluation of risk and prophylaxis of tumour lysis syndrome (tls) in adults and children with malignant diseases: An expert tls panel consensus. *Br J Haematol*, 2010, 149(4), 578-86.

[49] Pulte, D; Jansen, L; Gondos, A; et al. Survival of adults with acute lymphoblastic leukemia in Germany and the United States. *PLoS One*, 2014, 9, e85554.

In: Frontiers in Leukemia Pharmacotherapy
Editor: Lunawati L. Bennett
ISBN: 978-1-53614-960-9

Chapter 9

ACUTE PROMYELOCYTIC LEUKEMIA

Zachery R. Halford*, PharmD
Union University, College of Pharmacy, Jackson, Tennessee, US

ABSTRACT

Acute promyelocytic leukemia (APL) is a clinically and biologically distinct subtype of acute myeloid leukemia (AML) associated with unique challenges requiring specialized management. Over 98% of APL cases involve a translocation of the 15 and 17 chromosomes, resulting in the PML-RARA fusion gene that has become pathognomonic of the disease. The resulting protein contributes to leukemia by inhibiting differentiation and promoting hematopoietic precursor survival.

With the introduction of differentiating agents, acute promyelocytic leukemia transformed from an abysmal diagnosis to one of the most curable oncologic diseases in adults. This chapter highlights the epidemiology, clinical and pathological features, diagnosis, prognosis, and treatment approaches based on risk stratification. Management of relapsed and refractory disease is also discussed.

Keywords: Acute Promyelocytic Leukemia, cytopenias, induction, consolidation, maintenance, bone marrow transplantation, PML-RARA, ATRA, Arsenic trioxide

ABBREVIATIONS

AIDA	all-trans retinoic acid/Idarubicin regimen
AML	acute myeloid leukemia
APL	acute promyelocytic leukemia

---

* Corresponding Author Email: zhalford@uu.edu.

ATO	arsenic trioxide
ATRA	all-trans retinoic acid
CNS	central nervous system
COG	Children's Oncology Group
CR	complete remission
DIC	disseminated intravascular coagulopathy
DS	differentiation syndrome
FAB	French-American-British
FISH	fluorescence in situ hybridization
GO	gemtuzumab ozogamicin
HSCT	hematopoietic stem cell transplantation
MRD	minimal residual disease
NCCN	National Comprehensive Cancer Network
PCR	polymerase chain reaction
PML	*promyelocytic leukemia/retinoic acid receptor alpha*
RBC	red blood cell
RT-PCR	reverse transcriptase-polymerase chain reaction
WBC	white blood cell
WHO	World Health Organization

INTRODUCTION

Acute promyelocytic leukemia (APL) is a biologically distinct and particularly aggressive subtype of acute myeloid leukemia (AML) and is historically referred to as M3 AML based on the French-American-British (FAB) classification system. The vast majority of APL cases result from a translocation of the 15 and 17 chromosomes t(15;17)(q22;q12) characterized by the *promyelocytic leukemia/retinoic acid receptor alpha* (PML-RARA) fusion gene. This peculiar entity was first described in 1957 when the Norwegian hematologist LK Hillestad recognized APL as a unique disease [1]. Hillestad described APL as follows:

> "Most outstanding feature was its very rapidly downhill course of few weeks' duration, a white blood cell picture dominated by promyelocytes and severe bleeding caused mainly by fibrinolysis."

For several decades following the identification of APL as a clinically distinct entity, the disease ravaged thousands of patients each year and was widely considered the most deadly form of human leukemia. This paradigm of death and dismay was transformed with the discovery of differentiation agents; APL is now considered the most curable form of leukemia. A remarkable medical achievement accomplished by Chinese researchers trialing retinoic acid in patients with APL in the 1980's helped turn the tide and transform APL into a highly curable disease with excellent long-term outcomes [2].

EPIDEMIOLOGY

In the United States, APL is not a common malignancy, comprising only 5% to 10% of all AML cases each year. The age-adjusted annual incidence in the United States is 0.23 per 100,000 persons and a relatively young median age of diagnosis, 44 years of age, which is 23 years younger than the other AML subtypes [3]. Only 600-800 new cases of APL will be diagnosed each year in the United States and incidence does not vary based on gender. Similar to other variations of AML, patients receiving cytotoxic or immunosuppressant therapy may be diagnosed later on in life with APL. Approximately 1% to 2% of APL cases do not result from the t(15;17) translocation but instead arise from variant RARA mutations. APL appears to be more common in Hispanics than Caucasians.

CLINCAL FEATURES

APL can be viewed as a disease involving distinct morphological features (FAB M3 description), cytogenetic abnormalities, and coaguloapthies resulting in hemorrhagic diathesis. APL typically presents in middle-aged adults and is uncommon in children less than 10 years of age. Patients with APL will typically present with symptoms of pancytopenia, including infections of varying severity, gingival bleeding, epistaxis, weakness, fatigue, and possibly disseminated intravascular coagulopathy (DIC). At the time of diagnosis, patients with APL often display grave complications, especially catastrophic bleeds. The mass accumulation of promyelocytes within the marrow leads to severe anemia, thrombocytopenia, neutropenia, and profound coagulopathies with life-threatening implications requiring emergent care. Therefore, early diagnosis and management is imperative to reducing disease-related morbidity and mortality.

APL-associated coagulopathy is complex, involving both disseminated intravascular coagulopathy and hyperfibrinolysis. DIC is an oncologic emergency requiring immediate attention to reduce the risk of pulmonary or cerebrovascular hemorrhaging. Bleeding is often considered more concerning in APL than thrombosis and the mechanism of APL-associated coagulopathy is not completely understood. We do know, however, that a pro-coagulant state is created by the RARA gene activating tissue factor expression on the leukemic cells. Also, APL cell lysis results in the release of chromatin and phosphatidylserine, two cytokines responsible for thrombin generation and fibrin formation.

PATHOLOGIC FEATURES

Most APL patients do not present with significant leukemia in the peripheral blood; however, atypical promyelocytes can be easily identified in the bone marrow prior to a full molecular workup. There exist two distinct morphological variants: hypergranular and the granular forms. Hypergranular is the most common variant of APL, accounting for approximately 75% of cases [4]. The microgranular variant accounts for the other 25% of APL cases. Immunophenotyping can be performed to help identify immunophenotypic features. More importantly, APL patients should undergo molecular analysis using fluorescence in situ hybridization (FISH) testing to identify specific translocations, such as t(15;17)(q24.1;q21.2) or t(15;17)(q22;q12). Currently, reverse transcriptase polymerase chain reaction (RT-PCR) is considered by many to be the standard of care for confirming the diagnosis of APL due to its ability to detect measurable residual disease by identifying the PML breakpoint location. In less than 2% of APL cases, PML-RARA rearrangement is absent. These rare cases often test positive for a chromosome 17 abnormality involving only the RARA gene [5].

Table 1. Cytogenetic abnormalities in APL

Cytogenetics	Fusion Proteins	Proportion of APL	Prognosis
t(15;17)(q22;q21)	PML-RARA	98%	Excellent with favorable response to standard therapy
t(11;17)(q23;q21)	RARA-ZVTB16	1%	Poor due to treatment resistance
t(5;17)(q35;q21)	RARA-NPM	<1%	Good

APL = acute promyelocytic leukemia; PML-RARA = *promyelocytic leukemia/retinoic acid receptor alpha.*

DIAGNOSIS AND PROGNOSIS

APL diagnosis is confirmed with the identification of the PML-RARA fusion gene with or without other chromosomal translocations. Expedited FISH analysis is rapid and can often produce results within 2 to 3 days. Historically, APL frequently resulted in a relatively quick death even with conventional chemotherapy. If left untreated, patients with APL will likely die from catastrophic bleeding within the month. Fortunately, modern therapy with all-trans retinoic acid (ATRA) yields impressive cure rates and most patients experience long-term survival. Individuals who are under 30 years of age exhibit superior survival rates when compared to older adults. Similarly, patients presenting with a white blood cell (WBC) count $<10 \times 10^9$/L also tend to perform better.

Two clinical trials involving 217 total patients evaluated patient risk factors and relapse-free survival [6]. They found total WBC > 10,000/microL and a platelet count ≤ 40,000/microL to be the two most important risk factors. Multivariate regression analysis found that both platelet and initial leukocyte levels affected relapse-free survival. Based on these independent prognostic factors, the authors proposed a risk stratification system for APL. Additional studies are required to fully understand the prognostic implications of the various other cytogenetic abnormalities present in certain APL populations.

Table 2. APL risk stratification

Risk	Description	3-Year Relapse-Free Survival
Low	WBC ≤10,000/microL and platelets >40,000/microL	98%
Intermediate	WBC ≤10,000/microL and platelets ≤40,000/microL	89%
High	WBC >10,000/microL	70%

APL = acute promyelocytic leukemia; WBC = white blood cell.

TREATMENT OVERVIEW

The improvement of APL management over the last several decades is one of the great medical achievements of the 20th Century. Evolving from a death sentence to a highly curable disease, APL provides a promising model for future oncology research collaborations. The inclusion of ATRA in conjunction with risk stratification models significantly improved long-term survival.

Newly diagnosed APL requires immediate treatment due to its rapid progression and life-threatening complications. Treatment for APL consists of several phases, including remission induction, consolidation, and possible maintenance therapy. Despite long-term survival improvements, the 30-day mortality in patients with newly diagnosed APL is 10% to 20%, necessitating further education and improvements in early identification and management of APL complications.

Managing Early Complications

DIC is a life-threatening complication of APL and can result in pulmonary and intracerebral hemorrhaging, both of which are leading causes of early death following APL diagnosis [7]. Prior to the discovery of ATRA therapy, early hemorrhagic death occurred in approximately 20% of patients and was subsequently reduced to 10% following the introduction of therapeutic ATRA in 1988 [8]. With this in mind, early initiation of ATRA is critical to help avoid this complication of APL. Therefore, ATRA should be started as soon as APL is suspected, even if diagnostic studies have not been fully completed. Coagulopathies should be monitored closely following initial presentation and throughout induction therapy. Furthermore, invasive procedures, including central catheter placement, should be avoided during ongoing coagulopathies. Monitoring parameters include fibrinogen, D-dimer, platelet counts, and PT/aPTT. Platelet or RBC transfusions may be beneficial to help control overt bleeding. Several controversial treatment options exist for managing DIC complications, including heparin and recombinant factor VIIa.

Differentiation syndrome (DS) is a common complication occurring after initiation of ATRA and/or arsenic trioxide (ATO) therapy and can be fatal if not quickly reversed [9]. DS, also known as retinoic acid syndrome or cytokine storm, may occur in up to 25% of APL patients receiving a differentiation agent. The etiology of DS has not been fully elucidated but is thought to arise from the release of inflammatory cytokines resulting in capillary leak, edema, and hypotension. Most DS cases occur within a few days of treatment initiation and symptoms of DS include fever, acute respiratory distress, malignant effusions, hypoxemia, weight gain and edema, hypotension, and multi-organ dysfunction. Those APL patients developing DS will often present with leukocytosis as well. In patients who do develop DS, mortality rates may be as high as 30%. Even with aggressive treatment, fatality rates are approximately 5% [10]. Corticosteroids are the treatment of choice, with intravenous dexamethasone 10 mg twice daily for 3 days being the most common option. Common short-term complications of dexamethasone include hyperglycemia, insomnia, mania, ulceration, and immunosuppression. In severe cases of DS, ATRA and/or ATO should be temporarily discontinued until complete resolution of symptoms. Prophylactic corticosteroids is controversial and requires additional studies to confirm safety and efficacy.

Leukocytosis can also occur at initial presentation or shortly after starting induction therapy. Up to 50% of patients receiving initial ATRA therapy may experience hyperleukocytosis, defined as a total leukemia blood cell count >50,000 to 100,000/microL. Hyperleukocytosis results from a rapid maturation of leukemic cells and may result in leukostasis and death. Managing this acute complication is controversial and requires addition studies. Leukostasis is a medical emergency necessitating rapid WBC reduction via induction chemotherapy. Therapeutic leukapheresis is controversial and may be harmful due to its propensity to exacerbate coagulopathies and increase death. Some institutions advocate for rapid initiation of induction chemotherapy with daunorubicin and cytarabine.

Induction Therapy

Induction therapy in APL aims to reduce the initial leukemic burden from approximately one trillion cells (10^{12}) to one billion cells (10^9) with a marrow blast count <5%. This eradication of more than 99.9% of leukemic cells allows for restoration of normal hematopoiesis and clinical stability. The remaining leukemia cells make up the MRD, also known as "minimal residual disease" or "measurable residual disease," which has important prognostic and monitoring implications. MRD evaluation using cytometry allows for detection of one promyelocytic cell in 10,000 normal cells, which is far more sensitive and trustworthy than conventional morphological evaluation [11].

As with other acute leukemias, induction therapy for APL frequently involves multi-agent chemotherapy resulting in hematopoietic restoration and resolution of clinical signs and symptoms. Unlike the other acute leukemias, APL induction therapy involves ATRA to help promote terminal differentiation of the malignant promyelocyte.

ATRA was first suggested as a therapeutic option for APL by Huang et al. in Shanghai [12]. In early trials using ATRA, complete remission (CR) rates ranged between 80% and 90% and, unlike with conventional chemotherapy, coagulopathies improved and patients showed no signs of the typical myelosuppression, alopecia, nausea and vomiting, or infections commonly noted with other leukemia treatment [13]. ATRA is an orally available vitamin A analog that binds to nuclear receptors and decreases immature promyelocyte proliferation while also inducing terminal differentiation of the malignant clone into mature, functioning cells within the marrow. ATRA does not cross the blood-brain-barrier and can lead to various complications such as differentiation syndrome, headache, bone pain, dry mucous membranes, diarrhea, and elevated liver enzymes. Other vitamin A analogs have been studied but it appears ATRA is the most effective and remains the only Food and Drug Administration approved retinoic acid for the treatment of APL in the United States.

ATRA in combination with ATO was shown to be equally efficacious to ATRA and conventional chemotherapy in patients with low- or intermediate-risk APL. The APL0406 trial evaluated ATRA and ATO against ATRA and chemotherapy in 263 adult patients with low- or intermediate-risk patients [14]. ATRA and ATO were given daily until complete remission (CR) was obtained, followed by consolidation therapy. The ATO group showed similar rates of hematologic remission (100% versus 97%) and fewer deaths (0 versus 4) compared to the chemotherapy arm. The estimated four-year event-free survival rates (97% versus 80%) were improved with ATRA and ATO compared with ATRA and chemotherapy. Furthermore, ATRA and ATO displayed a better side effect profile compared to chemotherapy. ATO may result in higher rates of hepatotoxicity, QTc prolongation, and peripheral neuropathies. Fewer myelosuppressive complications were noted with ATO compared to conventional chemotherapy.

The specific induction regimen depends on risk stratification at the time of diagnosis. For low- and intermediate-risk APL, the National Comprehensive Cancer Network's (NCCN) guidelines recommend ATRA 45 $mg/m^2/day$ plus arsenic trioxide 0.15 mg/kg intravenous daily as their preferred regimen [15]. Besides ATRA and ATO, the other recommended regimen, according to the NCCN treatment guidelines, includes ATRA with idarubicin.

High-Risk APL

Approximately 30% of APL patients fall under the high-risk classification based on initial laboratory analysis (WBC > 10,000/microL at diagnosis). These high-risk patients will require more intensive induction and consolidation therapy compared to those with low- or intermediate-risk disease. Induction regimens historically included multi-agent chemotherapy with ATRA, cytarabine, and daunorubicin based on the PETHEMA LPA 99 trial [16]. The more recent APML4 trial showed induction therapy with just ATRA, idarubicin, and ATO could also be highly efficacious without excessive treatment-related complications [17]. Commonly employed regimens for remission induction are included in Table 3 [15].

The aforementioned induction regimens all offer excellent CR rates and the preferred option will depend on the patient's age, performance status, logistical concerns, and cardiovascular standing. In addition to these approved regimens, patients are also encouraged to consider enrolling in a clinical trial.

Gemtuzumab ozogamicin (GO), a CD33 antibody drug conjugate, has also shown some utility in treating high-risk APL and may be useful in certain situations. In 2010, the manufacturer removed GO from the market due to safety concerns (sinusoidal obstruction syndrome and anaphylaxis) and questionable efficacy in post-marketing analysis [18]. GO is no longer commercially available but can be obtained through the manufacturer's compassionate use program in patients who have exhausted other treatment options or in those with hyperleukocytosis not eligible for other cytoreductive strategies.

Table 3. Induction and consolidation therapy for high-risk APL [15]

Regimen	Induction	Consolidation
A	ATRA 45 mg/m^2 daily until CR Idarubicin 6-12 mg/m^2 days 2,4,6,8 ATO 0.15 mg/m^2 daily until CR	ATRA 45 mg/m^2 days 1-28, then 45 mg/m^2 x 7 days every 2 weeks ATO 0.15 mg/m^2 days 1-5 for 5 weeks
B	ATRA 45 mg/m^2 daily until CR ATO 0.15 mg/m^2 daily until CR	ATRA 45 mg/m^2 daily x 2 weeks every 4 weeks for 7 cycles ATO 0.15 mg/m^2 5 days/week for 4 weeks every 8 weeks x 7 cycles
C	ATRA 45 mg/m^2 daily until CR ATO 0.3 mg/m^2 on days 1-5 of week 1 and 0.25 mg/m^2 twice weekly in weeks 2-8	ATRA 45 mg/m^2 daily x 2 weeks every 4 weeks for 7 cycles ATO 0.3 mg/m^2 on days 1-5 of week one in courses 1-4 and 0.25 mg/m^2 twice weekly in weeks 2-4 of courses 1-4
D	**ATRA:** 45 mg/m^2 daily until CR Daunorubicin 50 mg/m^2 on days 3-6 Cytarabine 200 mg/m^2 continuous infusion for days 3-9	ATRA 45 mg/m^2 daily x 2 weeks every 4 weeks for 7 cycles ATO 0.15 mg/m^2 5 days/week for 5 weeks x 2 cycles Daunorubicin 50 mg/m^2 x 3 days for 2 cycles

APL = acute promyelocytic leukemia; ATO = arsenic trioxide; ATRA = all-trans retinoic acid; CR = complete remission; IV = intravenous.

Post-Remission Consolidation

The goal for post-remission consolidation in APL involves maintaining a CR and ensuring a durable molecular response by eradicating microscopic disease. Approximately 90% of newly diagnosed APL patients will achieve a CR following induction therapy. Unfortunately, disease recurrence is inevitable without further aggressive treatment targeting the malignant immature clone. A CR does not guarantee full eradication of and recovery from leukemia. Additional test are required in APL to determine molecular remissions, which are much more sensitive than standard morphological or cytogenetic evaluations. Bone marrow studies, typically occurring 4 to 6 weeks following induction therapy, are conducted to evaluate for a CR in APL. Once the patient displays count recovery, consolidation therapy can commence. If anthracycline-based therapy was used in induction, a follow-up echocardiogram is required prior to continue therapy in consolidation. Furthermore, ATO can result in QTc prolongation requiring frequent evaluation. These treatment-related complications should be addressed prior to initiating consolidation.

For patients receiving ATRA/ATO during induction therapy, guidelines recommend continued treatment with ATO-based consolidation. This recommendation includes those patients who cannot tolerate anthracycline therapy due to pre-existing cardiovascular complications. Several different treatment protocols with varying doses, schedules, and overall cycles exist for consolidation therapy. High-risk patients should receive the same regimen throughout consolidation and clinicians should refrain from mixing various dosing and scheduling schemes.

Most high-risk patients who can tolerate anthracycline-based therapy should be placed on a protocol containing ATRA along with cytarabine and either daunorubicin or idarubicin. There are no direct comparisons for these regimens among high-risk patients. APL appears to be especially sensitive to anthracycline therapy due to a lack of drug efflux pumps (p-glycoprotein) in premature promyelocytes. Ades prospectively evaluated the inclusion of cytarabine and found cytarabine improved long-term relapse-free rates (87% versus 71%) at 7 years follow-up [19]. The inclusion of cytarabine is permitted; however, additional long-term prospective studies are required to confirm its role in treating high-risk APL.

Common practice for high-risk APL includes 4 to 6 doses of intrathecal chemotherapy during consolidation to help eradicate any MRD sequestered in the central nervous system (CNS) [15]. Cytarabine, methotrexate, and hydrocortisone can be given together or alone based on the institution and treatment protocol.

For consolidation therapy, patients without cardiovascular complications should receive anthracycline-based therapy for several months to fully eradicate microscopic disease remaining after induction. In patients unable to tolerate daunorubicin or idarubicin, ATO is a reasonable option with growing evidence to support its use in post-remission consolidation as part of a "chemotherapy free" regimen.

Maintenance Therapy

Following consolidation, patients are assessed for complete molecular response using RT-PCR. Continued therapy following consolidation and sustained molecular remission is controversial due to questionable efficacy and persistent treatment-related complications. Maintenance therapy for 1 to 2 years is often included in modern APL protocols, but its importance remains questionable and requires additional studies. Prior to discovering ATRA, maintenance therapy with 6-mercaptopurine and methotrexate was shown to provide survival benefits in APL. Effective maintenance therapy is anomalous in AML, as all other subtypes do not benefit from continuous therapy following consolidation. A meta-analysis of nine clinical trials evaluating maintenance therapy versus observation in APL patients with a CR found no significant difference in overall survival [20]. Unfortunately, this Cochrane analysis displayed significant heterogeneity, limiting its generalizability and importance.

The NCCN guidelines recommend maintenance therapy with ATRA for PCR-negative patients as a reasonable treatment option based on several clinical trials [15,20]. High-risk patients appeared to benefit the most from sustained maintenance therapy following consolidation. For low-risk patients receiving maintenance therapy, routine PCR monitoring every 3 months is not required, as the risk of relapse is low in patients with a complete molecular remission in maintenance therapy. High-risk disease, older patients (>60 years), and those with prolonged treatment intervals during consolidation therapy warrant more intensive monitoring while undergoing maintenance therapy. If PCR evaluation is positive at any point following consolidation therapy, the patient is considered to have relapsed APL and will require further workup and intensive treatment.

RELAPSED/REFRACTORY APL

Relapse following a CR occurs in 10% to 15% of patients with APL and as high as 30% in high-risk disease. Most relapses occur within 3 years of initial diagnosis and involve various molecular abnormalities requiring further elucidation. A positive PCR test should be confirmed with a bone marrow evaluation to fully evaluate disease recurrence. Treatment following relapse or refractory disease should eradicate premature promyelocytes and obtain a complete molecular remission utilizing differentiation agents, high dose chemotherapy, and/or hematopoietic stem cell transplantation (HSCT). Clinicians must consider what APL therapy the patient initially received, how they responded to it, when relapse occurred, and what therapy will most likely result in molecular remission. Due to the wild success of modern APL therapy, few large-scale clinical trials exist evaluating relapsed or refractory disease.

Following confirmed relapse, treatment recommendations involve ATO therapy with the goal of achieving a second molecular remission. Single-agent ATO produces molecular remission in 70% to 80% of relapsed patients [22-24]. Re-treatment with ATO in patients who received ATO-based therapy for their initial induction/consolidation remains controversial. A small retrospective trial with 37 patients reported a second CR rate of 93% for patients receiving ATO-based chemotherapy with ATRA plus or minus an anthracycline [25]. The ability to penetrate the blood-brain barrier, a well-known sanctuary site for leukemic cells, is one potential benefit of ATO. Following re-induction with ATO and confirmed PCR-negative disease, consolidation therapy including additional ATO or HSCT should be considered. For patients treated with ATRA/ATO after initial diagnosis, The NCCN recommends using anthracycline-based therapy if relapse occurred within 6 months of initial CR [15].

If a CR cannot be obtained during induction therapy, consider pursing an allogeneic HSCT or anti-CD33 monoclonal antibody therapy with GO. Clinical trials involving GO have been too small to confidently evaluate the safety and efficacy in this specific patient population; however, the potential benefits must be weighed with safety concerns involving sinusoidal obstructive syndrome and anaphylactic reactions. Autologous HSCT may be preferred for most patients over allogeneic due to disparities in toxicity and cost. Conflicting data exist, but Chakrabarty evaluated 294 relapsed APL patients who received either autologous or allogeneic HSCT and found that 5-year disease-free survival (63% versus 50%) and overall survival (75% versus 54%) favored autologous transplantation [25]. They concluded that autologous HSCT yielded superior long-term results for APL patients in a second CR.

Some patients with relapsed APL will have residual disease in the (CNS), resulting in inevitable disease relapse if left untreated. Therefore, the NCCN recommends intrathecal chemotherapy for 4 to 6 doses during re-induction and consolidation [15]. Patients are also encouraged to enroll in a clinical trial, if possible.

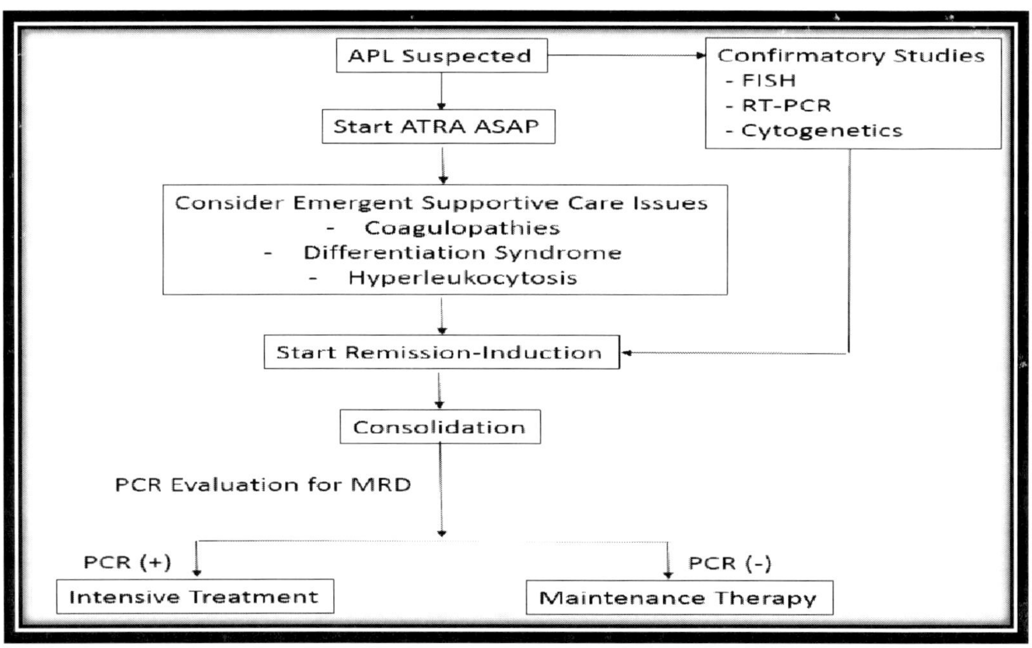

APL = acute promyelocytic leukemia; ASAP = as soon as possible; ATRA = all-trans retinoic acid; FISH = fluorescence in situ hybridization; MRD = minimal residual disease; RT-PCR = reverse transcriptase polymerase chain reaction.

Figure 1. Treatment Schematic for APL.

MANAGING PEDIATRIC APL

APL in pediatric patients is a rare occurrence and accounts for approximately 4% to 8% of all pediatric AML cases. Geography appears to play an important role in APL incidence, as studies from Italy and Africa report APL making up nearly 20% of their AML cases [26-28]. Historically, pediatric APL treatment reflects adult protocols utilizing differentiating agents, ATRA and ATO. The use of ATRA with anthracyclines (AIDA) achieves CR rates over 90% with an event-free survival rate of 70% for children with APL. In the CALGB 9710 trial, the addition of ATO further decreased the risk of relapse. The AAML0631 clinical trial conduced by the Children's Oncology Group (COG) incorporated ATO into consolidation cycles and reduced total anthracycline exposure compared to standard AIDA regimens [29]. Kutny reported that 3-year overall survival was 94% and event-free survival was 91%, which proved non-inferior when compared to the historical control arm receiving higher doses of anthracycline. They concluded that ATO in consolidation was well tolerated and allowed a significant reduction in cumulative anthracycline exposure while maintaining superb overall and event-free survival rates. The current COG trial attempts to further evaluate risk-stratifying methods and eliminate exposure to conventional chemotherapy for standard risk APL patients through the use of a "chemotherapy free" regimen of ATRA and ATO (NCT02339740). This study will also attempt to reduce exposure to conventional chemotherapy in high-risk APL patients. Enrollment began in 2015.

CONCLUSION

APL is a biologically and cytogenetically distinct AML subtype with aggressive behavior. APL is often described as M3 AML based on the French-American-British (FAB) classification system with the vast majority of cases resulting from a translocation of the 15 and 17 chromosomes t(15;17)(q22;q12) characterized by the PML-RARA fusion gene. In the United States, APL is not a common malignancy, encompassing approximately 10% of all AML cases each year with an average age of diagnosis of 44 years. A total of 600 to 800 new cases are diagnosed each year in the United States. APL will typically present with signs and symptoms of pancytopenia, including infections of varying severity, weakness, fatigue, gingival bleeding, epistaxis, and possibly DIC. At the time of diagnosis, hemorrhagic diathesis is a common complaint resulting in potentially catastrophic complications requiring emergent care. Coagulopathies and differentiation syndrome are common oncologic emergencies and appropriate monitoring and preventative measures are required to help reduce the risk early death.

ATRA and ATO are differentiation agents that promote terminal maturation of premature promyelocytes resulting in repopulation of bone marrow with normal, non-leukemic cells. The vast majority of APL patients can achieve a CR following induction therapy followed by a molecular remission from consolidation therapy. The introduction of differentiation agents into APL regimens provided a significant boost to inducing a CR with durable responses and are now considered the standard of care in low-risk patients. High-risk patients, based on initial WBC counts, may still require conventional chemotherapy in addition to differentiation agents. Patients with low-risk disease have long-term survival rates of 98% while high-risk patients experience long-term survival only 70% of the time. Compared to typical AML survival rates, these M3 AML patients do significantly better thanks to the discovery of ATRA and ATO.

References

[1] Hillested LK. Acute promyelocytic leukemia. *Acta Med Scand* 1957; 159(3):189-94.

[2] Lo-coco F, Cicconi L. History of acute promyelocytic leukemia: a tale of endless revolution. *Mediterr J Hematol Infect Dis* 2011;3(1):e2011067.

[3] Howlander NA, Krapcho M, Garshell J, et al. *SEER Cancer Statistics Review, 1975-2010*, National Cancer Institute. (http://seer.cancer.gov/csr//1975_2010/). Bethesda, MD; 2013.

[4] Sainty D, Liso V, Cantù-Rajnoldi A, et al. A new morphologic classification system for acute promyelocytic leukemia distinguishes cases with underlying PLZF/RARA gene rearrangements. *Blood* 2000; 96 (4):1287-1296.

[5] Arber DA, Orazi A, Hasserjian R, et al. The 2016 revision to the World Health Organization classification of myeloid neoplasms and acute leukemia. *Blood* 2016;127(20):2391-2405.

[6] Sanz MA, Lo Coco F, Martín G, et al. Definition of relapse risk and role of nonanthracycline drugs for consolidation in patients with acute promyelocytic leukemia: a joint study of the PETHEMA and GIMEMA cooperative groups. *Blood* 2000;96(4):1247-1253.

[7] Mantha S, Tallman MS, Soff GA. What's new in the pathogenesis of the coagulopathy in acute promyelocytic leukemia? *Curr Opin Hematol* 2016;23:121–126.

[8] Rodeghiero F, Avvisati G, Castaman G, et al. Early deaths and anti-hemorrhagic treatments in acute promyelocyticleukemia: a GIMEMA retrospective study in 268 consecutive patients. *Blood* 1990;75:2112–2117.

[9] Sanz MA, Montesinos P. How we prevent and treat differentiation syndrome in patients with acute promyelocytic leukemia. *Blood* 2014;123:2777–2782.

[10] Patatanian E, Thompson DF, et al. Retinoic acid syndrome: a review. *J Clin Pharm Ther* 2008;33(4):331.

[11] Carlson KS, Guzman ML. Is minimal residual disease monitoring clinically relevant in adults with acute myelogenous leukemia? *Curr Hematol Malign Rep* 2013;8(2):109-115.

[12] Huang M, Yu-Chen Y, Shu-Rong C, et al. Use of all-trans retinoic acid in the treatment of acute promyelocytic leukemia *Blood* 1988;72:567–578.

[13] Castaigne S, Chomienne C, Daniel MT, et al. All-trans retinoic acid as a differentiation therapy for acute promyelocytic leukemia. I. Clinical results. *Blood* 1990;76:1704–1713.

[14] Platzbecker U, Avvisati G, Cicconi L, et al. Improved Outcomes With Retinoic Acid and Arsenic Trioxide Compared With Retinoic Acid and Chemotherapy in Non-High-Risk Acute Promyelocytic Leukemia: Final Results of the Randomized Italian-German APL0406 Trial. *J Clin Oncol* 2017;35(6):605-612.

[15] *The NCCN Clinical Practice Guidelines in Oncology™ Acute Myeloid Leukemia* (Version 1.2018). National Comprehensive Care Network, Inc. Available at: www.NCCN.org. Accessed June 12, 2018.

[16] Sanz MA, Montesinos P, Vellenga E, et al. Risk-adapted treatment of acute promyelocytic leukemia with all-trans retinoic acid and anthracycline monochemotherapy: long-term outcome of the LPA 99 multicenter study by the PETHEMA Group. *Blood* 2008; 112:3130-3134.

[17] Iland HJ, Collins M, Hertzberg MS, et al. Final analysis of the Australasian leukaemia and lymphoma group (ALLG) APML4 trial: all-trans retinoic acid (ATRA), intravenous arsenic trioxide (ATO) and idarubicin as initial therapy for acute promyelocytic leukemia (APL). *Blood* 2014;124:375.

[18] McKoy JM, Angelotta C, Bennett CL, et al. Gemtuzumab ozogamicin-associated sinusoidal obstructive syndrome (SOS): an overview from the research on adverse drug events and reports (RADAR) project. *Leuk Res* 2007;31(5):599-604.

[19] Adès L, Chevret S, Raffoux E, et al. Long-term follow-up of European APL 2000 trial, evaluating the role of cytarabine combined with ATRA and Daunorubicin in the treatment of nonelderly APL patients. *Am J Hematol* 2013;88(7):556.

[20] Fenaux P, Chastang C, Chevret S, et al. A randomized comparison of all trans retinoic acid (ATRA) followed by chemotherapy and ATRA plus chemotherapy and the role of maintenance therapy in newly diagnosed acute promyelocytic leukemia. The European APL Group. *Blood* 1999;94:1192-1200.

[21] Muchtar E, Vidal L, Ram R, et al. The role of maintenance therapy in acute promyelocytic leukemia in the first complete remission. *Cochrane Database Syst Rev*. 2013;3:Cd009594.

[22] Lazo G, Kantarjian H, Estey E, et al. Use of arsenic trioxide in the treatment of patients with acute promyelocytic leukemia: the M.D. Anderson experience. *Cancer* 2003;97:2218-2224.

[23] Leoni F, Gianfaldani G, Annunziat M, et al. Arsenic trioxide therapy for relapsed acute promyelocytic leukemia: a bridge to transplantation. *Haematologica* 2002;87:485-489.

[24] Soignet SL, Frankel SR, Douer D, et al. United States multicenter study of arsenic trioxide in relapsed acute promyelocytic leukemia. *J Clin Oncol* 2001;19:3852-3860.

[25] Thiruganam R, George B, CHendamarai E, et al. Comparison of clinical outcomes of patients with relapsed acute promyelocytic leukemia induced with arsenic trioxide and consolidated with either an autologous stem cell transplant or an arsenic trioxide-based regimen. *Biol Blood Marrow Transplant* 2009;15:1479-1484.

[26] Testi AM, Biondi A, Lo Coco F, et al. GIMEMA-AIEOP AIDA protocol for the treatment of newly diagnosed acute promyelocytic leukemia (APL) in children. *Blood* 2005;106:447–53.

[27] de Botton S, Coiteux V, Chevret S, et al. Outcome of childhood acute promyelocytic leukemia with all-trans retinoic acid and chemotherapy. *J Clin Oncol* 2004;22:1404-1412.

[28] Testi AM, D'Angiò M, Locatelli F, et al. Acute promyelocytic leukemia (APL): comparison between children and adults. *Mediterr J Hematol Infect Dis* 2014; 6:e2014032.

[29] Kutny MA, Alonzo TA, Gerbing RB, et al. Arsenic trioxide consolidation allows anthracycline dose reduction for pediatric patients with acute promyelocytic leukemia: report from the children's oncology group phase III historically controlled tiral AAML0631. *J Clin Oncol* 2017;35:3021-3029.

In: Frontiers in Leukemia Pharmacotherapy
Editor: Lunawati L. Bennett
ISBN: 978-1-53614-960-9

Chapter 10

CHRONIC MYELOID LEUKEMIA

Zachery R. Halford,[*] PharmD and Elizabeth Sykes
Union University, College of Pharmacy, Jackson, Tennessee, US

ABSTRACT

Chronic myeloid leukemia (CML) is a myeloproliferative neoplasm characterized by myeloid cell proliferation and reduced apoptosis often resulting from a specific cytogenetic abnormality. The Philadelphia chromosome is a balanced reciprocal translocation resulting in the *BCR-ABL1* fusion gene and subsequent production of a constitutively active cytoplasmic tyrosine kinase. With approximately 5,000 new cases each year in the United States, CML accounts for nearly 15% of all leukemia cases. Median age of diagnosis is 55 years and nearly half of patients at diagnosis are considered symptomatic. Tyrosine kinase inhibitors (TKIs) dramatically altered the therapeutic landscape for managing CML, with overall survival estimates increasing from 6% in 1975 to over 90% in 2018. This chapter aims to highlight the epidemiology, etiology, pathogenesis, diagnosis, disease classification, prognostic factors, and general treatment approach for adult patients with CML. Particular interest will be placed on TKIs and their toxicity profiles.

Keywords: chronic myeloid leukemia, cytopenias, chronic phase, accelerated phase, blast phase, hematopoietic stem cell transplant, philadelphia chromosome, tyrosine kinase inhibitors, *BCR-ABL1*

[*] Corresponding Author Email: zhalford@uu.edu.

ABBREVIATIONS

AML	acute myeloid leukemia
AP	advanced phase
BCR-ABL1	breakpoint cluster region-Abelson murine leukemia
BP	blast phase
CCyR	complete cytogenetic response
CML	chronic myeloid leukemia
CP	chronic phase
EMR	early molecular response
FDA	Food and Drug Administration
FISH	fluorescence in situ hybridization
HSCT	hematopoietic stem cell transplantation
IFN-a	interferon-alpha
MCyR	major cytogenetic response
MPR	medication possession ratio
MRD	minimal residual disease
NCCN	National Comprehensive Cancer Network
PCR	polymerase chain reaction
Ph^-	Philadelphia chromosome negative
Ph^+	Philadelphia chromosome positive
qPCR	quantitative polymerase chain reaction
REMS	Risk Evaluation and Mitigation Strategy
RT-PCR	reverse transcriptase-polymerase chain reaction
SEER	Surveillance, Epidemiology, and End Results Program
TKI	tyrosine kinase inhibitor
WHO	World Health Organization

INTRODUCTION

Chronic myeloid leukemia (CML), also known as chronic myelogenous leukemia, is classified as a myeloproliferative neoplasm marked by increased proliferation of granulocytic cells resulting in bone marrow hyperplasia and accumulation of neoplastic cells [1]. CML was first identified in 1845, but little was known about the disease until Drs. Nowell and Hungerford discovered a small chromosome in metaphase preparation of marrow from patients with CML and thus initiated research into the Philadelphia chromosome [2]. The Philadelphia chromosome was later demonstrated to result from a translocation between chromosomes 9 and 22 [t(9;22)(q34;q11)] [3]. The unique translocation forms an abnormal gene product (*BCR-ABL1*), which is a constitutively active cytoplasmic tyrosine kinase, detectable in the peripheral blood, myeloid, erythroid, B-lymphoid cells, and megakaryocytes [3]. This dysregulated tyrosine kinase is implicated in the development of CML and is a primary target for the treatment of this disorder [1]. At the time of CML diagnosis, the white blood cell count is typically elevated with a median count of 150,000/μL. If left untreated, the typical course of CML is triphasic. Most patients will be diagnosed in the chronic phase (CP); however, the disease will fatally progress to an accelerated phase (AP) and blast phase (BP) if not properly managed. Prior to the discovery of TKIs, the median overall survival for CML was 3 to 7 years depending on treatment choice and comorbidities [1]. Survival is significantly longer with TKI therapy, with approximately 94% of healthy patients surviving 8 years from initial diagnosis [4].

EPIDEMIOLOGY

In the United States, CML accounts for 15% of all leukemias with an annual incidence of 1.5 cases per 100,000 individuals and a slight male preponderance. According to the American Cancer Society, it is estimated that 8,430 new cases of CML will be diagnosed and nearly 1,000 patients with CML will die in 2018 [1]. The median age at diagnosis is between 55 and 65 and is uncommon in children and adolescents. Since the advent of TKIs, the annual death rate of CML has declined from 10% to 20% down to 1% [1]. This impressive increase in survival has resulted in higher prevalence of CML within the United States, with some projections estimating 180,000 patients living with CML by 2030 [2].

ETIOLOGY

The Abelson murine leukemia (*ABL1*) gene on chromosome 9 coupled with the breakpoint cluster region (*BCR*) gene on chromosome 22 are fundamental to the pathogenesis of CML. This Philadelphia translocation was the first molecular abnormality identified in human malignancies [5]. The *BCR-ABL1* gene produces a constitutively active cytoplasmic tyrosine kinase that fuels cellular replication through activation of intracellular signals such as RAS, MYC, RAF, and STAT [6-8]. This newfound cytokine independence results in continuous cellular proliferation, altered differentiation, loss of apoptotic pathways, and eventual leukemogenesis. The *BCR-ABL1* fusion protein is identified in approximately 95% of patients with CML [5]. The development of CML is not associated with hereditary, familial, geographic, ethnic or economic status. There does appear, however, to be an association between CML and ionizing radiation exposure [5].

Clinical Presentation

CML is divided into 3 phases: CP, AP, and BP [5]. The CP is variable in length with nearly 90% of patients presenting in this phase. CML is usually discovered serendipitously on routine examination, with nearly 50% of patients appearing asymptomatic at the time of diagnosis. CML onset is usually slow and indolent, characterized by symptoms such as weakness, weight loss, sweating, bone pain, abdominal discomfort, and early satiety due to splenomegaly [5]. The hallmark of CP-CML is leukocytosis with white blood cell counts as high as 1,000,000 cells/mm^3 at diagnosis [9]. Anemia and thrombocytopenia may also develop. Anemia leading to weakness, fatigue, and dyspnea. Splenomegaly is the most common physical manifestation of CML occurring in up to 50% of cases [9]. Hepatomegaly and lymphadenopathy are rare occurrences in chronic phase CML. If patients with CP-CML are not treated appropriately, progression to AP or BP will occur within months to years.

Those with AP are characterized by splenomegaly, progressive myeloid maturation, and loss of drug efficacy resulting in lymphocytosis. AP-CML is relatively progressive, with a median survival of 18 months [10]. AP-CML is confirmed by an increase in basophil count and blastic cells in the blood or bone marrow. Approximately 5% to 10% of newly diagnosed patients are identified in AP-CML and these patients have a long-term survival rate of 75% with TKI therapy [11]. AP-CML is often associated with constitutional symptoms (fever, malaise, weight loss, and myalgias), hepatomegaly, splenomegaly, and worsening anemia. Once a patient progresses to AP-CML, successful treatment becomes more difficult due to increasing TKI resistance.

The blast crisis phase is a terminal phase of CML and resembles an acute leukemia, characterized by increasing number of blast cells in the blood. The World Health Organization (WHO) defines blast crisis as one or more of the following: greater than 20% blasts in the peripheral blood or bone marrow, extramedullary disease, or large clusters of blasts in the bone marrow [12]. Splenomegaly, bone aches, fever, bleeding, infections, and weight loss are common complaints. Most patients will naturally progress from CP-CML to AP-CMP and eventually BP-CML; however, up to 20% of BP-CML occurs without warning or clinically detectable prelude. Approximately 70% of patients in BP-CML have a myeloid or undifferentiated disease compared to 30% with a B-lymphoid histology [12].

Diagnosis

CML diagnosis is straightforward, requiring the documentation of the Philadelphia chromosome t(9;22)(q34;q11.2) via routine cytogenetic (karyotyping), fluorescent in situ hybridization (FISH) analysis, or molecular evaluation using polymerase chain reaction (PCR). A bone marrow aspiration and biopsy are required for morphological and cytogenetic analysis. Quantitative reverse transcriptase polymerase chain reaction (RT-PCR) is also required to help identify baseline *BCR-ABL1* mRNA transcripts. PCR testing can either be quantitative, evaluating the number of *BCR-ABL1* transcripts, or qualitative, assessing the presence of the *BCR-ABL1* transcript. Qualitative PCR is useful for initial diagnosis, with quantitative PCR (qPCR) finding utility in CML monitoring. Furthermore, qPCR testing is extremely sensitive and can detect one *BCR-ABL1* positive cell among 100,000 normal cells, therefore making it extremely useful in detecting minimal residual disease (MRD) [13, 14]. Due to the low cost, rapid turnaround, sensitivity, and ease of use, RT-PCR is becoming the diagnostic of choice in CML. Approximately 85% of CML patients have the hallmark t(9;22) translocation, but 5% will have variant translocations, and 10% will have additional chromosomal abnormalities such as trisomy 8, isochromosome 7, and additional mutations along the alternative 22nd chromosome [9]. Patients presenting with Ph^{-} variants display similar response and long-term survival rates as those with Philadelphia chromosome positive (Ph^{+}) disease [9]. Initial laboratory workup includes a complete blood count, comprehensive metabolic panel, and serum uric acid level.

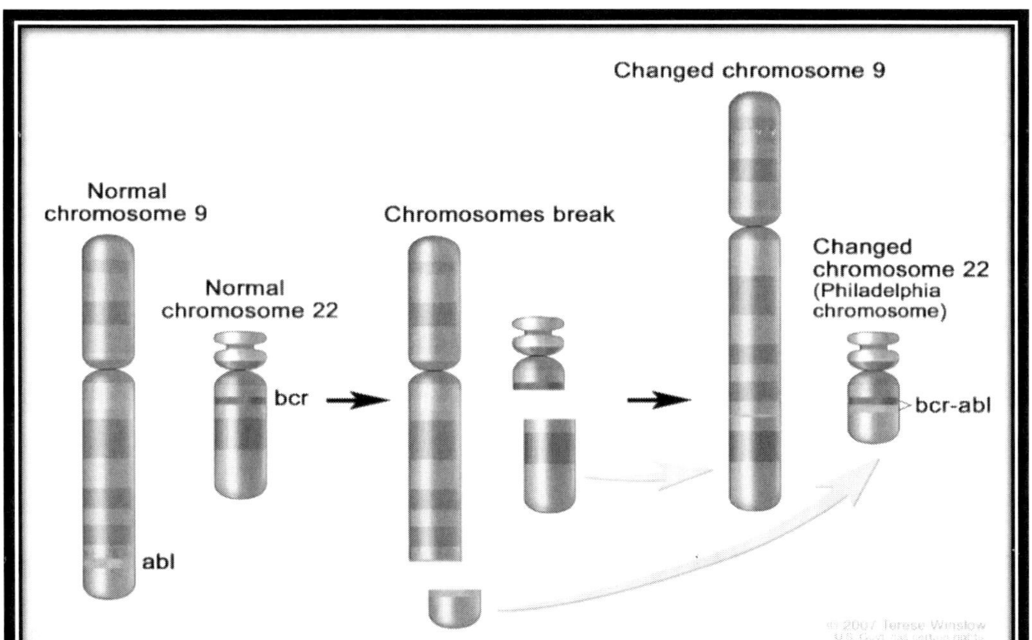

https://visualsonline.cancer.gov/details.cfm?imageid=7153. © 2007 Terese Winslow LLC, U.S. Govt. has certain rights.

Illustration 1. "Philadelphia Chromosome" Publication Year: 2007, Original Graphic.

Differential diagnosis of CML includes infection, myeloproliferative disorders (polycythemia vera, essential thrombocythemia, myelofibrosis), and chronic myelomonocytic leukemia. Clinicians must differentiate CML from leukemoid reactions. A physical exam and clinical history are useful for distinguishing the underlying etiology. A significant challenge arises in Ph$^-$ patients with splenomegaly and concordant leukocytosis. Patients who are Ph$^-$ with no evidence of *BCR-ABL1* transcripts are considered to have chronic myelomonocytic leukemia.

PROGNOSIS AND RISK STRATIFICATION

Long-term survival rates have improved dramatically in patients with CML over the last two decades, with the average CML patient now reaching a life expectancy similar to that of the general population [15]. The Surveillance, Epidemiology, and End Results (SEER) database conducted a trial evaluating 5,138 CML patients receiving TKI therapy and compared them to long-term survival rates for CML patients before TKI availability [16]. Five year overall survival rates for pre-imatinib patients and imatinib patients were dramatically different. For example, patients aged 15 to 44 years had a 5-year overall survival rate of 72% (pre-imatinib) compared to 86% (imatinib). Furthermore, those aged 75 to 84 years had a 5-year overall survival rate of 19% (pre-imatinib) compared to 36% (imatinib). The approval of TKI therapy in 2001 significantly altered the clinical landscape for managing patients with Ph$^+$ CML [16].

Due to various comorbidities, genetic mutations, age at diagnosis, and phases of CML disease, several risk classification systems have been established to help identify at-risk patients who might require more intensive therapy (Table 1). The Sokal prognostic score identifies four clinical variables: spleen size, age, platelet count > 700,000/microL, and blast percentage [17]. An online calculator is then used a sophisticated equation to calculate a Sokal score. The Hasford score adds eosinophilia and basophilia to the calculation [18]. Both of these devices were created prior to the discovery of imatinib and are rather cumbersome. An updated scoring option, the European Treatment and Outcome Study (EUTOS), was developed and validated using 2,060 CML patients receiving imatinib therapy [19]. Fortunately, the EUTOS score only incorporates two variables, percentage of basophils and spleen size, making it much more user friendly. The EUTOS scoring system may also be more predictive that either the Sokal or Hasford assessments; however, the predictive superiority over Sokal and Hasford were not duplicated in subsequent trials [20, 21]. According to the EUTOS score, patients are either low or high risk. Patients deemed high-risk show a 33% chance of failing to respond to initial imatinib therapy following CML diagnosis. Overall, once a patient has achieved a complete cytogenetic response (CCyR), all patients have an excellent long-term prognosis, regardless of initial risk stratification.

Table 1. Sokal and Hasford prognostic scores [17, 18]

Classification	Sokal Score	Hasford Score
Low	< 0.8	< 780
Intermediate	0.8 – 1.2	781 - 1480
High	> 1.2	> 1480

TREATMENT OVERVIEW

Without appropriate treatment, CML will inexorably result in disease progression and death. Prior to imatinib approval in 2001, treatment for CML was limited to interferon-alpha (IFN-a), busulfan, and hydroxyurea with only modest efficacy and significant treatment-related complications. Historically, the only curative option for patients with CML is allogeneic hematopoietic stem cell transplantation (HSCT) but recent studies now provide hope of obtaining deep and durable disease remissions without long-term TKI therapy. The goal, however, for most patients involves malignant clone eradication within the bone marrow resulting in a molecular remission followed by maintaining the patient in CP while minimizing treatment-related complications. TKIs dramatically altered the landscape by providing sustained molecular remissions with manageable toxicities. Finding targeted therapy with TKIs revolutionized CML treatment and improved 10-year overall survival rates from 20% to 90% [2]. With excellent long-term survival rates on TKIs, the National Comprehensive Cancer Network (NCCN) recommends starting newly diagnosed CML patients on one of the following first-line agents: imatinib, bosutinib, dasatinib, or nilotinib [22]. All CML patients on TKI therapy should receive comprehensive clinical and laboratory monitoring, including routine hematologic, cytogenetic, and molecular evaluations.

Disease monitoring is critical in determining a patient's disease status. Standard monitoring includes peripheral blood qPCR analysis. Bone marrow biopsy and cytogenetic evaluation are also important until a complete cytogenetic response has been documented. Treatment will vary based on the phase of CML designated at the time of diagnosis. The three primary treatment options include curative therapy with allogeneic hematopoietic stem cell transplantation (HSCT), disease control with TKI therapy, and palliative measures with or without chemotherapy [22].

Chronic Phase CML

Prior to the advent of TKIs, patients in the 1980s and 1990s would receive IFN-a-based or chemotherapy-based regimens with some advancing to allogeneic HSCT [23].

The reported 5-year overall survival rates for IFN-a-based regimens was approximately 57% with chemotherapy significantly less at 42%. IFN-a improved life expectancy by 20 months compared to chemotherapy. Allogeneic HSCT provided 5-year overall survival rates around 50% to 60% and were preferred in younger patients.

Currently, the two main treatment options for patients with CP-CML include TKI therapy or allogeneic HSCT [22]. The only reliable option for curing CML remains allogeneic HSCT, which is the preferred option for younger patients who develop resistance or intolerance to TKI therapy. No prospective, head-to-head clinical trial has compared allogeneic HSCT to TKI therapy in patients with chronic phase CML. However, based on historical controls, TKI therapy is the safer option resulting in fewer short- and long-term morbidity and mortality concerns. Therefore, despite the possibility of curing CML with allogeneic HSCT, initial treatment with TKI remains the standard of care [22].

Imatinib was the first TKI approved by the Food and Drug Administration (FDA) for the treatment of CP-CML. The IRIS trial randomized 1,106 patients to receive either imatinib 400 mg (n = 553) or IFN-a plus cytarabine (n = 553) [24]. The 5-year overall survival rates for imatinib patients was 89% with only 7% of patients progressing to AP-CML. Furthermore, 89% and 82% of patients experienced a major cytogenetic response (MCyR) and CCyR, respectively (Table 2). Among the 553 patients initially treated with IFN-a and cytarabine, 363 patients crossed over to imatinib therapy due to disease progression, intolerance to therapy, or poor initial response.

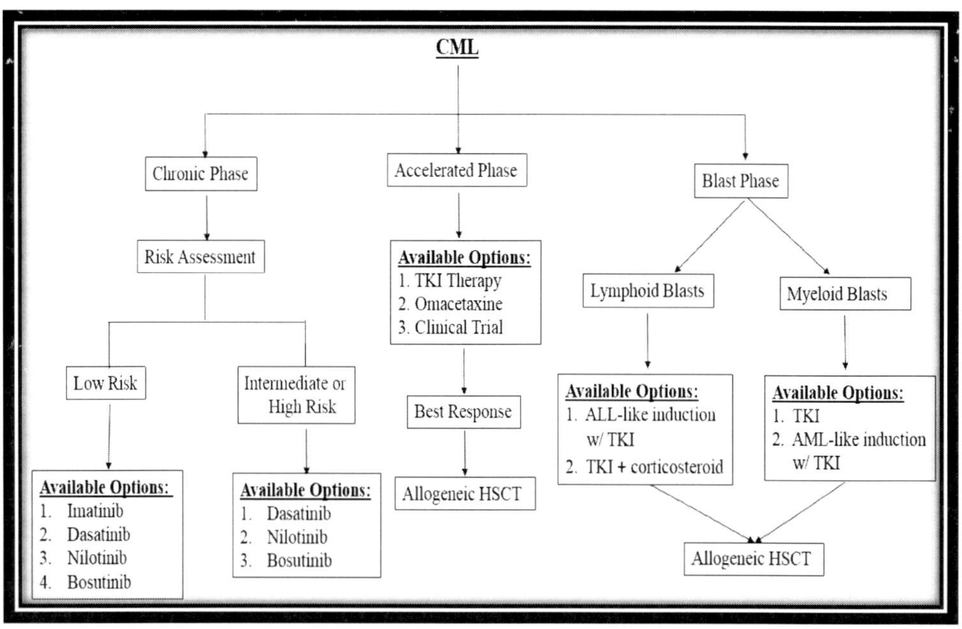

ALL = Acute lymphoblastic leukemia; AML = Acute myeloid leukemia; CML = Chronic myeloid leukemia; HSCT = Hematopoietic stem cell transplant; TKI = Tyrosine kinase inhibitor.

Figure 1. General Treatment Overview for CML.

Table 2. Long-term data from the IRIS trial [24]

Response Endpoint	Interferon + Cytarabine	Imatinib
CCyR at 18 months	15%	76%
MCyR at 18 months	35%	87%
FFP at 18 months	92%	97%
OS at 5 years	-	89%
CCyR at 5 years	-	87%
FFP at 8 years	-	92%
EFS at 8 years	-	81%

CCyR = complete cytogenetic response; EFS = event-free survival; FFP = freedom from progression; MCyR = major cytogenetic response; OS = overall survival.

The optimal imatinib dose was evaluated in several clinical trials [25, 26]. The TOPS trial evaluated imatinib 400 mg versus imatinib 800 mg in 476 patients with Ph+ CML. Major molecular response (MMR) rates were similar between imatinib 400 mg and imatinib 800 mg (51.6% versus 50.2%). There were no differences in event-free survival, progression-free survival, or overall survival between the different dosing regimens. Patients taking imatinib 800 mg daily did experience higher rates of adverse events. The FRENCH SPIRIT trial evaluated imatinib 600 mg against 400 mg daily and reported superior MMR rates in those receiving the higher dose, suggesting it could be the preferred dose moving forward [27]. Dose reductions secondary to treatment-related complications are common with high-dose imatinib. Currently, the NCCN guidelines list 400 mg daily as the recommended starting dose based on efficacy and toxicity findings [22].

Bosutinib is a second-generation TKI approved in 2012 by the FDA for the treatment of Ph+ CML in patients with resistance or intolerance to prior therapy. In 2017, the FDA granted accelerated approval for bosutinib in newly-diagnosed CP- CML based on an open-label, randomized, multicenter trial evaluating bosutinib 400 mg daily with imatinib 400 mg daily in 487 patients [28]. At 12 months, 47% of bosutinib patients experienced a MMR compared to 37% taking imatinib. Disease progression was reported in 2% of bosutinib and 3% of imatinib patients. No difference existed in event-free or overall survival. Standard dose for bosutinib is 400 mg once daily orally with food. Common adverse events included diarrhea, rash, nausea, thrombocytopenia, transaminitis, and abdominal pain.

Dasatinib was the first FDA-approved second-generation TKI for adult CML patients with resistance or intolerance to imatinib therapy. Following its 2006 approval, dasatinib is now approved as first-line therapy in both children and adults with newly-diagnosed Ph+ CP-CML, based on the DASISION trial. This phase III clinical trial compared dasatinib 100 mg daily with imatinib 400 mg daily in 519 newly-diagnosed CP- CML patients and found the CCyR (83% versus 78%) and MMR (76% versus 64%) to be significantly better in those receiving dasatinib (Table 3) [29]. Dasatinib led to more treatment discontinuations due to drug-related events (42% versus 17%) than imatinib, with the primary concerns revolving around pleural effusions, neutropenia, thrombocytopenia, and diarrhea.

Nilotinib 400 mg twice daily was initially FDA-approved in 2007 as an orally available TKI for the treatment of CP-CML in adult patients resistant or intolerant to prior therapy. It has since received approval for several other indications and is now a first-line option for adult and pediatric patients with newly diagnosed Ph^+ CML. The Evaluating Nilotinib Efficacy and Safety in Clinical Trials-Newly Diagnosed Patients (ENESTnd) trial compared various nilotinib doses (300 mg twice daily or 400 mg twice daily) with imatinib 400 mg once daily in 846 previously untreated Ph^+ CP-CML patients [30]. Nilotinib maintained higher rates of MMR at 5 years (77% versus 60%) regardless of dose (Table 4). The higher nilotinib dose provided superior rates of 5-year overall survival compared to imatinib (96% versus 92%). Fewer patients progressed to an accelerated or blast phase in the nilotinib arms (16 total) compared to imatinib (21). Lower rates of drug discontinuation were seen in nilotinib 300 mg and 400 mg compared to imatinib (19% versus 26% versus 38%, respectively). Nilotinib also appeared to have fewer treatment-related complications, with lower rates of nausea, vomiting, diarrhea, fluid retention, and muscle spasms. Cardiovascular complications were considerably more common and severe with nilotinib, particularly the 400 mg arm. QT prolongation (>30 ms) occurred in approximately 33% of patients. In 2010, the FDA issued a Risk Evaluation and Mitigation Strategy (REMS) to minimize the sequelae from QT prolongation in patients receiving nilotinib. This was retracted in 2013 and is no longer required for nilotinib prescribing or procurement; however, QT prolongation remains a concern requiring close monitoring and consideration. Nilotinib was also associated with an increased risk of vascular disease.

Table 3. Long-term data from the DASISION trial [29]

Response Endpoint	Dasatinib (n = 259)	Imatinib (n = 260)
CCyR at 12 months	83%	72%
MMR at 12 months	46%	28%
MMR achieved	52%	34%
Time to MMR	15 months	36 months
OS at 5 years	91%	90%
CCyR at 5 years	83%	78%
PFS at 5 years	85%	86%
MMR at 5 years	76%	64%

CCyR = complete cytogenetic response; MMR = major molecular response; OS = overall survival; PFS = progression free survival.

Table 4. Long-term data from the ERNESTnd trial [30]

Response Endpoint	Nilotinib 300 mg BID (n = 282)	Nilotinib 400 mg BID (n = 281)	Imatinib 400 mg daily (n = 283)
CCyR at 12 months	80%	78%	65%
MMR at 12 months	44%	43%	22%
CCyR at 24 months	87%	85%	77%
MMR at 24 months	71%	67%	44%
MMR at 5 years	77%	77%	60%
OS at 4 years	93%	97%	93%
PFS at 4 years	97%	98%	93%

CCyR = complete cytogenetic response; MMR = major molecular response; OS = overall survival; PFS = progression free survival.

Table 5. First-line tyrosine kinase inhibitor options for CML [22]

Drug	Dose	CCyR (%)	Concerns
Imatinib	400 mg daily	82	1. Lower rate of CCyR and MMR compared to other TKIs. 2. Fluid retention, diarrhea, myalgias, abdominal pain. 3. Take with food.
Bosutinib	400mg daily	79	1. Increased rates of gastrointestinal distress, diarrhea, and liver dysfunction. 2. Take with food.
Dasatinib	100 mg daily	83	1. Pleural effusion, thrombocytopenia, bleeding, drug interactions. 2. Take with or without food.
Nilotinib	300 mg twice daily	87	1. More medication adherence issues with a twice daily dosing schedule. 2. QT prolongation, vascular complications, dyslipidemia.

CCyR = complete cytogenetic response; CML = chronic myeloid leukemia.

Selecting a TKI for newly-diagnosed Ph^+ CP-CML is an important decision requiring careful consideration. The NCCN guidelines list imatinib, bosutinib, dasatinib, and nilotinib as category 1 options. Clinicians and patients should consider the following [22]:

1. For this specific patient, what is the desired goal of treatment? Older patients with multiple comorbidities might prefer an option with fewer toxicities at the expense of a deeper and more durable remission. Younger patients, on the other hand, might seek a deeper molecular remission in hopes of discontinuing TKI therapy.

2. What is the toxicity profile of the selected TKI? Nilotinib, for instance, has known cardiovascular complications and should be avoided in patients with cardiovascular disease. Dasatinib commonly leads to pleural effusions and might not be an ideal fit for patients with pre-existing lung disease.
3. What is the patient's risk score? A low-risk patient might be well-served receiving imatinib due to their minimal risk of progressing while on TKI therapy. A high-risk patient, however, might benefit more from a second-generation TKI that may provide superior rates of MMR and/or CCyR. The NCCN guidelines actually recommend second-generation TKIs over imatinib.
4. What agent is the clinician and patient most comfortable with? No TKI has a proven overall survival benefit when compared to other TKIs, so clinician comfort managing the various toxicities along with patient convenience are important considerations.

Allogeneic HSCT remains a curative option for certain CML patients; however, it is extremely toxic resulting in high rates of treatment-related morbidity and mortality. Despite these concerns, allogeneic HSCT is an option for treating certain patients with Ph^+ CP-CML. No prospective clinical trial has compared HSCT with TKI therapy. The European Group for Blood and Marrow Transplantation predict the five-year overall survival for allogeneic HSCT in low-risk patients to be approximately 60% to 80% [31]. Acute and chronic graft-versus-host-disease are common complications resulting from allogeneic HSCT and require extensive monitoring and prolonged courses of immunosuppressant therapy. Most guidelines and institutions recommend HSCT only in patients with inadequate control of CP-CML despite appropriate TKI therapy [22]. Overall, patients in chronic phase CML do extremely well on TKI therapy. The initial aim of TKI therapy is to achieve designated milestones (Table 7) [22].

MONITORING RESPONSE IN CML

Appropriate disease monitoring remains a critical component for long-term treatment success (Table 6). The NCCN guidelines recommend cytogenetic testing every three months until a CCyR has been established [22]. CCyR achievement within the first 12 months of TKI therapy is an established indicator of long-term success [32]. Following documentation of a CCyR, further cytogenetic testing is not needed unless qPCR analysis suggests a molecular relapse. RT-PCR should be conducted on peripheral blood every 3 months starting at the time of diagnosis and continued, at various intervals, indefinitely.

Early molecular response (EMR), defined as $\leq$ 10% *BCR-ABL1* international standard/scale (IS) after 3 and 6 months, is another prognostic factor useful in predicting long-term outcomes [33]. EMR will preferably appear at 3 months post-TKI initiation; however, it should appear no later than 6 months. Jabbour et al. evaluated the association between achievement of EMR and event-free survival in 435 newly diagnosed CML patient treated with imatinib or a second-generation TKI [32]. Patients achieving 3-, 6-, and 12-month CCyR showed significantly better 3-year event-free survival rates compared to those who did not meet these milestones (98%, 97% and 98% versus 83%, 72%, and 67%, respectively). This clinical trial also indicated second-generation TKIs attained higher rates of CCyR and MMR than imatinib.

Patients failing to achieve < 10% *BCR-ABL1* IS at 3 months and < 1% *BCR-ABL1* IS at 12 months should receive further evaluation for medication non-adherence, possible *BCR-ABL1* mutational abnormalities, and conversion to a second-generation TKI. If a proper response is not noted at 15 months, the patient is considered to be TKI resistant and HSCT evaluation is recommended.

Table 6. Monitoring parameters for CML [22]

Test	Recommendation
Bone Marrow Cytogenetics	1. Obtain at diagnosis 2. Repeat if failure to meet milestones 3. Repeat if hematologic or cytogenetic relapse
Quantitative PCR (qPCR)	1. Obtain at diagnosis 2. Every three months following TKI initiation. Once *BCR- ABL1* ≤ 1%, repeat every 3 months for 2 years then every 3 - 6 months thereafter. 3. Repeat in 1 - 3 months following a 1-log increase in *BCR-ABL1* transcript level with MMR

Table 7. Milestones for TKI Therapy in chronic phase CML [22]

Time From Initiation	Optimal *BCR-ABL1* (IS)	Warning *BCR-ABL1* (IS)	Failure *BCR-ABL1* (IS)
3 months	≤ 10%	> 10%	N/A
6 months	≤ 10%	N/A	> 10%
12 months	≤ 1%	> 1% - 10%	> 10%
>12 months	≤ 0.1%	0.1 - 1%	> 1%
Clinical Considerations	Continue to monitor response and side effects	1. Evaluate medication adherence and potential drug interactions 2. Mutational analysis	1. Evaluate medication adherence and potential drug interactions 2. Mutational analysis

Mechanisms of Resistance

Resistance to TKI therapy may result from amplified drug transporters and/or altered plasma protein binding of TKI agents and is often divided into either primary or secondary resistance [34, 35]. Primary resistance results when patients fail to respond to initial therapy. Secondary resistance, on the other hand, results when a patient responds to initial therapy but then eventually relapses. Primary and secondary resistance usually occur through different mechanisms. Medication non-adherence to TKI therapy may result in relapse and is therefore a confounding factor requiring careful evaluation. Furthermore, drug interactions with TKI therapy can also result in altered serum concentrations and possible disease relapse. Please see chapter 5 for more information on TKI drug interactions.

Primary resistance remains poorly understand; however, possible mechanisms include [34-36]:

1. Hematopoietic insufficiency resulting from an inadequate number of normal stem cells.
2. Inappropriate TKI trough levels leading to inadequate tyrosine kinase inhibition.
3. Aberrant expression of various drug transporters result in reduced intracellular levels of TKI.

Secondary resistance occurs most frequently from reactivation of *BCR-ABL1* signaling, typically resulting from point mutations in the *BCR-ABL1* kinase domain. These mutations are associated with a poor prognosis and increased likelihood of disease progression [37]. Branford et al. evaluated 144 CML patients receiving imatinib by testing for various point mutations [37]. Direct sequencing revealed 27 patients had detectable point mutations and 24 of the 27 patients had acquired TKI resistance. Müller evaluated 1,043 patients who had failed imatinib therapy [38]. Among the 1,043 patients, 39% had a pre-existing *BCR-ABL1* mutation. This study revealed 63 different point mutations affecting 49 amino acids. While some of these mutations confer significant TKI resistance, most result in only a moderate increase in resistance typically overcome with higher TKI doses and/or utilization of more potent agents such as dasatinib, nilotinib, and bosutinib [36]. One noteworthy mutation is the *BCR-ABL1* T315I abnormality, which is highly resistant to even potent TKIs such as nilotinib and dasatinib [39]. Future studies are required to fully elucidate the mechanisms behind these important mutations.

The NCCN guidelines currently recommend mutation analysis in CP-CML when any of the following parameters are met [22]:

1. Failure to reach appropriate milestones (Table 7).
2. Following either hematologic or cytogenetic relapse.
3. Disease progression to AP-CML or BP-CML.
4. 1-log increase in *BCR-ABL1* transcript levels with loss of MMR.

Proper mutational identification is imperative at the time of treatment failure in order to best select subsequent therapy. With four available TKIs for resistant CP-CML, special consideration needs to be taken with regards to mutational abnormalities, adverse event profile, patient comorbidities, and physician and patient comfort level with each available TKI.

Medication Non-Adherence

Patient adherence to TKI therapy is a significant driver of treatment relapse and considerable improvements are required in this arena. Poor medication adherence can have profound effects on resistance development and disease recurrence. The ADAGIO study highlighted the importance of proper medication adherence by showing that patients experiencing only a partial cytogenetic response reported taking approximately 75% of their doses whereas those with a CCyR reported taking over 90% of prescribed TKI doses [40]. According to a study conducted by Anderson evaluating TKI adherence in a cross-sectional retrospective chart review, approximately one-third of patients displayed medication non-adherence [41]. Poor TKI adherence is also associated with increased health care costs. Patients with a low medication possession ratio (MPR < 85%) used more healthcare resources resulting in higher expenditures compared to those with higher MPRs (≥ 85%). Possible risk factors for medication non-adherence include younger age, higher medication burden, higher copayment, treatment-related toxicities, male sex, decreased knowledge of disease state and treatment, and higher overall treatment doses. Healthcare professionals play a pivotal role in providing medication information and encouraging proper adherence. Various patient-reminder systems exist and range from simple pill boxes to sophisticated phone applications and text-reminders. Furthermore, prompt identification of adverse events should be a priority to help ensure long-term treatment adherence [42].

Second-Line Therapy

Patients with CML with either intolerance or resistance to initial TKI therapy will typically require treatment with a second-line TKI agent. Long-term data supports the notion that TKIs are generally well tolerated with mild adverse events usually managed without interruptions. Less than 5% of patients will show TKI-intolerance. More likely, CML treatment relapse results from resistant mechanisms previously described. Following treatment failure, patients should undergo a bone marrow biopsy to identify if the patient is still in CP-CML and to further evaluate clonal characteristics. Treatment with a second generation TKI (bosutinib, dasatinib, nilotinib) remains the preferred approach for managing imatinib resistance. Failure to achieve a cytogenetic or molecular response at 3, 6, or 12 months with second-line TKI treatment should result in allogeneic HSCT, if available and appropriate, or alternative therapy [22].

No robust clinical trial has been conducted directly comparing second-line TKI agents for treatment in CP-CML following initial treatment failure. Patients with non-T315I mutations who were intolerant or resistant to imatinib therapy can receive bosutinib, dasatinib, or nilotinib [22]. Selection should be based on adverse event profile and specific patient comorbidities. As researchers glean more information about *BCR-ABL1* mutations, select TKIs may gain preference depending on mutational analysis findings. For instance, nilotinib may have additional benefits in patients with the V299L or F317L mutations and ponatinib is preferred in patients exhibiting the T315I mutation [43].

Dasatinib

Several clinical trials have evaluated the efficacy of dasatinib in resistant or intolerant CP-CML with CCyR near 90% [44-46]. The CA180-034 clinical trial evaluated dasatinib 100 mg daily in imatinib-resistant or –intolerant patients with CML [46]. As highlighted in Table 8, rates of overall survival and progression-free survival were excellent. Overall, dasatinib was well tolerated with most complications resulting early in therapy. Pleural effusions were noted in 28% of patients and is a cause for concern leading to treatment discontinuation. Over the 7 year study, 66% of all patients experienced an infection, with 15% having on-study grade 3 or 4 infectious complications. Following imatinib failure, dasatinib is a reasonable treatment alternative. For those with either the *BCR-ABL1* T315I or F317I mutation, dasatinib displays limited activity and should be avoided [38].

Table 8. Dasatinib in second-line treatment [46]

Patients	OS at 7 years	PFS at 7 years
Imatinib-resistant (n = 124)	63%	39%
Imatinib-intolerant (n = 43)	70%	51%
All patients (n = 167)	65%	42%

OS = Overall survival; PFS = Progression-free survival.

Nilotinib

In uncontrolled clinical trials, nilotinib appears to be equally efficacious compared to dasatinib in imatinib-resistant or –intolerant patients. Giles reported overall survival and progression-free survival at 4 years to be 78% and 57%, respectively [47]. Overall, 59% of patients achieved MCR, with 45% obtaining a CCyR. Deeper molecular responses at 3 and 6 months resulted in long-term outcome improvements. Nilotinib discontinuation primarily resulted from disease progression (30%) or adverse events (21%). The most frequently occurring complications included rash (31%), pruritus (21%), and nausea (25%). Pleural effusions were uncommon (1%). Based on this clinical trial and others, nilotinib appears to be a safe and effective treatment option for patients with imatinib-resistant or intolerant CP-CML. Similar to dasatinib, nilotinib has no activity against *BCR-ABL1* T315I mutation and should not be used in that setting.

Bosutinib

Bosutinib is a dual tyrosine kinase inhibitor targeting the *ABL* and *SRC* pathways and can be used to treat imatinib-resistant or intolerant patients. Bosutinib is also effective in patients with known *BCR-ABL1* mutations, including Y253H, E255K/V, and F359C/V [48]. Like dasatinib and nilotinib, bosutinib should not be used to treat *BCR-ABL1* T315I mutations. Bosutinib appears to have similar response rates to dasatinib and nilotinib in CML patients with imatinib-resistant or intolerant disease [48]. The 4-year cumulative complete hematologic response rate was 74% in 117 patients. The overall survival rates ranged from 67% up to 87% depending on previous therapy. The most common non-hematologic complications included diarrhea (83%), nausea (48%), and vomiting (38%). Common hematologic complications included thrombocytopenia (39%), neutropenia (21%), and anemia (20%). Cardiac and vascular complications were reported in 15% and 6% of patients, respectively. In this particular trial, 28% of patients discontinued bosutinib therapy as a result of treatment-related complications [48]. Bosutinib is another viable treatment option for patients requiring second-line TKI therapy.

Table 9. Bosutinib in second-line treatment [48]

Patients	OS at 4 years	CCyR
Imatinib/Dasatinib-resistant (n = 38)	67%	22%
Imatinib/Dasatinib-intolerant (n = 50)	80%	40%
Imatinib/Nilotinib-resistant (n = 26)	87%	31%

CCyR = Complete cytogenetic response; OS = Overall survival.

Ponatinib

Ponatinib is an orally available TKI with activity against native and mutated *BCR-ABL1* proteins. Currently, ponatinib is the only TKI with demonstrated efficacy against the highly resistant *BCR-ABL1* T315I mutation. The FDA granted accelerated approval to ponatinib in 2012 for the treatment of adult patients resistant or intolerant to prior TKI therapy. The pivotal Ponatinib Ph^+ ALL and CML Evaluation (PACE) clinical trial was a phase II study evaluating safety and efficacy of ponatinib in 449 patients with CML or Ph^+ ALL resistant or intolerant to dasatinib or nilotinib [49]. Among the 267 evaluable patients with CML, 60% and 40% achieved MCyR and MMR, respectively. Among those who responded, the probability of maintaining MCyR for 5 years was 82%. Estimated 5-year overall survival was 73%. Common treatment-related complications included rash (47%), abdominal pain (46%), thrombocytopenia (46%), headache (43%), and constipation (41%). Arterial occlusive events are a major concern unique to ponatinib and occurred in 31% of patients leading to mandatory dose reductions and an FDA-issued black box warning. Ponatinib was also issued a risk REMS to help mitigate this concern. No prospective clinical trials have evaluated ponatinib with allogeneic HSCT in CML patients with the *BCR-ABL1* T315I mutation; however, retrospective reports suggest ponatinib may be superior, with 4-year overall survival rates of 73% compared to 56% with HSCT [50].

High Dose Imatinib

Dose escalation with imatinib has shown some utility in patients with primary resistance; however, those failing to achieve a hematologic remission or cytogenetic response on imatinib 400 mg are not likely to experience a benefit from increasing to 800 mg daily. Before the advent of second-generation TKIs, dose escalation with imatinib was a common practice in those with imatinib-tolerance. Higher imatinib doses provided a few different theoretical benefits, including increased trough levels, improved inhibition of *BCR-ABL1* mutations, and compensating for increased *BCR-ABL1* resulting from genomic amplification [51]. In a phase II, open-label trial evaluating 150 imatinib-resistant CML patients randomized to either dasatinib or high-dose imatinib, Kantarjian found significantly higher rates of CHR (93% versus 82%) and MMR (29% versus 12%) in dasatinib [52]. In addition, more patients maintained a cytogenetic response at 18 months (90% versus 74%). High-dose imatinib should be reserved for select patients with advanced stage CML.

Allogeneic HSCT

Allogeneic HSCT remains an important treatment option for various CML patients, including those who have progressed after at least two TKIs, those who harbor the *BCR-ABL1* T315I mutation, and in advanced stage CML. Overall, HSCT numbers have decreased since the introduction of TKIs; however, they remain an important option as 2% of patients develop resistance to TKIs each year and therefore require alternative therapy such as allogeneic transplantation [9]. Eligibility for HSCT varies from institution to institution and availability of matched donors remains a major limitation. For patients with resistance or intolerance to TKIs, two main treatment options exist: continued therapy on a second-generation TKI or allogeneic HSCT. Patients faced with this decision should receive a transplant consultation to discuss donor selection, cost considerations, short- and long-term complications, and alternative options. Scoring systems have been devised to help identify appropriate CML patients requiring allogeneic HSCT [31]. The Chronic Leukemia Working Party of the European Group for Blood and Marrow Transplantation system incorporates age, disease stage, HLA matching, and time from diagnosis.

For some patients, especially those who are younger, allogeneic HSCT is an attractive consideration because it is the only available curative option, with some transplant studies showing 5-year survival rates as high as 80% [31]. It is possible that these survival rates are even higher with recent advances in HLA-matching and supportive care for allogeneic HSCT. The ideal transplant patient is relatively young (< 40 years) with an HLA-matched sibling donor, in the chronic phase, and without significant co-morbidities. Patients entering transplantation perform better if they are CP-CML with a low leukemic burden.

Treatment-related morbidity and mortality resulting from HSCT are real concerns, with Gratwohl showing transplant-related mortality rates ranging from 20% to 73% depending on various risk factors [31]. One ongoing clinical question is treating post-HSCT patients with TKIs to help prevent relapse. The NCCN recommends considering one year of TKI therapy following HSCT in patients with previous AP-CML or BP-CML [22]. Overall, allogeneic HSCT remains an important treatment option for select patients who display resistance or intolerance to TKI therapy. Most CML relapses following HSCT occur within 3 to 5 years. Effective *BCR-ABL1* transcript monitoring is important for early detection of disease recurrence. For those who experience a post-transplant relapse, several treatment options exist, including donor leukocyte infusion, resumption of TKI therapy, another allogeneic HSCT, or IFN-a.

Management of Advanced Stage CML

Most newly diagnosed patients will present in CP-CML, with only 10% to 15% of patients showing characteristics of AP- or BP-CML. Typical progression involves CP-CML evolving to AP-CML before finally resulting in blast crisis and death. Various definitions for AP- and BP-CML exist. According to the NCCN, their adopted definition of AP-CML includes the presence of any of the following [22]:

1. Peripheral blood myeloblasts ≥ 15% and < 30%
2. Peripheral blood myeloblasts and promyelocytes ≥ 30%
3. Peripheral blood basophils ≥ 20%
4. Platelets < 100,000/microL, unrelated to therapy
5. Additional clonal cytogenetic abnormalities in Ph^+ cells

BP-CML, according to the NCCN, includes ≥ 30% blasts in the blood, marrow, or both. This is slightly different from the WHO criteria, which regards ≥ 20% blasts as diagnostic for blast crisis. BP-CML can also be diagnosed in patients with extramedullary blastic infiltrates (e.g., sarcoma or chloroma). Treatment for advanced stage CML is dependent on multiple factors such as patient age, disease stage, previous therapy, co-morbidities, availability of a clinical trial, patient preference, and financial constraints. The ultimate treatment goal for advanced stage CML is to revert the patient back to Cp-CML before proceeding to curative therapy with allogeneic HSCT. For newly diagnosed *de novo* advanced stage CML, treatment may include standard TKI therapy, similar to CP-CML, followed by careful evaluation for eventual allogeneic HSCT. For patients who progressed from CP-CML to advanced stage CML while on TKI therapy, more aggressive treatment is required. These individuals should be placed on a clinical trial whenever possible in conjunction with allogeneic HSCT. Bridge therapy is often required to reduce disease burden prior to transplantation. The primary indicator of long-term success in patients with advanced stage CML undergoing allogeneic HSCT is the phase in which they receive transplantation. For instance, patients who receive bridge therapy and revert to CP-CML before receiving allogeneic transplantation have 4-year disease-free survival rates as high as 80% compared to 30% to 40% for those who are transplanted while in AP-CML [31].

Imatinib, bosutinib, dasatinib, nilotinib, and ponatinib have all demonstrated activity in advanced stage CML [29, 48, 50, 53-55]. A paucity of data exists evaluating which TKI is preferred in the setting of advanced stage CML. Most institutions currently utilize second-generation TKIs in this setting based on extrapolated data from various clinical trials suggesting deeper and faster cytogenetic responses with the non-imatinib TKIs. With higher rates of resistance, using highly potent TKI therapy makes sense and may provide patients with better long-term survival than imatinib therapy. Similar to CP-CML management, choice of agent should be based on side effect profile along with patient co-morbidities. Generic imatinib is now available in the United States and may be an option for patients unable to afford second-generation TKIs. In these patients opting for imatinib therapy, higher doses should be considered [56].

BCR-ABL1 mutational analysis is a critical component required to select subsequent therapy in patients progressing from CP-CML to advanced stage disease while on TKI therapy. For example, patients with the *BCR-ABL1* F317L mutation will likely response better to nilotinib than imatinib or dasatinib [57]. There are no randomized clinical trials comparing second-generation TKIs in relapsed or refractory CML and extrapolated response rates appear similar.

Omacetaxine mepesuccinate is a reversible protein synthesis inhibitor with proven efficacy against TKI-resistant CML regardless of *BCR-ABL1* mutational status [58]. The CML202 study evaluated 62 CP-CML patients with *BCR-ABL1* T315I mutation and demonstrated a CCyR in 16% of patients. The median progression-free survival was 8 months with an overall survival of 30 months. In advanced stage CML, omacetaxine was evaluated in 51 patients with AP-CML and TKI resistance [59]. The median progression-free survival and overall survival were 5 and 18 months, respectively. Omacetaxine results in myelosuppression but is otherwise well tolerated.

Lymphoid and myeloid blast crisis are the two major forms of blast crisis exists in CML. Myeloid blast crisis accounts for nearly 70% of cases and lymphoid blast crisis along with undifferentiated or mixed lineage cases accounting for the remaining 30%. The current treatment paradigm for managing myeloid blast crisis is TKI therapy with or without chemotherapy followed by allogeneic HSCT. AML-like induction therapy does not appear to be advantageous compared to other available treatment options and is reserved for select patients who develop myeloid blast crisis while on TKI therapy [60]. Two-year survival following allogeneic HSCT can be as high as 65% in patients who were transplanted after reverting back to CP-CML. For those myeloid blast patients who remained in the blast phase, two-year survival rates following transplantation were significantly worse at 25% [61]. Overall treatment plans vary, and when feasible, the patient should be reverted back to CP-CML using TKI therapy with subsequent allogeneic HSCT. Lymphoid blast crisis respond well to chemotherapy regimens utilized in Ph^+ ALL, such as HYPER-CVAD along with a TKI [62]. A CCyR was noted in 58% of patients with a median overall survival of 17 months. Most cases of lymphoid blast crisis occur in patients already receiving TKI therapy. When this occurs, switching TKIs to improve response rates is a reasonable consideration. For patients in blast crisis who fail initial therapy alternative treatment strategies should include switching TKI agents based on mutational analysis and adverse event profile. Clinical trials should also be considered in these patients as well.

Overall, clinicians are seeing fewer cases of advanced CML due to treatment improvements and mutational analysis. Treating advanced stage CML is difficult and every attempt should be made to return the patient to CP-CML followed by allogeneic HSCT in eligible patients.

Discontinuing TKI Therapy

Patients customarily continue TKI therapy indefinitely despite exorbitant financial cost and noteworthy treatment-related toxicities. The rationale for extended treatment durations involved early *in vitro* analysis of CML stem cells showing continued proliferation even in the presence of *BCR-ABL1* inhibition. Furthermore, researchers believed that MRD remained even in patients showing PCR negativity for *BCR-ABL1* transcripts using the most sensitive qPCR assays. However, recent studies have shown that up to 40% of select patients in a CMR can discontinue TKI therapy and maintain the possibility of treatment-free remission. The STOP imatinib (STIM1) trial was the first attempt to evaluate this possibility [35, 63]. The STIM1 trial evaluated 100 patients in CMR for at least 2 years with a median follow-up of 77 months following imatinib discontinuation. The molecular recurrence-free survival was 43% and 38% at 6 and 60 months, respectively. Other analogous trials evaluating TKI discontinuation in CML have found similar results, with most patients relapsing within 6 months of discontinuation [36-39]. Fortunately, relapsed patients frequently returned to CMR following resumption of TKI therapy. Some studies have reported concerning toxicities, including musculoskeletal pain and pruritus, resulting from TKI discontinuation in up to 40% of patients [39].

With long-term data lacking, TKI discontinuation should be pursued under the auspices of a clinical trial whenever possible. With this in mind, TKI discontinuation appears to be safe in select patients following a thorough discussion of the potential risks and benefits. The NCCN guidelines do outline principles for selecting potentially eligible patients suitable for TKI cessation [22]. All of the following parameters must be met in order to qualify for TKI discontinuation:

1. At least 18 years old.
2. Currently in chronic phase with no past history of accelerated or blast phase CML.
3. On appropriate TKI therapy for at least 3 years.
4. Prior evidence of quantifiable *BCR-ABL1* transcript.
5. Stable molecular response for at least 2 years (at least 4 tests performed at 3 month increments).
6. Access to reliable qPCR testing with the appropriate sensitivity.
7. Monthly molecular monitoring for at least one year, then every 6 months for the second year, and then every 12 weeks thereafter.

8. Immediate resumption of TKI within 4 weeks of relapse.
9. Discuss TKI discontinuation with a CML Specialty Center to discuss risks and benefits.

For the vast majority of patients, CML continues to be managed as a chronic disease state requiring long-term treatment and support. Currently, based on the above parameters, TKI discontinuation would be expected in only 10% to 15% of newly diagnosed patients [64]. However, for these select few, significant benefit can be derived from foregoing these expensive and potentially toxic agents.

FUTURE STRATEGIES

Most CML patients respond extremely favorably to first-line TKI therapy with quick, durable, and deep molecular remissions. Unfortunately, a certain subset of patients show early development of TKI resistance and *BCR-ABL1* mutations resulting in disease resistance and progression to advanced stage CML. Future strategies must account for these high-risk patients by incorporating new investigational agents into existing archetypes. Investigational strategies include checkpoint inhibitors, hedgehog inhibitors, JAK2 inhibitors, stem cell poisons, and cancer vaccines. Another future goal includes increasing the number of patients who can safely discontinue TKI therapy altogether while maintaining deep molecular remissions. With increasing prevalence, the cost of managing CML continues to skyrocket, leaving a significant burden on the healthcare system. Finding patients who can safely discontinue therapy would help ease this financial burden.

CONCLUSION

Chronic myeloid leukemia is a myeloproliferative disorder typically resulting from the development of the Philadelphia translocation and subsequent oncoprotein production. CML is a triphasic disease with most patients presenting in CP-CML and 10% to 15% appearing in more advanced stages. Prior to 2000, CML was treated with busulfan, IFN-a, and hydroxyurea, leading to poor long-term outcomes and eventual death. Allogeneic HSCT remains the primary curative treatment option, but unfortunately confers significant morbidity and mortality concerns. Following the discovery of TKIs, the therapeutic landscape for CML shifted substantially, resulting in 10-year survival rates in excess of 90% for those receiving first-line TKI therapy [4]. Patients diagnosed with CP-CML should receive treatment with a *BCR-ABL1* TKI in hopes of obtaining and maintaining a MMR. CML will typically require long-term treatment with TKI and subsequent monitoring to ensure deep and sustained molecular remissions.

References

[1] Siegel, RL; Miller, KD; Jemal, A. Cancer statistics, 2018. *CA Cancer J Clin*, 2017, 68(1), 7-30.

[2] Huang, X; Cortes, J; Kantarjian, H. Estimations of the increasing prevalence and plateau prevalence of chronic myeloid leukemia in the era of tyrosine kinase inhibitor therapy. *Cancer*, 2012, 118(12), 3123–3127.

[3] Mandanas, RA; Leibowitz, DS; Gharehbaghi, K; et al. Role of p21 RAS in p210 bcr-abl transformation of murine myeloid cells. *Blood*, 1993, 82(6), 1838–1847.

[4] Saussele, S; Krauss, MP; Hehlmann, R; et al. Impact on comorbidities on overall survival in patients with chronic myeloid leukemia: results of the randomized CML study IV. *Blood*, 2015, 126, 42-49.

[5] Faderl, S; Talpaz, M; Estrov, Z; et al. The biology of chronic myeloid leukemia. *N Engl J Med*, 1999, 341(3), 164.

[6] Mandanas, RA; Leibowitz, DS; Gharehbaghi, K; et al. Role of p21 RAS in p210 bcr-abl transformation of murine myeloid cells. *Blood*, 1993, 82(6), 1838–1847.

[7] Sawyers, CL; Callahan, W; Witte, ON. Dominant negative MYC blocks transformation by ABL oncogenes. *Cell*, 1992, 70(6), 901–910.

[8] Shuai, K; Halpern, J; Hoeve, J; et al. Constitutive activation of STAT5 by the BCR-ABL oncogene in chronic myelogenous leukemia. *Oncogene*, 1996, 13(2), 247–254.

[9] Jabbour, E; Kantarjian, HM. Chronic myeloid leukemia: 2018 update on diagnosis, therapy and monitoring. *Am J Hematol*, 2018, 93, 442-459.

[10] Kantarjian, HM; Dixon, D; Keating, MJ; et al., Characteristics of accelerated disease in chronic myelogenous leukemia *Cancer*, 1988, 61, 1441-1446.

[11] Kantarjian, H; O'Brien, S; Jabbour, E; et al., Improved survival in chronic myeloid leukemia since the introduction of imatinib therapy: a single-institution historical experience. *Blood*, 2012, 119, 1981.

[12] Arber, DA; Orazi, A; Hasserjian, R; et al. The 2016 revision to the World Health Organization classification of myeloid neoplasms and acute leukemia. *Blood*, 2016, 127, 2391.

[13] Kantarjian, HM; Talpaz, M; Cortes, J; et al. Quantitative polymerase chain reaction monitoring of BCR-ABL during therapy with imatinib mesylate (STI571; gleevec) in chonric-phase chronic myelogenous leukemia. *CLin Cancer Res*, 2003, 9, 160-166.

[14] Hughes, TP; Ambrosetti, A; Barbu, V; et al. Clinical value of PCR in diagnosis and follow-up of leukaemia and lymphoma: report of the third Workshop of the Molecular Biology/BMT study group. *Leukemia*, 1991, 5(6), 448.

[15] Bower, H; Björkholm, M; Dickman, PW; et al. Life Expectancy of Patients With Chronic Myeloid Leukemia Approaches the Life Expectancy of the General Population. *J Clin Oncol*, 2016 Aug, 34(24), 2851-2857.

[16] Brunner, AM; Campigotto, F; Sadrzadeh, H; et al. Trends in all-cause mortality among patients with chronic myeloid leukemia: a Surveillance, Epidemiology, and End Results database analysis. *Cancer*, 2013, 119(14), 2620-2629.

[17] Sokal, JE; Cox, EB; Baccarani, M; et al. Prognostic discrimination in "good-risk" chronic granulocytic leukemia. *Blood*, 1984 Apr, 63(4), 789-99.

[18] Hasford, J; Pfirrmann, M; Hehlmann, R; et al. A new prognostic score for survival of patients with chronic myeloid leukemia treated with interferon-alfa. Weiting committee for the collaborative CML prognostic factors project group. *J Natl Cancer Inst*, 1998, 90(11), 850.

[19] Hasford, J; Baccarani, M; Hoffmann, V; et al. Predicting complete cytogenetic response and subsequent progression-free survival in 2060 patients with CML on imatinib treatment: the EUTOS score. *Blood*, 2011, 118(3), 686.

[20] Marin, D; Ibrahim, AR; Goldman, JM. European treatment and outcome study (EUTOS) score for chronic myeloid leukemia still requires more confirmation. *J Clin Oncol*, 2011, 29, 3944-3945.

[21] Jabbour, E; Cortes, J; Nazha, A; et al. EUTOS score is not predictive for survival and outcome in patients with early chronic phase chronic myeloid leukemia treated with tyrosine kinase inhibitors: a single institution experience. *Blood*, 2012, 119, 4524-4526.

[22] *The NCCN Clinical Practice Guidelines in Oncology™ Chronic Myeloid Leukemia* (Version 4.2018). National Comprehensive Cancer Network, Inc. Available at, www.NCCN.org. Accessed, June 10, 2018.

[23] Silver, RT; Woolf, SH; Hehlmann, R; et al. An evidence-based analysis of the effect of busulfan, hydroxyurea, interferon, and allogeneic bone marrow transplantation in treating chronic phase of chronic myeloid leukemia: developed for the American Society of Hematology. *Blood*, 1999, 94(5), 1517-1536.

[24] Druker, BJ; Guilhot, F; O'Brien, S; et al. Five-year follow-up of patients receiving imatinib for chronic myeloid leukemia. *N Eng J Med*, 2006, 355, 2408-2417.

[25] Baccarani, M; Druker, BJ; Branford, S; et al. Long-term response to imatinib is not affected by the initial dose in patients with Philadelphia chromosome-positive chronic myeloid leukemia in chronic phase: final update from the Tyrosine Kinase Inhibitor Optimization and Selectivity (TOPS) study. *Int J Hematol*, 2014, 99, 616-624.

[26] Hehlmann, R; Muller, MC; Lauseker, M; et al. Deep molecular is reached by the majority of patients treated with imatinib, predicts survival, and is achieved more quickly by optimized high-dose imatinib: results from the randomized CML study IV. *J Clin Oncol*, 2014, 32, 415-423.

[27] Preudhomme, C; Guilhot, J; Nicolini, FE; et al. Imatinib plus peginterferon alfa-2a in chronic myeloid leukemia. *N Eng J Med*, 2010, 363, 2511-2521.

[28] Cortes, JE; Gambacorti-Passerini, C; Deininger, MW; et al. Bosutinib versus imatinib for newly diagnosed chronic myeloid leukemia: results from the randomized BFORE trial. *J Clin Oncol*, 2018, 36, 231-237.

[29] Cortes, JE; Saglio, G; Kantarjian, HM; et al. Final 5-year study results of DASISION: the dasatinib versus imatinib study in treatment-naïve chronic myeloid leukemia patients trial. *J Clin Oncol*, 2016, 34, 2333-2340.

[30] Hochhaus, A; Saglio, G; Hughes, TP; et al. Long-term benefits and risks of frontline nilotinib vs imatinib for chronic myeloid leukemia in chronic phase: 5-year update of the randomized ENESTnd trial. *Leukemia*, 2016 May, 30(5), 1044-54.

[31] Gratwohl, A; Hermans, J; Goldman, JM; et al. Risk assessment for patients with chronic myeloid leukaemia before allogeneic blood or marrow transplantation. Chronic Leukemia Working Party of the European Group for Blood and Marrow Transplantation. *Lancet*, 1998, 352(9134), 1087.

[32] Jabbour, E; Kantarjian, H; O'Brien, S; et al. The achievement of an early complete cytogenetic response is a major determinant for outcomes in patients with early chronic phase chronic myeloid leukemia treated with tyrosine kinase inhibitors. *Blood*, 2011, 118, 4541-4546.

[33] Hanfstein, B; Muller, MC; Hehlmann, R; et al. Early molecular and cytogenetic response is predictive for long-term progression-free and overall survival in chronic myeloid leukemia (CML). *Leukemia*, 2012, 26, 2096-2102.

[34] Thomas, J; Wang, L; Clark, PE; et al. Active transport of imatinib into and out of cells: implications for drug resistance. *Blood*, 2004, 104, 3739-3745.

[35] Hegedus, C; Ozvegy-Laczka, C; Apati, A; et al. Interactions of nilotinib, dasatinib, and bosutinib with ABCB1 and ABCG2: implications for altered anti-cancer effects and pharmacologic properties. *Br J Pharmacol*, 2009, 158, 1153-1164.

[36] Milojkovic, D; Apperley, J. Mechanisms of Resistance to Imatinib and Second-Generation Tyrosine Inhibitors in Chronic Myeloid Leukemia. *Clin Cancer Res*, 2009, 15(24), 7519.

[37] Branford, S; Rudzki, Z; Walsh, S; et al. Detection of BCR-ABL mutations in patients with CML treated with imatinib is virtually always accompanied by clinical resistance, and mutations in the ATP phosphate-binding loop (P-loop) are associated with a poor prognosis. *Blood*, 2003, 102(1), 276-83.

[38] Müller, MC; Cortes, JE; Kim, DW; et al. Dasatinib treatment of chronic-phase chronic myeloid leukemia: analysis of responses according to preexisting BCR-ABL mutations. *Blood*, 2009, 114(24), 4944-53.

[39] Lee, TS; Potts, SJ; Kantarjian, H; et al. Molecular basis explanation for imatinib resistance of BCR-ABL due to T315I and P-loop mutations from molecular dynamics simulations. *Cancer*, 2008, 112(8), 1744.

[40] Noens, L; van Lierde, MA; De Brock, R; et al. Prevalence, determinants, and outcomes of nonadherence to imatinib therapy in patients with chronic myeloid leukemia: the ADAGIO study. *Blood*, 2009, 113, 5401-5411.

[41] Anderson, KR; Chambers, CR; Lam, N; et al. Medication adherence among adults prescribed imatinib, dasatinib, or nilotinib for the treatment of chronic myeloid leukemi. *J Oncol Pharm Pract*, 2015, 21(1), 19-25.

[42] Jabbour, EJ; Kantarjian, H; Eliasson, L; et al. Patient adherence to tyrosine kinase inhibitor therapy in chronic myeloid leukemia. *Am J Hematol*, 2012, 87, 687-691.

[43] Cortes, JE; Pinilla-Ibarz, J; leCoutre, P; et al. A phase 2 trial of ponatinib in Philadelphia chromosome-positive leukemias. *N Eng J Med*, 2013, 369, 1.

[44] Hochhaus, A; Baccarani, M; Deininger, M; et al. Dasatinib induces durable cytogenetic responses in patients with chronic myelogenous leukemia in chronic phase with resistance or intolerance to imatinib. *Leukemia*, 2008, 22(6), 1200.

[45] Shah, NP; Guilhot, F; Cortes, JE; et al. Long-term outcome with dasatinib after imatinib failure in chronic-phase chronic myeloid leukemia: follow-up of a phase 3 study. *Blood*, 2014 Apr, 123(15), 2317-24.

[46] Shah, NP; Rousselot, P; Schiffer, C; et al. Dasatinib in imatinib-resistant or –intolerant chronic-phase, chronic myeloid leukemia patients: 7-year follow-up of study CA180-034. *Am J Hematol*, 2016 Sep, 91(9), 869–874.

[47] Giles, FJ; le Coutre, PD; Pinilla-Ibarz, J; et al. Nilotinib in imatinib-resistant or imatinib-intolerant patients with chronic myeloid leukemia in chronic phase: 48-month follow-up results of a phase II study. *Leukemia*, 2013, 27, 107-112.

[48] Cortes, JE; Khoury, HJ; Kantarjian, H; et al. Long-term bosutinib for chronic phase chronic myeloid leukemia after failure of imatinib plus dasatinib and/or nilotinib. *Am J Hematol*, 2016, 91(12), 1206-1214.

[49] Cortes, JE; Kim, DW; Pinilla-Ibarz, J; et al. A phase 2 trial of ponatinib in Philadelphia chromosome-positive leukemias. *N Engl J Med*, 2013, 369, 1.

[50] Nicolini, FE; Basak, GW; Kim, DW; et al. Overall survival with ponatinib versus allogeneic stem cell transplantation in Philadelphia chromosome-positive leukemias with the T315I mutation. *Cancer*, 2017, 123(15), 2875.

[51] Druker, BJ. Circumventing resistance to kinase-inhibitor therapy. *N Eng J Med*, 2006, 354(24), 2594.

[52] Kantarjian, H; Paquini, R; Levy, V; et al. Dasatinib or high-dose imatinib for chronic-phase chronic myeloid leukemia resistant to imatinib at a dose of 400 to

600 mg daily: two-year follow-up of a randomized phase 2 study (START-R). *Cancer*, 2009, 115(18), 4136-4147.
[53] Kantarjian, H; Shah, NP; Hochhaus, A; et al. Dasatinib versus imatinib in newly diagnosed chronic-phase chronic myeloid leukemia. *N Engl J Med*, 2010, 362(24), 2260.
[54] Saglio, G; Kim, DW; Issaragrisil, S; et al. Nilotinib versus imatinib for newly diagnosed chronic myeloid leukemia. *N Engl J Med*, 2010, 362(24), 2251.
[55] Gurion, R; Gafter-Gvili, A; Vidal, L; et al. Has the time for first-line treatment with second generation tyrosine kinase inhibitors in patients with chronic myelogenous leukemia already come? Systematic review and meta-analysis. *Haematologica*, 2013 Jan, 98(1), 95-102.
[56] Kantarjian, HM; O'Brien, S; Cortes, JE; et al. Treatment of philadelphia chromosome-positive, accelerated-phase chronic myelogenous leukemia with imatinib mesylate. *Clin Cancer Res*, 2002, 8(7), 2167.
[57] Soverini, S; Hochhaus, A; Nicolini, FE; et al. BCR-ABL kinase domain mutation analysis in chronic myeloid leukemia patients treated with tyrosine kinase inhibitors: recommendations from an expert panel on behalf of European LeukemiaNet. *Blood*, 2011, 118(5), 1208.
[58] Cortes, J; Lipton, JH; Rea, D; et al. Phase 2 study of subcutaneous omacetaxine mepesuccinate after TKI failure in patients with chronic-phase CML with T315I mutation. *Blood*, 2012, 120, 2573-2580.
[59] Khoury, HJ; Cortes, J; Baccarani, M; et al. Omacetaxine mepesuccinate in patients with advanced chronic myeloid leukemia with resistance or intolerance to tyrosine kinase inhibitors. *Leuk Lymphoma*, 2015, 56, 120-127.
[60] Sacchi, S; Kantarjian, HM; O'Brien, S; et al. Chronic myelogenous leukemia in nonlymphoid blastic phase: analysis of the results of first salvage therapy with three different treatment approaches for 162 patients. *Cancer*, 1999, 86(12), 2632.
[61] Armand, P; Kim, HT; Logan, BR; et al. Validation and refinement of the Disease Risk Index for allogeneic stem cell transplantation. *Blood*, 2014, 123(23), 3664.
[62] Strati, P; Kantarjian, H; Thomas, D; et al. HCVAD plus imatinib or dasatinib in lymphoid blastic phase chronic myeloid leukemia. *Cancer*, 2014 Feb, 120(3), 373-80.
[63] Thomas, J; Wang, L; Clark, PE; et al. Active transport of imatinib into and out of cells: implications for drug resistance. *Blood*, 2004, 104, 3739-3745.
[64] Apperley, JF. Twist it but don't spin it. *Blood*, 2013, 122(4), 470.

In: Frontiers in Leukemia Pharmacotherapy
Editor: Lunawati L. Bennett
ISBN: 978-1-53614-960-9

Chapter 11

CHRONIC LYMPHOCYTIC LEUKEMIA

Zachery R. Halford*, PharmD
Union University, College of Pharmacy, Jackson, Tennessee, US

ABSTRACT

Chronic lymphocytic leukemia (CLL) is the most common adult leukemia in the United States with approximately 21,000 new cases and 4,500 deaths estimated for 2018. Accumulation of incompetent clonal B lymphocytes characterizes this chronic leukemia and results in lymphadenopathy, lymphocytosis, "B" symptoms, and eventually anemia, thrombocytopenia, and death. Most patients initially diagnosed with CLL appear asymptomatic and experience prolonged survival. The only known cure for this indolent disease remains allogeneic hematopoietic stem cell transplantation (HSCT); however, few patients are viable transplant candidates. Other common treatment options include chemoimmunotherapy and tyrosine kinase therapy.

This chapter highlights the epidemiology, clinical presentation, disease classification, pathologic features, diagnosis, staging, prognostic factors, and general treatment options for various risk stratifications. Emerging treatment options for relapsed and refractory disease are also discussed.

Keywords: lymphoproliferative disorders, B lymphocytes, cytopenias, chronic lymphocytic leukemia, ibrutinib, fludarabine-based chemotherapy, Richter's transformation, Bruton's tyrosine kinase, small lymphocytic lymphoma

* Corresponding Author Email: zhalford@uu.edu.

Abbreviations

BR	bendamustine and rituximab
CLL	chronic lymphocytic leukemia
FCR	fludarabine, cyclophosphamide, and rituximab
FDA	Food and Drug Administration
FISH	fluorescence in situ hybridization
HSCT	hematopoetic stem cell transfusion
IGHV	immunoglobulin heavy chain variable region gene
MBL	monoclonal B cell lymphocytosis
NCCN	National Comprehensive Cancer Network
SLL	small lymphocytic lymphoma

Introduction

Chronic lymphocytic leukemia (CLL) and Small lymphocytic lymphoma (SLL) are lymphoproliferative disorders of monomorphic B-cell lymphocytes found in the bone marrow, peripheral blood, and lymphoid organs [1]. Both CLL and SLL are different manifestations of the same basic disease and require similar treatment strategies. CLL/SLL are characterized by leukemic cells accumulating in the peripheral blood and bone marrow leading to various acute and chronic complications depending on overall staging and rate of proliferation. CLL is typically described as dysfunctional B cells in the blood, bone marrow and lymphoid tissue; whereas SLL will primarily exist in the marrow and lymphoid tissue. Chronic lymphocytic lymphocytes are CD19 positive B cell clones co-expressing CD5, CD23, and, to a lesser degree, CD20. CLL and SLL are generally considered to be indolent diseases with some patients living 10-20 years following diagnosis. Some patients, however, develop much more aggressive disease and die rapidly following diagnosis. Therefore, the clinical progression of CLL is variable, with some survival times ranging from 2-20 years and a median overall survival of nearly 10 years. Treatment options continue to improve, and those with CLL now have life expectancies approaching that of the general population.

Epidemiology

CLL is the most common variation of leukemia in the United States with an estimated 20,940 new cases diagnosed in 2018 and an estimated 4,510 deaths [2]. Incidence rates in the European Union are similar to the United States with nearly 4 to 6 cases per 100,000 person years. Increasing incidence occurs with older populations and more than 70% of CLL cases are in patients over 65 years. The median age of diagnosis in the United States is 72 years of age and males have a greater predisposition for acquiring CLL than females with a ratio of 1.5-2.0:1 [3]. CLL incidence varies by race and location, with a higher incidence in Caucasians compared to African Americans or Hispanics. Furthermore, CLL is rare in Asian countries such as China and Japan where the incidence is roughly one tenth that of the United States. Genetic factors may help explain these discrepancies.

Molecular studies surrounding CLL tend to show the genetic determinants of developing CLL are consistent regardless of geographic location. While CLL is not normally hereditary, first-degree relatives are three to eight times more likely to develop a lymphoid malignancy than those in the general population [4]. Approximately 12% of patients diagnosed with CLL report a family history of lymphoproliferative disorders [5]. It is becoming increasingly apparent that family history is an important risk factor in the development of CLL and warrants additional genome-associated studies to identify the pathogenic connection and underlying susceptibility genes. Currently, no known environmental or occupational risk factor will predispose someone to CLL. For instance, atomic bomb and radiation studies showed a significant increase in the development of various forms of leukemia among those with radiation exposure, but CLL was not one of them [6].

Clinical Presentation

CLL is often diagnosed serendipitously with patients undergoing routine lab monitoring during their annual check-up. Most patients diagnosed with CLL will feel normal and relatively healthy with no specific leukemia symptoms present. Other patients may have a wide array of symptoms including painless cervical lymphadenopathy that wax and wane over time along with laboratory abnormalities. Approximately 5% to 10% of patients will present with "B" symptoms common to lymphoma patients; these include drenching night sweats, persistent fevers, unilateral weight loss, and extreme fatigue [7]. Advanced CLL may present with fatigue, chronic infections, and intolerance to physical exercise. Infections result from immune defects in cell-mediated and humoral immunity. Recurring infections in advanced CLL are the primary cause of disease- or treatment-related death.

Lymphadenopathy is the most common presenting sign or symptom, with 50% to 90% of newly diagnosed CLL patients showing evidence of this complication. Cervical and supraclavicular nodes are most commonly enlarged with varying shapes and sizes. In some cases, adjacent lymph nodes may become congruent and form one large lymphoid mass. CLL may also present with splenomegaly resulting in a large painless and non-tender lymphoid organ. Approximately 25% to 55% of newly diagnosed CLL patients will have splenomegaly [8]. Similarly, about a quarter of newly diagnosed CLL patients will also present with mild, non-tender hepatomegaly. Leukemia cutis, the infiltration of the skin by malignant lymphocytes, can occur in up to 5% of newly diagnosed CLL patients. These lymphoid lesions may present as papules, macules, ulcers, blisters or plaques.

Laboratory abnormalities are frequently noted at presentation with lymphocytosis being the most common. The absolute blood lymphocyte threshold for diagnosing CLL is B lymphocytes >5 x 10^9/L [7]. Most patients, however, will present with counts significantly higher than this, some even presenting with a white blood cell count over 100 x 10^9/L. Other bone marrow abnormalities may be discovered at the time of diagnosis, including various cytopenias and hypogammaglobulinemia. Autoimmune hemolytic anemia, autoimmune thrombocytopenia, and agranulocytosis may occur in patients with CLL. Clinicians must evaluate for anemia and thrombocytopenia at diagnosis to help determine staging and treatment as cytopenias play an important prognostic role in managing CLL. Elevations in lactate dehydrogenase, uric acid, beta-2 microglobulin, electrolytes, and transaminases should also be evaluated upon diagnosis.

Pathologic Features

A peripheral blood smear is required for patients with suspected CLL in order to perform morphological and immunophenotypic analysis. B lymphocytes in CLL are small and mature cells with a dense nucleus. Prolymphocytes, which are relatively uncommon, appear as larger lymphocytes. Flow cytometry evaluation is critical for identifying B cell-associated antigens such as CD19, CD20, and CD23. The presence of CD5 antigen presumes T-cell disease. Levels of other surface antigens may be evaluated; however, most cases of CLL will be monoclonal and easily identifiable through standard flow cytometry. Unlike acute leukemias, a bone marrow aspirate and biopsy are not required for the diagnosis of CLL. A lymph node biopsy can help distinguish between CLL and SLL.

Some patients with CLL can experience histologic transformation resulting in a separate lymphoproliferative disorder such as an aggressive lymphoma (Richter's transformation), prolymphocytic leukemia, Hodgkin lymphoma, or multiple myeloma. Richter's transformation is the most common reported development with 3% to 7% of CLL cases resulting in a terminal transformation. Richter's transformation may occur suddenly with clinical deterioration and worsening "B" symptoms. Patients experiencing a Richter's transformation are less likely to survive and often die within the year. These transformations may be exacerbated by chemotherapy, especially anthracyclines or purine analogues.

DIAGNOSIS

In order to secure a CLL diagnosis, clinicians must obtain a complete blood count with differential, peripheral blood sample for immunophenotyping and morphologic evaluation [7]. The 2008 International Workshop on Chronic Lymphocytic Leukemia standardized the diagnostic criteria for CLL by updating the 1996 Working Group guidelines [7]. The diagnosis of CLL now requires the presence of at least 5 x 10^9/L clonal B cells in the peripheral blood sample along with flow cytometry verification of B cell clonality (CD19, CD20, and CD23).

In patients with suspected CLL who have less than 5 x 10^9/L clonal B cells and no evidence of other disease manifestations are determined to have monoclonal B cell lymphocytosis (MBL), which is a relatively new classification for individuals with an abnormal B-cell population and similar immunophenotype to CLL but who do not meet diagnostic criteria. Patients with MBL will commonly show normal cytogenetics and favorable molecular lesions. The average progression from MBL to diagnosable CLL is 1.1% per year [8]. Individuals who have do not meet the B cell cutoff but display lymphadenopathy are diagnosed with SLL following histologic evaluation.

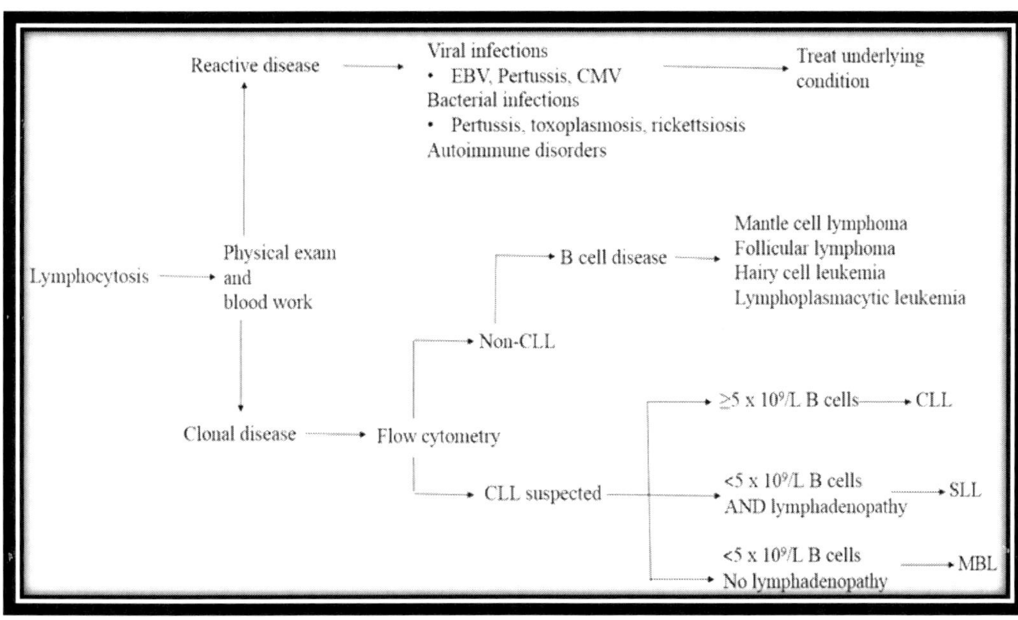

CLL = chronic lymphocytic leukemia; MBL = monoclonal B cell lymphocytosis; SLL = small lymphocytic lymphoma.

Figure 1. CLL Diagnostic Workup.

Lymphocytosis and lymphadenopathy may result from several distinct causes and require careful consideration while evaluating the differential diagnosis. Clinicians must first distinguish between clonal causes of lymphocytosis and reactive causes such as infections (Epstein Barr Virus, pertussis, CMV, etc). Various lymphoproliferative disorders leading to lymphocytosis include monoclonal B lymphocytosis, mantle cell lymphoma, follicular lymphoma, hairy cell leukemia, and lymphoplasmacytic lymphoma. Flow cytometry is especially useful for distinguishing CLL from these various other lymphoproliferative disorders.

STAGING

There are currently two co-existing staging methods in place for CLL; the Rai staging system and the Binet staging system [9, 10]. These methods are inexpensive, simple, and rely solely on a physical exam and routine laboratory analysis. Rai was initially developed in 1975 and divided patients into one of five groups centered on overall survival. Based on this criteria, it became clear over time that three primary cohorts of patients existed and researchers later revised the Rai staging system to reflect these various risk stratifications [11].

The Binet staging system utilizes five distinct sites of involvement including inguinal, cervical, and axillary lymph nodes as well as the spleen and liver. Based on a physical exam and laboratory analysis, patients are then classified as having stage A, B, or C disease. Impressive advancements have been made in identifying other risk factors and staging concerns that require consideration beyond what these two systems allow. Therefore, further staging methods are being evaluated to more accurately predict treatment outcomes and long-term survival based on clinical staging and genetic abnormalities.

Table 1. Rai staging system [9]

Stage	Description	% Patients at Diagnosis	Median Survival (mo)
0	Lymphocytosis in the peripheral blood without lymphadenopathy	25%	150
I	Stage 0 but with lymphadenopathy	50%	101
II	Positive for hepatosplenomegaly		71
III	Positive for anemia (Hg < 11 g/dL)	25%	19
IV	Positive for thrombocytopenia (<100,000)		

Table 2. Revised Rai staging system [11]

Stage	Description	Comparison
Low risk	Lymphocytosis in the peripheral blood without lymphadenopathy	Rai stage O
Intermediate risk	Positive for lymphadenopathy and/or hepatosplenomegaly	Rai stage I,II
High risk	Positive for anemia and/or thrombocytopenia	Rai stage III, IV

Table 3. Binet staging system [10]

Stage	Description	Median Survival (months)
A	No anemia/thrombocytopenia and less than 3 lymphoid sites involved	Similar to age-matched cohorts
B	No anemia/thrombocytopenia and 3 or more lymphoid sites	84
C	Positive for anemia and/or thrombocytopenia	24

PROGNOSTIC FACTORS

Clinical staging may be the most important prognostic factor, however, other important cconsiderations are required to help guide treatment decisions. Immunoglobulin heavy chain variable region gene (IGHV) mutational status along with cytogenetic abnormalities and serum markers are other noteworthy prognostic markers. IGHV status is an important predictor of survival with wild-type showing inferior survival outcomes compared to those with mutated IGHV [12]. IGVH mutation status testing is encouraged by the National Comprehensive Cancer Network (NCCN) due to its reproducibility and availability [13]. Fluorescence in situ hybridization (FISH) testing can identify cytogenetic abnormalities in up to 80% of patients with CLL. The most common abnormalities include 13q deletion (55%), 11q deletion (18%), trisomy 12 (16%), 17p deletion (7%) and 6q deletion (7%). Del(11q) is frequently associated with disease progression and reduced overall survival (~80 months). Conversely, del(13q) is a positive prognostic indicator and is associated with prolonged overall survival (greater than 10 years). A loss of TP53 gene is linked to del(17p) and confers a worse prognosis with significantly diminished overall survival (32 months) and possible chemotherapy resistance [14]. The CLL4 trial evaluated these cytogenetic abnormalities and their effect on treatment outcomes [15]. The study identified three risk groups based on independent risk factors predicting progression-free survival. The greatest risk factor for poor outcomes identified in these patients was loss of TP53. Unmutated IGVH and elevated B-2 microglobulin were also independent risk factors for poor overall survival. Clinicians should also evaluate the lymphocyte doubling time defined as the number of months it takes to double the absolute lymphocyte count. The doubling time can be a surrogate marker for rate of disease progression.

An international consortium developed the CLL International Prognostic Index (CLL-IPI) based on data from 3,472 treatment-naïve patients in various countries including the United States [16]. Five independent prognostic factors were identified and included TP53 dysfunction, serum B-2 microglobulin, clinical stage, age, and immunoglobulin heavy chain variable gene (IGHV) mutational status. Evaluating these independent risk factors, a four tiered stratification system was developed to highlight overall survival differences. The 5-year overall survival rates were significantly different for all four groups: low (93%), intermediate (79%), high (63%), and very high (23%). The CLL-IPI system also helps facilitate treatment decisions. Several other somatic mutations have been identified and include TM, MYD88, SF3B1, ZYM3, MAPK1, DDX3X, ZAP70, etc. These mutations can affect the cell-cycle and DNA repair pathways in addition to intracellular signaling. Further evaluation is needed to identify treatment implications of these various cytogenetic abnormalities.

In addition to these commonly employed prognostic tools, clinicians must also take into consideration the patient's overall health. With a diagnosis typically occurring in elderly patients, comorbidities are common and require thoughtful consideration due to the rigors of conventional treatment strategies in patients with CLL. Multiple comorbidities are another independent risk factor for adverse outcomes compared to otherwise healthy individuals with newly diagnosed CLL [17].

Table 4. Prognostic considerations in CLL

Positive Prognosticators
Del (13q)
Low Rai or Binet scoring
Mutated IGHV status
Lymphocyte doubling time > 12 months
Negative Prognosticators
High Rai or Binet scoring
Del(11q)
TP53 mutations
Unmutated IGHV status
Mutated B-2 microglobulin
Lymphocyte doubling time < 12 months

CLL = chronic lymphocytic leukemia; IGHV = immunoglobulin heavy chain variable region gene.

Table 5. CLL International prognostic index (CLL-IPI) [16]

Risk Factor	Description	Score
Del(17p) and/or P53 mutation	Presence of either mutation	4
IGHV mutation status	Unmutated (>98% homology)	2
B2-microglobulin	>3.5 mg/L	2
Clinical staging	Rai stage I-IV Or Binet stage B-C	1
Age	>65 years	1

CLL = chronic lymphocytic leukemia; IGHV = immunoglobulin heavy chain variable region gene.

Table 6. CLL International Prognostic Index (CLL-IPI) Risk Groups [16]

Total Score	Overall Risk	Median Survival (months)	5-year Overall Survival
0-1	Low	Not reached	93%
2-3	Intermediate	104	79%
4-6	High	63	63%
7-10	Very High	31	23%

TREATMENT OVERVIEW

At initial presentation, CLL is a heterogeneous and complicated disease. CLL will naturally progress over time from early to intermediate and finally to an advanced stage. Treatment with chemotherapy and targeted therapy can alter this natural progression and improve quality of life and overall survival. The overarching goal of CLL treatment hinges on achieving and maintaining disease remission while minimizing treatment-related complications. Not all patients, however, require initial treatment following diagnosis, primarily due to the indolent nature of CLL. Certain CLL cohorts have similar survival rates to their age-matched demographic, suggesting a watch-and-wait approach is superior to conventional cytotoxic chemotherapy in low-risk, asymptomatic patients. Furthermore, allogeneic HSCT is the only viable cure for patients with CLL and all other treatment options remain palliative with the goal of relieving symptoms and prolonging life. Several prospective clinical trials evaluating immediate versus delayed treatment failed to show a survival difference in those receiving early treatment [18]. In summary, these trials support a conservative treatment strategy for most patients with early-stage disease. For advanced or symptomatic patients, several treatment options are available depending on performance status and patient preference. These options include conventional chemotherapy with fludarabine-based regimens, single agent chlorambucil, monoclonal antibodies targeting CD20, and bruton's tyrosine kinase inhibitors (e.g., ibrutinib). In general, the traditional paradigm for dealing with CLL surrounds treating patients who have become symptomatic or have disease-related cytopenias. Potential symptoms indicating treatment include severe fatigue, persistent "B" symptoms, progressive lymphadenopathy, hepatosplenomegaly, autoimmune hemolytic anemia, idiopathic thrombocytopenic purpura, and paraneoplastic complications.

Treating Asymptomatic, Early-Stage CLL/SLL

Approximately 25% of newly diagnosed CLL patients will have asymptomatic, early-stage disease. The standard of care in these patients is observation rather than immediate treatment. A meta-analysis of over 2,000 Rai stage I or II patients evaluated immediate versus delayed treatment and found that 10-year overall survival rates did not differ between the two options (44% versus 47%) [18]. This approach, however, may change as researchers discover additional genetic mutations affecting treatment response and overall survival.

During the observation period, routine blood counts at three-month intervals are recommended along with standard clinical examinations. After the first 12 months of observation, a doubling time can be calculated and a clear clinical decision regarding their disease progression can be made. In addition, symptomatology can also be assessed. If patients become symptomatic or if their absolute lymphocyte count doubled in the past 12 months, treatment initiation may be recommended.

For patients with localized SLL, involved-field radiation alone may be preferred to systemic chemotherapy or observation. Unfortunately, no prospective clinical trials have compared radiation therapy to chemotherapy or observation in localized SLL. As SLL is similar to indolent non-Hodgkin lymphoma, data was extrapolated from these patients, showing radiation therapy as a preferred option in localized disease. The NCCN guidelines recommend a watch-and-wait approach unless they become symptomatic or experience progressive cytopenias [13].

Treating Symptomatic or Advanced CLL/SLL

For patients with symptomatic or high-risk CLL/SLL, treatment should be offered to help ameliorate symptoms and lengthen overall survival. Pre-treatment evaluation including staging, performance status, patient preference, and comorbidities are recommended prior to initiating therapy. There is currently no preferred treatment regimen for patients with symptomatic or advanced CLL/SLL. Therapeutic options are numerous and may include chemotherapy, monoclonal antibodies, tyrosine kinase inhibitors, lenalidomide, and allogeneic bone marrow transplantation. Current NCCN guidelines recommend several category 1 options for first line treatment.

Table 7. First-line therapy in CLL

Age <65 and otherwise healthy	Age ≥65 or younger with significant comorbidities	Frail patient with comorbidities
Fludarabine + Cyclophosphamide + Rituximab (FCR)*	Chlorambucil + Obinutuzumab*	Chlorambucil + Obinutuzumab*
Bendamustine ± CD20 MAB	Ibrutinib*	Ibrutinib*
Ibrutinib	Bendamustine ± CD20 MAB	Chlorambucil + Rituximab or Ofatumumab

*NCCN Category I recommendation.

Chlorambucil has been a staple CLL option for decades and remains a viable chemotherapeutic option in combination with anti-CD20 monoclonal antibody therapy. More specifically, chlorambucil in combination with obinutuzumab is a first-line option for treating elderly patients or younger patients with significant comorbidities. A study evaluated 781 symptomatic patients with comorbidities and found that the combination of chlorambucil/obinutuzumab resulted in superior improvement in progression-free survival compared to rituximab monotherapy or chlorambucil monotherapy (27 months versus 16 months versus 11 months, respectively) [19]. Grade 3 or higher toxicities included neutropenia (35%), hypersensitivity reactions (21%), thrombocytopenia (11%), and infections (11%). Based on this trial, NCCN lists combination chlorambucil and obinutuzumab as a category 1 recommendation for elderly patients or younger individuals with significant comorbidities.

Ibrutinib (Imbruvica®) is an orally administered irreversible inhibitor of Bruton's tyrosine kinase approved by the Food and Drug Administration (FDA) in 2014 for the treatment of relapsed/refractory CLL. It also gained FDA approval in 2015 as first-line therapy in patients with chromosome 17p deletion. Ibrutinib potently inhibits Bruton's tyrosine kinase, which serves as an integral component of the cell-signaling pathway. Inhibition of this pathway reduces malignant B cell survival and results in a decreased B cell proliferation rate. Historically, chlorambucil was the treatment of choice for elderly patients or those with significant comorbidities. The RESONATE-2 trial evaluated 269 elderly CLL treatment-naïve patients who received either ibrutinib daily until progression or chlorambucil as initial therapy [20]. Ibrutinib resulted in significantly longer progression-free survival than the chlorambucil arm (median, not reached versus 18.9 months). Ibrutinib also led to significant improvements in overall survival at 24 months

(98% versus 85%) and response rates (86% versus 35%). Another phase III clinical trial compared ibrutinib to ofatumumab, a CD20-directed monoclonal antibody, and found overall response rates (43% versus 4.1%) and 12-month overall survival (90% versus 81%) were significantly improved with ibrutinib [21]. Overall, ibrutinib is a fairly well tolerated treatment option with some noteworthy toxicities including bleeding, liver dysfunction, diarrhea, fatigue, and vomiting. Ibrutinib is also a cytochrome P450 substrate and is contraindicated in patients taking strong inhibitors or inducers of CYP3A4. The current NCCN recommendations place ibrutinib as a category 1 agent in all CLL patients requiring treatment [13]. Additional prospective studies are required for younger patients without del(17q) or TP53 mutations.

Fludarabine-based regimens are commonly employed in younger CLL patients with few, if any, significant comorbidities. One frequently used regimen includes fludarabine, cyclophosphamide, and rituximab (FCR) which was studied in a large, international, phase III clinical trial evaluating FCR against fludarabine and cyclophosphamide [22]. The FCR regimen resulted in higher response rates (90% versus 80%) and longer progression-free survival (57 months versus 33 months). Prolonged neutropenia is a common complication in FCR requiring careful monitoring and consideration. Other concerning toxicities with FCR include infectious complications, infusion reactions, nausea/vomiting, hemorrhagic cystitis, infertility, leukemogenesis, and alopecia. FCR is the preferred treatment option for younger patients with standard risk CLL [13].

Bendamustine-based combinations are an acceptable alternative to FCR or chlorambucil/obinutuzumab in older patients with comorbidities. Compared to FCR, bendamustine is well tolerated but with slightly worse response rates (38% versus 47%) and 2-year progression-free survival (78% versus 85%). However, when compared to chlorambucil, bendamustine with rituximab (BR) demonstrated superior response rates [23].

Chlorambucil-based regimens are an alternative to ibrutinib therapy in elderly and/or frail patients with comorbidities. Furthermore, older patients at high risk for bleeding or those taking anticoagulants should consider chlorambucil over ibrutinib due to the bleeding risk inherent with ibrutinib therapy. Combination chlorambucil and obinutuzumab result in significantly higher response rates and progression-free survival but this efficacy benefit must be weighed against the higher rates of treatment-related complications such as infusion reactions and myelosuppression. Obinutuzumab is an anti-CD20 monoclonal antibody that stimulates cell death via actin reorganization, homotypic adhesion, and complement-dependent cytotoxicity. When compared to the original anti-CD20 monoclonal antibody, rituximab, obinutuzumab in combination with chlorambucil showed superior overall response rates (78% versus 65%) and progression-free survival (27 months versus 15 months) and is therefore preferred to chlorambucil/rituximab therapy [24].

Ofatumumab is another anti-CD20 monoclonal antibody with an FDA approved indication in CLL. The COMPLEMENT-1 trial evaluated 447 adults with treatment-naïve CLL not eligible for fludarabine-based treatment randomized to ofatumumab plus chlorambucil or chlorambucil alone [25]. Combination therapy with ofatumumab resulted in higher overall response rates (82% versus 69%), longer progression-free survival (22 months versus 13 months) and better duration of response (22 months versus 13 months). However, both regimens exhibited similar overall survival at 3 years (85% versus 83%). Infusion reactions were common in the ofatumumab group (67%) despite pre-medication. Both groups lost 13% of patients due to adverse events leading to study withdrawal.

Lenalidomide monotherapy was shown in the CLLM1 study to be an effective maintenance option following initial therapy [26]. This trial evaluated 89 patients with a poor outcome following first-line chemoimmunotherapy. A poor outcome was described as minimal residual disease levels $\geq 10^{-2}$ or $\geq 10^{-4}$ to 10^{-2} with either an unmutated IGHV, 17p deletion or TP53 mutation. Lenalidomide was compared to placebo and greater progression-free survival rates were seen with maintenance lenalidomide. Larger prospective trials are currently needed to substantiate these findings and the NCCN currently offers maintenance lenalidomide therapy for these high risk patients as a viable option [13].

Treating Relapsed/Refractory CLL

Following initial therapy, CLL patients are followed at routine intervals to monitor for disease relapse and late-effects of chemotherapy. Relapse is defined as disease recurrence following a partial or complete disease remission that lasted at least six months. Refractory CLL occurs when the patient fails to achieve a partial or complete remission following initial therapy. Relapse patients, particularly those with late relapses following years of disease-free status, are much more likely to experience successful retreatment than patients who are refractory to initial therapy. Confirmatory evaluation needs to be completed including a physical exam, complete blood count with differential, and flow cytometry before the patient officially has relapsed/refractory disease.

Once the diagnosis is confirmed, treatment options should be considered if the patient is symptomatic with active disease. Treatment may include chemoimmunotherapy with similar regimens as initial therapy, namely FCR or BR. Other viable options include targeted therapy with oral Bruton's tyrosine kinase inhibitors such as ibrutinib. Similar to initial treatment decisions, finding the most appropriate salvage regimen depends on patient desires, clinician comfort, financial constraints, performance status, genetic abnormalities, and co-morbidities. In addition to these elements, clinicians should also consider the quality and duration of initial response. With early relapses or refractory disease, patients may be considered to have aggressive disease requiring a more aggressive approach. The average time to progression with initial FCR is approximately 57 months [27]. Combination BR has a median progression-free-survival of approximately 34 months and chlorambucil with obinutuzumab showed a time to progression of 27 months [28, 29]. Patients receiving these regimens who relapsed before the median PFS interval or those who relapsed within two to three years of treatment initiation are considered to have "early relapse" and preference should be given to novel targeted therapy rather than conventional chemoimmunotherapy.

The resonate clinical trial compared the safety and efficacy of ibrutinib to ofatumumab monotherapy in 391 patients with relapsed/refractory disease [30]. Ibrutinib significantly improved overall response rates (90% versus 25%), progression-free survival (76% versus 8%) at 18 months, and overall survival (86% versus 77%) at 18 months. Even patients with historically poor cytogenetic abnormalities, del(17p) or del(11q) experienced benefit while on ibrutinib monotherapy.

Idelalisib is a small molecule oral inhibitor of phosphoinositide 3'-kinase delta (PI3Kδ), which is highly expressed in malignant B cells. Inhibition of PI3Kδ results in apoptosis of the malignant clone by interfering with the PI3Kδ-AKT signaling pathway. Idelalisib 150 mg twice daily is the FDA approved dose for relapsed/refractory CLL. One clinical trial evaluated idelalisib and rituximab with rituximab and placebo in relapsed/refractory patients [31]. This phase III study found the idelalisib group displayed superior overall response rates (81% versus 13%), 12-month overall survival (92% versus 80%), and progression-free survival. Black box warnings for idelalisib include severe diarrhea, colitis, pneumonitis, intestinal perforation, and hepatotoxicity. Additionally, idelalisib is metabolized by cytochrome P450 3A4 and has the potential to interact with strong inducers or inhibitors. Idelalisib has also shown the potential to exacerbate infectious risks in relapse/refractory CLL patients and therefore warrants close evaluation and consideration prior to initiation. Anti-infective prophylaxis for herpes simplex virus, pneumocystis jirovecii pneumonia, and cytomegalovirus reactivation are encouraged for all patients on idelalisib therapy [13].

Venetoclax is an orally available small molecule inhibitor of the BCL-2 protein which is overexpressed in CLL and contributes to tumor cell survival and chemotherapy resistance. Venetoclax is titrated over 5 weeks from 20 mg daily to a maintenance dose of 400 mg daily that's administered until disease progression or unacceptable toxicity. Venetoclax was FDA approved in 2016 and is currently indicated for CLL/SLL patients with or without del(17p) who have failed at least one prior therapy. The MURANO trial evaluated 389 patients with relapsed or refractory CLL who were randomly assigned to two years of venetoclax plus six month of rituximab or six months of bendamustine plus rituximab [33]. The venetoclax arm resulted in higher progression-free survival (85%

versus 36%) and overall survival (92% versus 87%) at two years. Venetoclax and rituximab showed higher rates of grade 3 or 4 neutropenia and tumor lysis syndrome occurred in 3.1% of patients. Diarrhea, anemia, thrombocytopenia, nausea, fatigue, and respiratory tract infections were also commonly noted.

Table 8. Treatment regimens for relapsed/refractory CLL

Age <65 and otherwise healthy	Older patients or those with significant comorbidities
Preferred Treatment Options	Preferred Treatment Options
Ibrutinib	Ibrutinib
Idelalisib + rituximab	Idelalisib + rituximab
Venetoclax + rituximab	Venetoclax + rituximab
Alternative Treatment Options	Alternative Treatment Options
Acalabrutinib	Acalabrutinib
Bendamustine + rituximab	Chlorambucil + rituximab
FCR	Reduced-dose FCR
Idelalisib or venetoclax monotherapy	Idelalisib or venetoclax monotherapy
Obinutuzumab	Obinutuzumab

CLL = chronic lymphocytic leukemia; FCR = fludarabine, cyclophosphamide, rituximab.

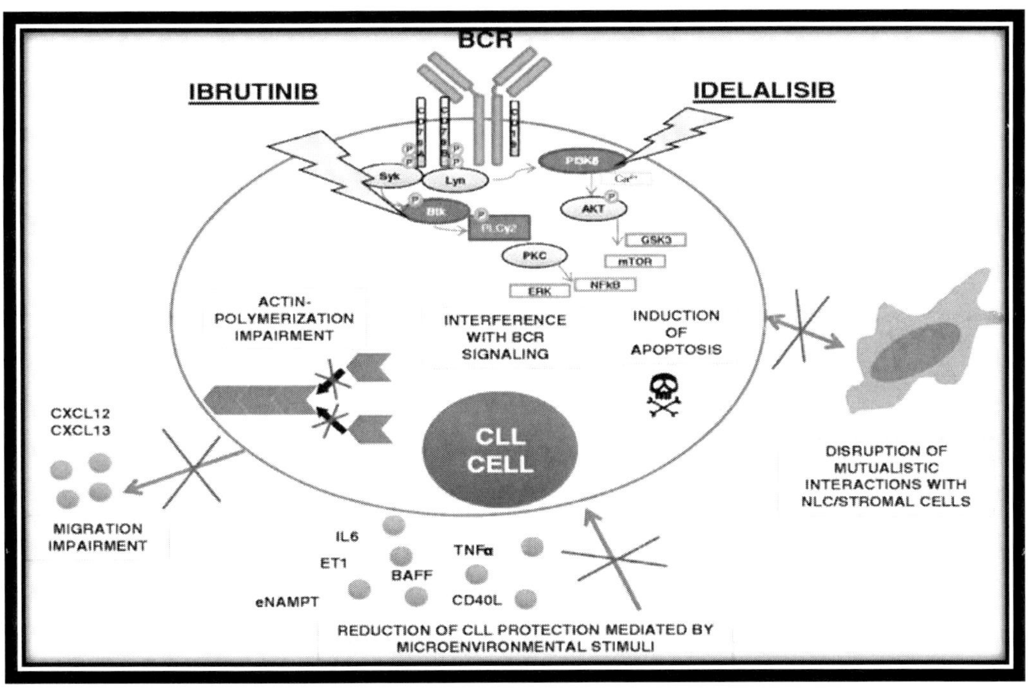

Ibrutinib and Idelalisib interfer with the B-cell receptor (BCR) signaling cascade by inhibiting the bruton's tyrosine kinase (Btk) and PI3Kδ molecules, respectively. Both agents induce pro-apoptotic signaling, leading to cell death.

Figure 2. Mechanisms of Action in CLL for Ibrutinib and Idelalisib [32].

Along with the preferred treatment options for relapsed/refractory CLL mentioned above, several other regimens exist and have shown efficacy following initial disease progression. These regimens include fludarabine-based therapy, bendamustine-based therapy, anti-CD20-based therapy, chlorambucil-based therapy, and allogeneic HSCT. The median age at diagnosis for CLL is 72 years, making bone marrow transplantation relatively uncommon due to the frequently occurring treatment-related complications. This treatment, however, is the only possible cure for patients with CLL/SLL. For younger patients with more aggressive disease, transplant eligibility should be evaluated especially with those fostering high-risk genetic factors such as chromosome 11 and 17 abnormalities.

Richter's Transformation

First described in 1928 by Maurice Richter, CLL may develop into an aggressive large-cell lymphoma often categorized as diffuse large B cell lymphoma. Estimated incidence of Richter's transformation is 2% to 9% with a median time to progression from initial CLL/SLL diagnosis between two to four years [34]. The acquisition of new cytogenetic abnormalities and the loss of common CLL immunophenotypic features helps explain the histologic evolution into a diffuse lymphoma. The development of a Richter's transformation is a poor prognostic factor with few patients experiencing long-term survival. Standard treatment following a Richter's transformation is dependent on the histologic lymphoma subtype, patient preference, performance status, and previous treatment.

CONCLUSION

CLL is a chronic lymphoproliferative disorder resulting in the accumulation of malignant and malfunctioning B cells. CLL is currently the most common leukemia diagnosed in adults and is generally considered to be incurable. CLL is a heterogeneous disease with varying outcomes; however, most patients will progress from an indolent disease to a more aggressive phenotype with the potential to undergo a Richter's transformation. The Rai or Binet staging systems are often used to group patients based on their overall prognosis with flow cytometry and FISH aiding the initial stratification. Patients with asymptomatic, early-stage disease do not require active treatment but instead should be routinely monitored until symptoms occur or the disease becomes more aggressive. Numerous genetic abnormalities are thought to drive the development and progression of CLL including del(17p) and TP53 mutations. Chemoimmunotherapy is the standard first-line therapy for most CLL/SLL patients depending on their age, performance status, and cytogenetic profile.

REFERENCES

[1] Swerdlow SH, Campo E, Harris NL, et al. *WHO Classification of Tumours of Haematopoietic and Lymphoid Tissues.* 2008 IARC Press, Lyon.

[2] Siegel RL, Miller KD, Jemal A. Cancer statistics, 2018. *CA Cancer J Clin* 2018;68:7-30.

[3] Noone AM, Howlader N, Krapcho M, et al. *SEER Cancer Statistics Review*, 1975-2015, National Cancer Institute. Bethesda, MD, https://seer.cancer.gov/csr/1975_2015/, based on November 2017 SEER data submission, posted to the SEER web site, May 2018.

[4] Goldin LR, Pfeiffer RM, Li X, et al. Familial risk of lymphoproliferative tumors in families of patients with chronic lymphocytic leukemia: results from the Swedish Family-Cancer Database. *Blood* 2004;104(6):1850–1854.

[5] Mauro FR, Giammartini E, Gentile M, et al. Clinical features and outcome of familial chronic lymphocytic leukemia. *Haematologica* 2006;91(8):1117–1120.

[6] Schubauer-Berigan MK, Daniels RD, Fleming DA, et al. Chronic lymphocytic leukaemia and radiation: findings among workers at five US nuclear facilities and a review of the recent literature. *Br J Haematol* 2007;139(5):799.

[7] Hallek M, Cheson BD, Catovsky D, et al. Guidelines for the diagnosis and treatment of chronic lymphocytic leukemia: a report from the International Workshop on Chronic Lymphocytic Leukemia updating the National Cancer Institute-Working Group 1996 guidelines. *Blood* 2008;111(12):5446.

[8] Rawstron AC, Bennett FL, O'Connor SJ, et al. Monoclonal B-cell lymphocytosis and chronic lymphocytic leukemia. *N Engl J Med* 2008; 359:575–583.

[9] Rai KR, Sawitsky A, Cronkite EP, et al. Clinical staging of chronic lymphocytic leukemia. *Blood* 1975;46(2):219.

[10] Binet, JL, Auquier A, Dighiero G, et al. A new prognostic classification of chronic lymphocytic leukemia derivedfrom a multivariate survival analysis. *Cancer* 1981;48:198–206.

[11] Rai KR. A critical analysis of staging in CLL. In: Chronic Lymphocytic Leukemia: Recent Progress and future Direction. *1987 UCLA Symposia on Molecular and Cellular Biology, New Series,* Vol. 59. Gale RP, Rai KR (Eds). Alan R Liss, New York 1987. p. 253.

[12] Damle RN, Wasil T, Fais F, et al. Ig V gene mutation status and CD38 expression as novel prognostic indicators in chronic lymphocytic leukemia. *Blood* 1999;94:1840-1847.

[13] *The NCCN Clinical Practice Guidelines in Oncology™ Chronic Lymphocytic Leukemia* (Version 5.2018). National Comprehensive Care Network, Inc. Available at: www.NCCN.org. Accessed May 28, 2018.

[14] Dohner H, Stilgenbauer S, Benner A, et al. Genomic aberrations and survival in chronic lymphocytic leukemia. *N Engl J Med* 2000;343:1910-1916.

[15] Oscier D, Wade R, Davis Z, et al. Prognostic factors identified three risk groups in the LRF CLL4 trial, independent of treatment allocation. *Haematologica* 2010;95:1705-1712.

[16] International CLL-IPI working group. An international prognostic index for patients with chronic lymphocytic leukaemia (CLL-IPI): a meta-analysis of individual patient data. *Lancet Oncol* 2016;17(6):779.

[17] Goede V, Cramer P, Busch R, et al. Interactions between comorbidity and treatment of chronic lymphocytic leukemia: Results of German Chronic Lymphoctyic Leukemia Study Group Trials. *Haematologica* 2014;99:1095-1100.

[18] Chemotherapeutic options in chronic lymphocytic leukemia: a meta-analysis of the randomized trials. CLL Trialists' Collaborative Group. *J Natl Cancer Inst* 1999;91(10):861-868.

[19] Goede V, Fischer K, Busch R, et al. Obinutuzumab plus chlorambucil in patients with CLL and coexisting conditions. *N Eng J Med* 2014;370:1101-1111.

[20] Burger JA, Tedeschi A, Barr PM, et al. Ibrutinib as initial therapy for patients with chronic lymphocytic leukemia. *N Engl J Med* 2015;373(25):2425-2437.

[21] Byrd JC, Brown JR, O'Brien S; RESONATE Investigators. Ibrutinib versus ofatumumab in previously treated chronic lymphocytic leukemia. *N Eng J Med* 2014;371:213–223.

[22] Fischer K, Bahlo J, Fink AM, et al. Long-term remissions after FCR chemoimmunotherapy in previously untreated patients with CLL: Updated results of the CLL8 trial. *Blood* 2016;127:208-215.

[23] Knauf WU, Lissitchkov T, Aldaoud A, et al. Bendamustine compared with chlorambucil in previously untreated patients with chronic lymphocytic leukemia: updated results of a randomzed phase III trial. *Br J Haematol* 2012;159(1):67-77.

[24] Goede V, Fischer K, Busch R, et al. Obinutuzumab plus chlorambucil in patients with CLL and coexisting conditions. *N Engl J Med* 2014;370(12):1101.

[25] Hillmen P, Tadeusz R, Jannsens A, et al. Chlorambucil plus ofatumumab versys chlorambucil alone in previously untreated patients with chronic lymphocytic leukemia. *Lancet* 2015;385(9980):1873-1883.

[26] Fink AM, Bahlo J, Robrecht S, et al. Lenalidomide maintenance after first-line therapy for high-risk chronic lymphocytic leukaemia (CLLM1): final results from a randomised, double-blind, phase 3 study. *Lancet Haematol* 2017;4:e475-e486.

[27] Fischer K, Bahlo J, Fink AM, et al. Long-term remissions after FCR chemoimmunotherapy in previously untreated patients with CLL: updated results of the CLL8 trial. *Blood* 2016;127(2):208-215.

[28] Fischer K, Cramer P, Busch R, et al. Bendamustine in combination with rituximab for previously untreated patients with chronic lymphocytic leukemia: a multicenter phase II trial of the German Chronic Lymphocytic Leukemia Study Group. *J Clin Oncol* 2012 Sep;30(26):3209-3216.

[29] Goede V, Fischer K, Busch R, et al. Obinutuzumab plus chlorambucil in patients with CLL and coexisting conditions. *N Engl J Med* 2014;370(12):1101.

[30] Brown JR, Hillmen P, O'Brien S, et al. Extended follow-up and impact of high-risk prognostic factors from the phase 3 RESONATE study in patients with previously treated CLL/SLL. *Leukemia* 2018;32(1):83. Epub 2017.

[31] Furman RR, Sharman JP, Coutre SE, et al. Idelalisib and rituximab in relapsed chronic lymphocytic leukemia. *N Eng J Med* 2014;370:997–1007.

[32] Maffei R, Fiorcari S, Martinelli S, et al. Targeting neoplastic B cells and harnessing microenvironment: the "double face: of ibrutinib and idelalisib. *J Hematol Oncol* 2015;8:60.

[33] Seymour JF, Kipps TJ, Eichhorst B, et al. Venetoclax-Rituximab in Relapsed or Refractory Chronic Lymphocytic Leukemia. *N Engl J Med* 2018;378(12):1107.

[34] Tsimberidou AM, Keating MJ. Richter syndrome: biology, incidence, and therapeutic strategies. *Cancer* 2005;103(2):216.

In: Frontiers in Leukemia Pharmacotherapy
Editor: Lunawati L. Bennett
ISBN: 978-1-53614-960-9

Chapter 12

PEDIATRIC ACUTE MYELOID LEUKEMIA

Zachery R. Halford*, PharmD
Union University, College of Pharmacy, Jackson, Tennessee, US

ABSTRACT

Acute leukemias are the most frequently occurring pediatric malignancy, accounting for nearly 1 out of every 3 childhood cancers. Compared to adult cancers, childhood leukemia is a rare occurrence with only 4,824 new cases expected in 2018. Pediatric acute myeloid leukemia (AML) is even less common, with approximately 800 new cases per year in the United States. The 5-year overall survival rate for pediatric AML is 66% for children and adolescents younger than 15 years. Standard treatment for AML includes intensive chemotherapy, lasting 6 to 12 months, with or without allogeneic hematopoietic stem cell transplantation (HSCT). The goal of AML treatment involves obtaining a complete remission (CR) followed by eradication of minimal residual disease (MRD).

This chapter evaluates the epidemiology, etiology, pathogenesis, clinical signs and symptoms, diagnosis, prognostic factors, staging, risk stratification, and treatment options for pediatric AML. Current and future therapies with some discussion on historical aspects of treating acute leukemias are emphasized and explored. Several clinical trials are discussed along with their implications on managing acute childhood leukemia.

Keywords: children, pediatric, acute myeloid leukemia, cytopenias, induction, consolidation, hematopoietic stem cell transplantation, FLT3

* Corresponding Author Email: zhalford@uu.edu.

ABBREVIATIONS

ALL	acute lymphocytic leukemia
AML	acute myeloid leukemia
APL	acute promyelocytic leukemia
ATO	arsenic trioxide
ATRA	all-trans retinoic acid
CNS	central nervous system
COG	Children's Oncology Group
DIC	disseminated intravascular coagulopathy
DS	Down syndrome
FAB	French-American-British
FDA	Food and Drug Administration
FISH	fluorescence in situ hybridization
FLAG	fludarabine, cytarabine, filgrastim regimen
FLT3	FMS-like tyrosine kinase 3 ligand
HiDAC	high-dose cytarabine
HSCT	hematopoietic stem cell transplantation
MLL	mixed lineage leukemia
MRD	minimal residual disease
PCR	polymerase chain reaction
PML-RARA	promyelocytic leukemia/retinoic acid receptor alpha
t-AML	treatment-related acute myeloid leukemia
TMD	transient myeloproliferative disorder
WBC	white blood cell
WHO	World Health Organization

INTRODUCTION

Acute leukemias make up nearly 30% of all childhood malignancies, making them the most frequently diagnosed pediatric cancer in the United States. AML accounts for only 20% of childhood acute leukemias with approximately 800 cases each year [1]. Unlike adult patients, children are rarely diagnosed with chronic leukemias and the vast majority of leukemia cases are of the acute variety.

Acute leukemia is characterized by a malignant proliferation of immature hematopoietic cells that accumulate in the bone marrow and frequently result in pancytopenia. Both AML and acute lymphoblastic leukemia (ALL) are heterogeneous diseases with various subtypes based on morphological and cytogenetic features.

Despite substantial progress in the treatment of AML over the past several decades, nearly 40% of patients will die from either disease recurrence or treatment-related complications. Survival improvements stemmed from advances in risk stratification, MRD identification, targeted therapy, allogeneic HSCT, and management of supportive care needs.

EPIDEMIOLOGY

Among children 15 and younger, leukemia is the most frequently diagnosed malignancy with ALL occurring roughly four times as frequently as AML. While ALL is often diagnosed between the ages of 2 and 4 years, AML peak incidence in children occurs at 1 to 2 years of age with a nadir around 9 years before progressing upwards again as patients reach adulthood. The incidence of AML is estimated to be approximately seven cases per million people per year in the United States. Over the past two decades, epidemiological studies showed no significant increase or decline in overall incidence of AML [1]. Caucasians are less likely to develop AML than African American children (4.8 million versus 5.8 million cases per million) and Hispanic children carry the highest incidence. Pediatric AML often occurs *de novo* and is rarely preceded by myelodysplastic syndrome. Only 10% of AML cases are M3 (acute promyelocytic leukemia) with promyelocytic leukemia – retinoic acid receptor alpha (PML-RARA) gene positivity. Children with trisomy are at significantly higher risk of developing acute leukemia, with some studies showing a 20-fold increase in risk [2]. Leukemogenesis in Down syndrome is associated with the development of somatic mutations involving the GATA1 gene, an X-linked transcription factor essential for cellular differentiation and maturation [3]. Other genetic disorders are also associated with an increased risk for developing AML, including Blood syndrome, Fanconi anemia, Blackfan-Diamond anemia, neurofibromatosis, and Noonan syndrome [4].

Siblings of children affected with leukemia are at a two- to four-fold increase of acquiring an acute leukemia in the first decade of life compared to children without affected siblings. When leukemia occurs in an identical twin, the sibling has a 20% chance of also acquiring the leukemia. This risk is even greater when the identical twin develops leukemia within the first year of life. Twins with concordant leukemia have been identified through various molecular studies. This phenomenon may result from chimeric fusion gene development *in utero* [5].

Etiology and Pathogenesis

Most cases of pediatric AML arise in children with no known genetic predisposition or relevant family history. Evidence exists linking leukemia to genetic mutations affecting ploidy and chromosomal structural integrity including translocations, inversions, point mutations and deletions. A few discernable etiological factors have been identified with leukemogenesis; however, most cases of acute leukemia in children are lacking recognizable etiologic causes and are considered spontaneous [6]. Several potential associations exist between leukemia and magnetic field exposure, early infection, and parenteral use of medications and illicit drugs, but most data emanates from small case-reports requiring further research. Ionizing radiation and chemical exposure with mutagenic agents are known risk factors in the development of leukemia. For example, survivors of the Nagasaki and Hiroshima atomic bombs experienced a 20-fold increase in leukemia incidence. Following this exposure, the peak incidence of leukemia occurred between 6 to 8 years and remained elevated for the next 20 years compared to unexposed individuals [7]. An assortment of chemical exposures have been associated with leukemogenesis, including benzene, herbicides and pesticides, and petroleum products.

Treatment-related AML (t-AML) is often associated with regimens containing topoisomerase II inhibitors, a known genotoxin, with some studies showing rates of t-AML as high as 12% in patients treated for ALL with high cumulative doses of etoposide [8]. Children exposed to leukemogenic agents such as cyclophosphamide, ifosfamide, etoposide, melphalan, and chlorambucil have an increased risk of developing a secondary leukemia, with a peak incidence of 4 to 5 years after initial treatment, but some cases were reported as far out as 10 years [8].

Genome-wide mapping showed pediatric AML patients have less genetic alterations than those with other malignancies. Fortunately, these studies did identify a few novel lesions worthy of consideration and exploration – mainly mutations in IDH1 and IDH2, which occur in up to 10% of cases [9]. Infant leukemia is a particularly troublesome leukemia subtype resulting from the mixed lineage leukemia (MLL) gene occurring in 5% to 10% of all pediatric leukemia cases and 60% to 70% of all infant cases [10]. Germ-line mutations have recently been discovered in several genes, including TP53, GATA2, CEBPA, and RUNX1, indicating a familial predisposition to AML development [11]. Moreover, AML is a highly molecularly diverse and heterogeneous disease with a multitude of distinct chromosomal alterations. It appears that some cases of AML require only a single cytogenetic irregularity, but most complete leukemic transformations require a series of genetic mutations.

Epigenetic lesions, such as promoter silencing through hypermethylation, are frequently gaining traction as important components in the development of AML. Furthermore, epigenetic changes controlling histone, DNA methylation, and nucleosome positioning are commonly mutated in both myeloid and lymphoid malignancies and are potential therapeutic targets requiring further research.

Clinical Presentation

Children with acute leukemia may present with various signs and symptoms consistent with anemia, thrombocytopenia, and/or neutropenia and reflect the depth and breadth of leukemic burden. Pallor, fatigue, fever, gingival bleeding, ecchymoses, infection, and petechiae are common manifestations of early leukemia [12]. Persistent fevers occur in one-third of patients and likely result from pyrogen release from the leukemic cells or macrophages/lymphocytes attacking the leukemic blast. Fevers may also result from ongoing infectious complications. The severity of cytopenias is dependent on the degree to which leukemic cells have overtaken the bone marrow and oppressed normal hematopoiesis. Bone pain, arthralgia, and myalgia are also common due to leukemic infiltration [12]. Extramedullary involvement may include the spleen, liver, lymph nodes, and central nervous system (CNS). Hepatosplenomegaly occurs in roughly half of all new AML patients with lymphadenopathy, leukemia cutis, and gingival hypertrophy also occurring from leukemic infiltration. Unlike ALL, testicular involvement is rare in AML. Patients diagnosed with AML will frequently have elevated lactate dehydrogenase levels accompanied by hyperuricemia and/or hyperphosphatemia. Only 2% to 5% of AML patients will initially test positive for leukemic blasts within the cerebral spinal fluid [12]. Disseminated intravascular coagulopathy (DIC) can occur in certain AML subtypes, especially in acute promyelocytic leukemia (M3). Tumors containing AML blasts may arise in a variety of anatomical sites. These chloromas may occur in the orbit or periorbital regions leading to ptosis.

Hyperleukocytosis and leukostasis occur when the peripheral WBC count reaches levels greater than 100,000 to 200,000/mL. The leukemic cells occlude normal blood flow throughout the vasculature and result in an accumulation of blast cells in the small vessels causing tissue hypoxia, infarction, and hemorrhaging. Hyperleukocytosis is an oncologic emergency requiring immediate medical attention. Tumor lysis syndrome is another oncologic emergency frequently associated with AML and high WBC counts. Hyperuricemia, hyperkalemia, hyperphosphatemia, and hypocalcemia are all metabolic derangements resulting from the destruction of leukemic blasts.

Diagnosis and Disease Classification

AML is a heterogeneous disease with various morphological, immunophenotypic, and genetic abnormalities [13]. A bone marrow biopsy is required for leukemic blast analysis using a combination of morphology, immunophenotyping, cytogenetic, cytochemical, and molecular evaluations. The historic French-American-British (FAB) classification system incorporating M0 through M7 subtypes has mostly been replaced with the World Health Organization's (WHO) classification system incorporating karyotype and molecular abnormalities [13]. The WHO classification system does not provide classifications for specific infant AML subtypes that can occur with the following known genetic alterations: *HLXB9-MNX1*, t(11;12)(p15;p13)/*NUP98-KDM5A* and t(1;22)(p13;q13)/*RBM15-MKL1*. AML is distinguished from ALL by cytochemistry and immunophenotyping typically conducted as soon as possible. Fluorescence in situ hybridization (FISH) helps determine the FAB subtype augmented with polymerase chain reaction (PCR) to detect translocations, fusion genes, or chromosomal deletions. Patients with suspected extramedullary disease should have radiographic evaluations completed for the concerning site(s). CNS involvement requires confirmatory cytologic evaluation including the presence of leukemia cells within the cerebrospinal fluid.

Table 1. World Health Organization classification of AML [13]

AML with recurrent genetic abnormalities
AML with t(8;21)(q22;q21);RUNX1-RUNX1T1 AML with inv(16)(p13.1q22) or t(16;16)(p13.1;q22);CBFB-MYH11 APL with PML-RARA AML with t(9;11)(p21.3;q23.3);MLLT3-KMT2A AML with t(6;9)(p23;q34.1);DEK-NUP214 AML with inv(3)(q21.3q26.2) or t(3;3)(q21.3;q26.2); GATA2, MECOM AML (megakaryoblastic) with t(1;22)(p13.3;q13.3);RBM15-MKL1 AML with BCR-ABL1 (provisional entity) AML with mutated NPM1 AML with biallelic mutations of CEBPA AML with mutated RUNX1 (provisional entity)
AML with myelodysplasia-related changes
Therapy-related myeloid neoplasms
AML, not otherwise specified
AML with minimal differentiation AML without maturation AML with maturation Acute myelomonocytic leukemia Acute monoblastic/monocytic leukemia Pure erythroid leukemia Acute megakaryoblastic leukemia Acute basophilic leukemia Acute panmyelosis with myelofibrosis
Myeloid sarcoma
Myeloid proliferations related to Down syndrome
Transient abnormal myelopoiesis Myeloid leukemia associated with Down syndrome

AML = acute myeloid leukemia.

PROGNOSIS AND RISK STRATIFICATION

Historically, AML stratification revolved around morphologic and cytogenetic features. More recently, however, initial response to induction therapy and MRD status were incorporated into risk stratification protocols. No consensus exists for risk stratification of pediatric AML, with various cooperative groups using differing criteria for favorable, intermediate and high-risk classification. Multiple recurring mutations exist in pediatric AML, several of which have prognostic implications requiring analysis for full diagnostic evaluation. Risk stratification plays an important role in selecting appropriate treatment protocols.

Favorable risk AML includes patients with inv(16)/t(16;16), t(8;21) cytogenetic features, NPM or CEBPα mutation regardless of monosomy 7, monosomy 5, or del5q and regardless of MRD at end of induction I. Other favorable risk AML includes negative MRD ($< 0.1\%$) at the end of induction I with no high-risk features.

Intermediate risk AML includes cases lacking cytogenetic or molecular abnormalities that would classify the patient as either favorable or high risk. The most important risk factor for these patients involves their initial response to induction chemotherapy and MRD status following induction therapy using flow cytometry. If MRD positive, these patients become high-risk and carry a significantly worse overall prognosis, with approximately 60% of patients relapsing [14]. The Children's Oncology Group (COG) categorizes AML patients without any poor or favorable molecular markers as favorable risk.

High risk AML can arise from several distinct molecular or cytogenetic abnormalities. FMS-like tyrosine kinase 3 ligand (FLT3) positivity, presence of monosomy 7, monosomy 5, or del(5q) result in a poor prognosis. FLT3 activating mutation is one of the most commonly occurring somatic abnormalities found in pediatric AML, with nearly 10% to 15% of patients testing positive. Other high-risk features include evidence of residual AML (MRD $\geq 0.1\%$) at end of induction I or clinical or radiographic evidence of progressive extramedullary disease [15].

TREATMENT OVERVIEW

Treatment goals include obtaining a CR followed by full eradication of the leukemic clone while minimizing potential acute and long-term complications. The pillars of AML treatment include high-dose multi-agent chemotherapy and aggressive supportive care. Prior to 1970, AML cure rates were abysmal and disheartening. As researchers began grasping basic concepts for successfully treating ALL in the 1950s and 1960s, these principles were carried over to the smaller pediatric AML population. Induction chemotherapy followed by cranial radiation and prolonged maintenance were initially trialed in the 1970s. Researchers quickly learned that shorter treatment durations without cranial radiation or prolonged maintenance could provide CR and long-term survival in 25% of AML patients [16]. Dose-intensification, risk stratification, and HSCT have since increased long-term survival rates. Pediatric AML patients now have cure rates of 50% to 60% [17-25]. Unfortunately, conventional AML treatment come at a significant cost, resulting in various short- and long-term complications. Current treatment includes remission-induction chemotherapy followed by post-remission consolidation and, in some cases, allogeneic HSCT.

Treatment for pediatric AML usually consists of two courses of intensive induction chemotherapy using multi-agent regimens followed by either cytarabine-based post-remission consolidation or allogeneic HSCT. According to the U.S. National Library of Medicine (www.clinicaltrials.gov), there are currently 28 recruiting or soon-to-be-recruiting clinical trials for pediatric AML in the United States. Patients and parents should be encouraged to consider enrolling in a clinical trial whenever possible.

Induction

Once AML is confirmed, induction therapy should be initiated. The goal of induction therapy is to obtain a CR with high-dose, multi-agent chemotherapy. A CR is defined as the presence of < 5% blasts within the bone marrow in conjunction with trilineage hematopoietic recovery and no signs or symptoms of extramedullary disease. Recent protocols incorporate minimal residual disease into remission status and base treatment progression on the resulting levels. Standard Induction chemotherapy involves concomitant anthracycline (daunorubicin, doxorubicin, idarubicin, or mitoxantrone) with cytarabine. Some pediatric protocols enlist etoposide as a third leukemocidal agent. Complete remission rates following these regimens range from 70% to 90% in pediatric patients [17-25]. Most induction protocols will incorporate two courses of induction therapy typically completed over two to three months. Depending on the patient's initial risk stratification, treatment might be more intense for those with high-risk disease than patients with favorable risk factors. Most protocols require sequential cycles of induction chemotherapy. Remission status assessment typically follows the second induction course of chemotherapy. Assessing initial response is an important component of AML treatment with significant prognostic implications. Children with detectable disease following induction therapy are nearly 5 times more likely to relapse than those with a favorable induction response [15].

Induction chemotherapy is intense and requires routine hospitalization for significant stretches of time, with some patients requiring prolonged admissions lasting weeks to months. The extended period of pancytopenia is classic for pediatric AML treatment and poses significant risks for infection and bleeding. In addition, chemotherapy often damages the gastrointestinal tract, along with other organs, leading to an increase in vulnerability to infections. Aggressive supportive care measures are a critical component of total care in these highly susceptible patients.

Dose-intensification, risk stratification, early identification, rapid diagnosis, and improved supportive care have all helped to improve remission rates in pediatric AML. Although the standard cytarabine, anthracycline, and now etoposide regimens remain successful, a great deal of room exist for improvement and refinement [26]. Most notably, no targeted treatment currently provides a survival benefit when given as part of induction therapy. Perhaps this will change with the Children Oncology Group (COG) AAML1031 study evaluating up-front bortezomib and sorafenib for certain patient populations (NCT#01371981, NSC#681239).

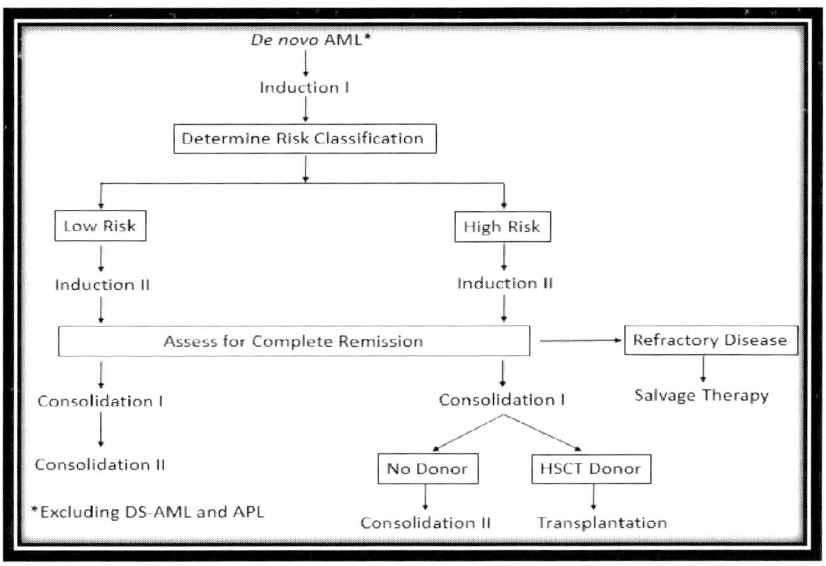

AML = acute myeloid leukemia; APL = acute promyelocytic leukemia; DS = Down syndrome; HSCT = hematopoietic stem cell transplant.

Figure 1. Example Treatment Schema for Pediatric AML.

Table 2. Example induction regimen [26]

Drug	Dose	Schedule
Cytarabine	100 mg/m^2/dose IV every 12 hours OR 3.3 mg/kg/dose IV every 12 hours for those <0.6 m^2	Days 1-10
Daunorubicin	50 mg/m^2/dose IV OR 1.7 mg/kg/dose for those < 0.6 m^2	Days 1, 3, 5
Etoposide	100 mg/m^2/dose IV OR 3.3 mg/kg/dose for those < 0.6 m^2	Days 1-5

Table 3. Clinical trials in pediatric AML [17-25]

Study	Patients (n)	CR (%)	Overall Survival (%)	Event-Free Survival (%)	HSCT Available
AIEOP	161	79	42	25	Yes
EORTC-58872	108	77	56	41	No
LAME-91	268	90	60	48	No
BFM-87	307	75	49	41	No
NOPHO 93	219	91	64	49	Yes
POG 9421	565	90	53	36	No
AML-BFM 2004	521	-	74	55	No
AML-2002	482	87	67	55	Yes
AAML03P1	340	83	66	53	Yes
MRC AML 2004	564	90	63	54	Yes

AML = acute myeloid leukemia; CR = complete remission; HSCT = hematopoietic stem cell transplant.

Post-Remission Consolidation

Without post-remission consolidative therapy, nearly all pediatric patients with AML will succumb to their aggressive disease. Therefore, following both induction courses, patients will then receive additional intensive chemotherapy to consolidate and maintain disease remission. Optimal consolidation therapy has yet to be determined but most current regimens utilize high-dose cytarabine (HiDAC) with or without subsequent allogeneic HSCT. In patients not receiving transplantation, post-remission treatment lasts for nearly 6 months with most protocols. For patients with high-risk AML, an allogeneic HSCT might be the best option for obtaining a long-term remission and avoiding disease recurrence. Unfortunately, even with aggressive allogeneic HSCT, these high-risk patients do poorly with 5-year overall survival rates around 40% to 50% [27].

An important question pertaining to post-remission consolidation surrounds the ideal number of chemotherapy cycles for pediatric AML patients. Studies have suggested that one or two cycles is all that is required prior to undergoing a bone marrow transplantation; however, not all patients will be transplant eligible. Gibson et al. suggests three consolidation cycles are no better than two, with no difference noted in event-free survival or overall survival [25]. Results suggest a ceiling of benefit with conventional high-dose chemotherapy and highlight a need for novel agents that target specific cytogenetic abnormalities.

Post-consolidation maintenance therapy was not shown to be efficacious in pediatric AML, except for those with the M3 subtype requiring ATRA. The POG-8101 study incorporated a 2-year maintenance schedule and found no difference between two different maintenance regimens [28]. Furthermore, the LAME-89 trial used 18 months of maintenance therapy and found patients receiving maintenance had significantly lower overall survival rates than those who did not receive post-consolidation maintenance [19].

Allogeneic Hematopoietic Stem Cell Transplant

Bone marrow transplant is an appealing option for AML patients because it offers several potential benefits, including dose-intensification as well as graft-versus-leukemia effect. Unfortunately, treatment-related morbidity and mortality following allogeneic HSCT are real and present dangers requiring close monitoring and long-term management. Frequently identified complications following allogeneic transplantation are direct organ damage to the liver, kidneys, lungs, skin, and gastrointestinal tract. Furthermore, long-term effects include graft-versus-host-disease, growth delays, sterility, and increased rate of secondary malignancies.

The ideal bone marrow transplantation is with a syngeneic donor; however, this is a rare occurrence and most clinicians are eager to find an HLA-matched sibling donor. Without a sibling donor, matched unrelated donors are still useful and encouraged, with some studies showing little to no difference in long-term survival [29, 30]. These studies are somewhat antiquated, as improvements in supportive care and graft-versus-host-disease management have significantly changed over the last 10 to 20 years. Randomized trials using biologic randomization have consistently shown matched related donors improve long-term outcomes compared to intensive chemotherapy regardless of risk stratification. Therefore, some investigators will offer HSCT to all AML patients when a matched sibling donor is available. Other investigators will not recommend allogeneic HSCT in lower risk patients and reserve this option only for disease relapse. The optimal timing for undergoing HSCT remains unknown and requires further elucidation. Aside from this controversy, most clinicians agree that allogeneic transplantation should be offered in very-high risk AML (monosomy 5 or 7, del (5q), 3q abnormalities, acute megakaryoblastic leukemia without the t(1;22)/*OTT-MAL)* and those with poor initial response to induction therapy.

Table 4. Example consolidation regimen [26]

Drug	Dose	Schedule
High-Dose Cytarabine (HiDAC)	1000 mg/m^2/dose IV every 12 hours OR 33 mg/kg/dose IV every 12 hours for those <0.6 m^2	Days 1 - 5
Etoposide	150 mg/m^2/dose IV OR 5 mg/kg/dose for those < 0.6 m^2	Days 1 - 5

Haploidentical transplantation, where one parent is the stem cell donor, continues remains an experimental option. Autologous HSCT avoids graft-versus-host-disease and provides for dose-intensification, but currently appears less efficacious, even when considering treatment-related complications, than allogeneic transplantation. The immune-mediated anti-leukemic effect following allogeneic HSCT appears to play a major role in producing superior event-free and overall survival benefits.

CNS-Directed Therapy

Pediatric patients with AML, including those without detectable CNS disease, should receive prophylactic CNS-directed therapy using intrathecal chemotherapy throughout the induction and consolidation phases. Common intrathecal chemotherapy includes cytarabine, methotrexate, and/or hydrocortisone. CNS involvement occurs in 5% to 10% of pediatric AML patients at diagnosis and is not considered a poor risk factor due to early identification and effective CNS-penetrating agents such as high-dose cytarabine. For those without detectable CNS disease, single-agent cytarabine is the most frequently utilized agent, with each treatment cycle requiring one intrathecal dose. Some institutions, including St. Jude's Research Hospital, found superior treatment outcomes with triple intrathecal therapy when compared to single-agent cytarabine [31]. Cytarabine is dosed based on patient age, with a range of 20 mg up to 70 mg. Intrathecal chemotherapy is preferred over cranial radiation due to fewer late-effects, including secondary malignancies, growth deficits, and cognitive disabilities.

Acute Promyelocytic Leukemia (APL)

APL is a biologically and genetically distinct subtype of AML and confers excellent long-term outcomes due to differentiation therapy such as all-trans retinoic acid (ATRA) and arsenic trioxide (ATO). A hallmark cytogenetic abnormality found in APL is the PML-RARA fusion protein that results from a translocation of the 15th and 17th chromosome. This fusion protein represses transcriptional activity, thus inhibiting cellular maturation and differentiation. The discovery of differentiation agents revolutionized APL treatment, with most pediatric patients experiencing CR and event-free survival rates of 95% and 75%, respectively [32]. With the inclusion of ATRA and ATO, APL is the most curable form of AML in both adults and children. See the APL chapter for more information.

AML and Down Syndrome

Children with Down syndrome (DS) have a ~20-fold increased risk of acquiring an acute leukemia compared to children without DS [2, 33]. Infants with DS are also at an increased risk for developing transient myeloproliferative disorder (TMD), which looks and acts like acute megakaryoblastic leukemia (M7). Children with DS have a 400-fold increase in risk for developing M7 AML. Fortunately, most DS patients who develop TMD will experience a spontaneous resolution without any treatment. For the 25% of DS patients who do not experience resolution of TMD and require treatment, chemotherapy is the preferred option.

Interestingly, patients with DS-associated AML display superior results following treatment than children without DS, possibly due to leukemic cells of DS-AML showing an increased sensitivity to cytarabine and daunorubicin therapy compared to other children [34]. Because of this increased chemotherapy sensitivity, these DS-AML patients experience excellent outcomes without intensive chemotherapy. One multicenter trial evaluated 204 patients with DS-AML who received less intense chemotherapy than standard protocols. Five-year event free and overall survival rates were 90% and 93%, respectively, which is significantly better than your average pediatric AML patient [34]. Also of note, patients with DS have higher rates of treatment-related complications and cannot typically tolerate standard AML regimens due to profound cytopenias and cardiotoxicity. Therefore, cooperative treatment groups, such as the COG, have created specific treatment protocols for patients with DS-AML.

Supportive Care

As previously mentioned, AML patients are at significant risk of acquiring disease- and/or treatment-associated complications. Anticipatory measures are critical for prolonging life and ensuring appropriate supportive care during and following intensive chemotherapy treatment. Upon initial diagnosis, patients with AML are at significant risk for developing tumor lysis syndrome, leukostasis, disseminated intravascular coagulopathy, and infectious complications. Improvements in supportive care have helped reduce early death rates in acute leukemias to approximately 2% [35]. AML patients are frequently at risk for developing severe infections secondary to the profound and prolonged neutropenia characteristic of intensive chemotherapy. Bacterial, fungal, and viral infections are all possible pathogens in this population. Following chemotherapy, bacteria can translocate into the blood stream through mucosal barrier disruptions. Streptococci is a common pathogen in AML due to heightened risk with HiDAC therapy and prolonged neutropenia [36]. Pediatric patients with AML have a 25% chance of developing streptococcal shock syndrome and acute respiratory distress syndrome. No consensus exists on prophylactic antibiotics in this patient population.

With increasing rates of long-term survival following treatment for pediatric AML, researchers are beginning to take note of important late-effects resulting from treatments such as etoposide, anthracyclines, and allogeneic transplantation. Most current AML protocols use 300 to 400 mg/m^2 of cumulative anthracycline dosing which results in cardiac complications in 3% to 5% of patients [37]. Therefore, AML patients require routine echocardiographic evaluation during and following anthracycline treatment. In addition, secondary neoplasms occur in approximately 1.7% of pediatric AML patients [38]. The COG published Long-Term Follow-Up Guidelines for survivors of childhood, adolescent and young adult cancers, outlining specific monitoring requirements for pediatric patients. These guidelines provide recommendations for screening and managing late-effects that potentially arise following treatment for childhood cancer. They also serve to raise awareness of potential long-term complications and standardize the follow-up care survivors receive. These guidelines (www.survivorshipguidelines.org) are useful not only for the oncologist but also for primary care physician who may be responsible for care years after the patient completes therapy.

Relapsed/Refractory AML

Unfortunately, up to 30% of pediatric AML patients will relapse following initial treatment and only 33% of these relapsed patients will experience long-term survival following subsequent therapy. These poor survival rates are exacerbated in specific patients with high-risk features. For patients relapsing within a year of initial treatment, survival rates are less than 20% [39]. Patients with relapsed or refractory disease typically respond poorly to subsequent chemotherapy and experience shorter remissions. There is no current standard for treating relapsed or refractory AML, most studies demonstrate that high-dose cytarabine regimens are useful in obtaining a subsequent remission. Cytarabine will frequently be given in combination with mitoxantrone, fludarabine, or etoposide. Some clinicians prefer the FLAG regimen containing fludarabine, cytarabine, and filgrastim. Some institutions will also incorporate idarubicin along with FLAG to produce a more durable remission at the risk of increased toxicity [40]. Regardless of the chemotherapy regimen selected, long-term survival rates are poor and allogeneic HSCT should be used whenever possible to help improve disease-free survival. Significant improvements are needed for this patient population and long-term survival rates remain poor with few groundbreaking therapies on the horizon.

FUTURE THERAPIES

Next-generation sequencing helps interrogate AML and provide a better understanding of the various genetic and epigenetic abnormalities in pediatric AML. This deeper understanding may produce future molecular targets that can be exploited using novel agents. An excellent example of this concept is the FLT3 mutation identified as one of the first genomic lesions found in pediatric AML. This mutation is now targetable using FLT3-inhibitors. Several small trials have evaluated sorafenib, quizartinib, midostaurin, and lestaurtinib in AML with mixed results [41-44]. A first-generation FLT3-inhibitor, midostaurin, showed benefit and second-generation agents seek to build on that promise. FLT3 remains an important target in AML due to its relative frequency and poor outcomes. Additional studies are required to further investigate this molecular target.

CPX-351 is a liposomal-encapsulated combination of daunorubicin and cytarabine approved in 2017 by the FDA for the treatment of newly diagnosed therapy-related AML or AML with myelodysplasia-related changes. In a phase III clinical trial in older patients (60-75 years old), CPX-351 was compared to the traditional "7+3" regimen and researchers found higher rates of overall survival with CPX-351 [45]. This novel formulation has yet to be studied in pediatric patients but future COG studies will likely evaluate its role in pediatric AML.

Gemtuzumab ozogamicin is an antibody-drug conjugate targeting CD33 initially approved for treating relapsed/refractory acute leukemias. The surface antigen CD33 is found on the majority of pediatric AML patients and is thought to be a poor prognostic indicator [26]. Pediatric studies showed gemtuzumab ozogamicin to be a safe and potentially efficacious option in combination with conventional chemotherapy. Future COG studies plan to incorporate Gemtuzumab ozogamicin in upfront therapy to help improve survival rates in high-risk patients.

CONCLUSION

Acute leukemia is the most commonly diagnosed malignancy in children, with AML occurring in approximately 20% of leukemia cases. Most AML cases are considered spontaneous with no known precipitating factors. Overall survival rates for acute leukemias have risen across the board over the last several decades but significant improvements are still required for several common subtypes of childhood AML. Common presenting signs and symptoms include persistent fevers, lethargy, hepatosplenomegaly, infections, and bleeding. An initial workup typically reveals anemia and thrombocytopenia while WBC counts may be suppressed, normal, or elevated. Other potential complications include tumor lysis syndrome, disseminated intravascular coagulopathy, and hyperleukocytosis. A bone marrow biopsy is required for initial diagnosis along with pathologic review of the morphology, immunohistochemistry, and molecular abnormalities.

Following diagnosis, treatment should commence as soon as possible with remission induction chemotherapy for two sequential cycles typically involving cytarabine, anthracycline, and etoposide. Once a CR is confirmed and MRD evaluated, patients can embark on post-remission consolidation therapy for two to three cycles depending on risk stratification and institutional protocol. Children with AML should be treated on a clinical trial whenever possible to augment current care and improve future therapy. Allogeneic HSCT is a preferred option for certain AML populations, especially in those with matched sibling donors with high-risk features. CNS prophylaxis with intrathecal chemotherapy is a standard treatment component and is given throughout induction and consolidation. Children with Down syndrome or APL (M3) do exceptionally well compared to other AML subtypes due to their unique biological characteristics that significantly affect prognosis and available treatment options.

Despite improving cure rates, with some low-risk AML patients experiencing long-term survival rates of 70%, outcomes for children with unfavorable cytogenetic features and those with refractory disease remain poor. Additional treatment options targeting specific genetic abnormalities are required in the future to help overcome chemotherapy resistance and disease progression. Patients receiving AML treatment with intensive chemotherapy are extremely susceptible to short- and long-term complications and require close monitoring and excellent supportive care.

REFERENCES

[1] Noone, AM; Howlader, N; Krapcho, M; et al. *SEER Cancer Statistics Review, 1975-2015*, National Cancer Institute. Bethesda, MD, https://seer.cancer.gov/csr/1975_2015/, based on November 2017 SEER data submission, posted to the SEER web site, April 2018.

[2] Xavier, AC; Taub, JW. Acute leukemia in children with Down syndrome. *Haematologica*, 2010, 95, 1043-1045.

[3] Wechsler, J; Greene, M; McDevitt, MA; et al. Acquired mutations in GATA1 in the megakaryoblastic leukemia of Down syndrome. *Nat Genet*, 2002, 32(1), 148-52.

[4] Bhatia, S; Neglia, JP. Epidemiology of childhood acute myelogenous leukemia. *J Pediatr Hematol Oncol*, 1995, 17, 94-100.

[5] Maia, AT; Ford, AM; Jalali, GR; et al. Molecular tracking of leukemogenesis in a triplet pregnancy. *Blood*, 2001, 98, 478-482.

[6] Spector, LG; Ross, JA; Robison, LL; Bhatia, S. Epidemiology and etiology. Pui CH *Childhood leukemias.* 2nd ed. 2006; Cambridge University Press Cambridge, UK 48-66.

[7] Kato, I; Tajima, K; Hirose, K; et al. A descriptive epidemiological study of hematopoietic neoplasms in Japan. *Jpn J Clin Oncol*, 1985, 15, 347–364.

[8] Smith, MA; Rubinstein, L; Ungerleider, RS. Therapy-related acute myeloid leukemia following treatment with epipodophyllotoxins: estimating the risk. *Med Pediatr Oncol*, 1994, 23(2), 86-98.

[9] Andersson, AK; Miller, DW; Lynch, JA; et al. IDH1 and IDH2 mutations in pediatric acute leukemia. *Leukemia.*, 2011, 25(10), 1570-1577.

[10] Biondi, A; Cimino, G; Pieters, R; Pui, CH. Biological and therapeutic aspects of infant leukemia. *Blood*, 2000, 96, 24-33.

[11] Owen, C; Barnett, M; Fitzgibbon, J. Familial myelodysplasia and acute myeloid leukaemia—A review. *Br. J. Haematol.*, 2008, 140, 123–132.

[12] Rubnitz, JE; Gibson, B; Smith, FO. Acute myeloid leukemia. *Hematol Oncol Clin North Am*, 2010, 24, 35-63.

[13] Arber, DA; Orazi, A; Hasserjian, R; et al. The 2016 revision to the World Health Organization classification of myeloid neoplasms and acute leukemia. *Blood*, 2016, 127, 2391-2405.

[14] Loken, MR; Alonzo, TA; Pardo, L; et al. Residual disease detected by multidimensional flow cytometry signifies high relapse risk in patients with de novo acute myeloid leukemia: a report from Children's Oncology Group. *Blood.*, 2012 Aug, 120(8), 1581-8.

[15] Sievers, EL; Lange, BJ; Alonzo, TA; et al. Immunophenotypic evidence of leukemia after induction therapy predicts relapse: results from a prospective Children's Oncology Group study of 252 patients with acute myeloid leukemia. *Blood*, 2003, 101, 3398-2406.

[16] Kersey, JH. Fifty years of studies of the biology and therapy of childhood leukemia. *Blood*, 1997, 90, 4243–4251.

[17] Amadori, S; Testi, AM; Arico, M; et al. Prospective comparative study of bone marrow transplantation and postremission chemotherapy for childhood acute myelogenous leukemia. The Associazione Italiana Ematologia ed Oncologia Pediatrica Cooperative Group. *J Clin Oncol*, 1993, 11, 1046–1054.

[18] Behar, C; Suciu, S; Benoit, Y; et al. Mitoxantrone-containing regimen for treatment of childhood acute leukemia (AML) and analysis of prognostic factors: results of the EORTC Children Leukemia Cooperative study 58872. *Med Pediatr Oncol*, 1996, 26, 173–179.

[19] Perel, Y; Auvrignon, A; Leblanc, T; et al. Impact of addition of maintenance therapy to intensive induction and consolidation chemotherapy for childhood acute

myeloblastic leukemia: results of a prospective randomized trial, LAME 89/91. Leucamie Aique Myeloide Enfant. *J Clin Oncol*, 2002, 20, 2774–2782.

[20] Creutzig, U; Ritter, J; Zimmermann, M; et al. Improved treatment results in high-risk pediatric acute myeloid leukemia patients after intensification with high-dose cytarabine and mitoxantrone: results of Study Acute Myeloid Leukemia-Berlin-Frankfurt-Munster 93. *J Clin Oncol*, 2001, 19, 2705–2713.

[21] Stine, KC; Becton, D; Van Houten, G; et al. Genetic randomization to allogeneic bone marrow transplant in first remission pediatric acute myeloid leukemia patients, Pediatric Oncology Group 9421. *Blood*, 004, 104, 178a.

[22] Creutzig, U; Zimmermann, M; Bourquin, JP; et al. Randomized trial comparing liposomal daunorubicin as induction for pediatric acute myeloid leukemia; results from Study AML-BFM 2004. *Blood.*, 2013, Jul 4, 122(1), 37-43.

[23] Pession, A; Masetti, R; Rizzari, C; et al. Results of the AIEOP AML 2002/01 multicenter prospective trial for the treatment of children with acute myeloid leukemia. *Blood.*, 2013, Jul 11, 122(2), 170-8.

[24] Cooper, TM; Franklin, J; Gerbing, RB; et al. AAML03P1, a pilot study of the safety of gemtuzumab ozogamicin in combination with chemotherapy for newly diagnosed childhood acute myeloid leukemia: A report from the Children's Oncology Group. *Cancer*, 2012, 118, 761–769.

[25] Gibson, BE; Webb, DK; Howman, AJ; et al. Results of a randomized trial in children with Acute Myeloid Leukaemia: medical research council AML12 trial. *Br J Haematol*, 2011 Nov, 155(3), 366-76.

[26] Gamis, AS; Aplenc, R; Alono, T; et al. Gemtuzumab ozogamicin (GO) in children with de novo acute myeloid leukemia (AML), improves event-free survival (EFS) by reducting relapse risk-results from the randomized phase III Children's Oncology Group (COG) trial, AAML0531. *Blood*, 2013, 122(21), 355.

[27] Kelly, MJ; Horan, JT; Alonzo, TA; et al. Comparable survival for pediatric acute myeloid leukemia with poor-risk cytogenetics following chemotherapy, matched related donor, or unrelated donor transplantation. *Pediatr Blood Cancer*, 2014, Feb, 61(2), 269-75.

[28] Steuber, CP; Civin, C; Krischer, J; et al. A comparison of induction and maintenance therapy for acute nonlymphocytic leukemia in childhood: results of a Pediatric Oncology Group study. *J Clin Oncol*, 1991, 9, 247–258.

[29] Mayer, RJ; Davis, RB; Schiffer, CA; et al. Intensive postremission chemotherapy in adults with acute myeloid leukemia. Cancer and Leukemia Group B. *N Engl J Med*, 1994, 331, 896–903.

[30] Mayer, RJ. Intensive chemotherapy versus allogeneic bone marrow transplantation in first remission acute myeloid leukemia. *Bone Marrow Transplant*, 1990, 6[Suppl 6], 48–51.

[31] Rubnitz, JE; Inaba, H; Dahl, GV; et al. Minimal residual disease-directed therapy for childhood acute myeloid leukemia: results of the AML02 multicenter trial. *Lancet Oncol*, 2010, 11, 543-552.
[32] Mann, G; Reinhardt, D; Ritter, J; et al. Treatment with all-trans retinoic acid in acute promyelocytic leukemia reduces early deaths in children. *Ann Hematol*, 2001, 80, 417–422.
[33] Rabin, KA; Whitlock, JA. Malignancy in children with trisomy 21. *Onologist*, 2009, 14(2), 164-173.
[34] Taub, JW; Berman, JN; Hitzler, JK; et al. Improved outcomes for myeloid leukemia of Down syndrome: a report from the Children's Oncology Group AAML0431 trial. *Blood*, 2017, 129(25), 3304.
[35] Pui, CH; Carroll, WL; Meshinchi, S; Arceci, RJ. Biology, risk stratification, and therapy of pediatric acute leukemias: an update. *J Clin Oncol*, 2011, 29, 551-565.
[36] Gamis, AS; Howell, WB; DeSwarte-Wallace, J; et al. Alpha hemolytic streptococcal infection during intensive treatment for acute myeloid leukemia: a report from the Childrens cancer group study CCG-2891. *J Clin Oncol*, 2000, 18(9), 1845-1855.
[37] Creutzig, U; Diekamp, S; Zimmermann, M; et al. Longitudinal evaluation of early and late anthracycline cardiotoxicity in children with AML. *Pediatr Blood Cancer*, 2007 Jun, 48(7), 651-62.
[38] Mulrooney, DA; Dover, DC; Li, S; et al. Twenty years of follow-up among survivors of childhood and young adult acute myeloid leukemia: a report from the Childhood Cancer Survivor Study. *Cancer*, 2008, 112(9), 2071-9.
[39] Sander, A; Zimmerman, M; Dworzak, M; et al. Consequent and intensified relapse therapy improved survival in pediatric AML: results of relapse treatment in 379 patients of three consecutive AML-BFM trials. *Leukemia*, 2010, 24(8), 1422-1428.
[40] Virchis, A; Koh, M; Rankin, P; et al. Fludarabine, cytosine arabinoside, granulocyte-colony stimulating factor with or without idarubicin in the treatment of high risk acute leukaemia or myelodysplastic syndromes. Br. *J Haematol*, 2004, 124, 26–32.
[41] Cheuk, Him Man; Tsz, Kan Fung; Christa, Ho; et al. Sorafenib treatment of FLT3-ITD+ acute myeloid leukemia: favorable initial outcome and mechanisms of subsequent nonresponsiveness associated with the emergence of a D835 mutation. *Blood*, 2012, 119, 5133-5143.
[42] Smith, BD; Levis, M; Beran, M; et al. Single-agent CEP-701, a novel FLT3 inhibitor, shows biologic and clinical activity in patients with relapsed or refractory acute myeloid leukemia. *Blood*, 2004, 103, 3669-3676.
[43] Fischer, T; Stone, RM; Deangelo, DJ; et al. Phase IIB trial of oral midostaurin (PKC412), the FMS-like tyrosine kinase 3 receptor (FLT3) and multi-targeted kinase inhibitor, in patients with acute myeloid leukemia and high-risk

myelodysplastic syndrome with either wild-type or mutated FLT3. *J Clin Oncol*, 2010, 28, 4339-4345.

[44] Cortes, JE; Kantarjian, H; Foran, JM; et al. Phase I study of quizartinib administered daily to patients with relapsed or refractory acute myeloid leukemia irrespective of FMS-like tyrosine kinase 3-internal tandem duplication status. *J Clin Oncol*, 2013, 31, 3681-3687.

[45] Lancet, JE; Uy, GL; Cortes, JE; et al. Final results of a phase III randomized trial of CPX-351 versus 7+3 in older patients with newly diagnosed high risk (secondary) AML. *J Clin Oncol*, 2016, 34, 7000.

In: Frontiers in Leukemia Pharmacotherapy
Editor: Lunawati L. Bennett
ISBN: 978-1-53614-960-9

Chapter 13

PEDIATRIC ACUTE LYMPHOBLASTIC LEUKEMIA

Zachery R. Halford**, PharmD
and Danya Horchi
Union University, College of Pharmacy, Jackson, Tennessee, US

ABSTRACT

Acute lymphoblastic leukemia (ALL), the most common childhood malignancy, results from a series of mutational events occurring primarily in precursor lymphoblasts preventing maturation and normal hematopoiesis. ALL is a genetically diverse disease typically manifesting with signs and symptoms consistent with anemia, thrombocytopenia, and neutropenia. Significant progress has been made over the past 50 years in the identification, diagnosis, risk stratification, treatment, and overall management of these patients. Cure rates for pediatric ALL is 80% to 90%. Advances in genomic and epigenomic screening has improved our understanding of childhood leukemia and provides insights into potential targetable lesions.

This chapter aims to highlight the epidemiology, etiology, pathogenesis, diagnosis, disease classification, prognostic factors, and general treatment approach for pediatric patients with acute lymphoblastic leukemia. Emerging treatment options will also be discussed for patients with relapsed and/or refractory disease.

Keywords: acute lymphoblastic leukemia, cytogenetics, cytopenias, induction, consolidation, maintenance, bone marrow transplantation, Philadelphia chromosome, tyrosine kinase inhibitors, pediatrics, chimeric antigen receptor, bispecific t-cell engager

* Corresponding Author Email: zhalford@uu.edu.

Abbreviations

6-MP	6-mercaptopurine
ALL	acute lymphocytic leukemia
AML	acute myeloid leukemia
ANC	absolute neutrophil count
AYA	adolescents and young adults
BiTE	bispecific T-cell-engager
CAR-T	chimeric antigen receptor t-cells
CD	cluster of differentiation
CNS	central nervous system
CR	complete remission
DIC	disseminated intravascular coagulopathy
FDA	Food and Drug Administration
FISH	fluorescence in situ hybridization
HSCT	hematopoietic stem cell transplantation
LBL	lymphoblastic lymphomas
MRD	minimal residual disease
MPAL	mixed phenotype acute leukemia
NCCN	National Comprehensive Cancer Network
PCR	polymerase chain reaction
Ph^+	Philadelphia chromosome positive
SEER	Surveillance, Epidemiology and End Results program
TDT	terminal deoxytransferase
TKI	tyrosine kinase inhibitor
TPMT	thiopurine S-methyltransferase
URD	unrelated donor
WBC	white blood cell
WHO	World Health Organization

Introduction

ALL is a heterogeneous hematological disorder characterized by immature blood cell proliferation within the bone marrow. These immature cells, known as lymphoblasts, become invasive and suppress normal hematopoiesis. This suppression of normal cell growth leads to a disruption of the bone marrow, often resulting in anemia, thrombocytopenia, and neutropenia [1]. Leukemia accounts for nearly 1 out of 3 pediatric malignancies, making it the most common cancer in childhood. Among the different types of leukemia, acute lymphocytic leukemia (ALL) is the most prominent, accounting for 3 out of 4 pediatric leukemia diagnoses [2]. Acute myeloid leukemia (AML) is the second most common form of leukemia in children and adolescents, with approximately 1 out of 5 childhood leukemias being AML [2]. While the peak age of ALL diagnosis is between 1 and 4 years, ALL can also occur in adults [3, 4]. Despite similar incidences, long-term survival between children and adults differs significantly with pediatric survival rates near 90% compared to approximately 40% in adults [3]. The survival rate in children has increased dramatically over the last several decades. For instance, survival rates in 1975 were only 60% [4]. A series of survival improvements resulted from chemotherapy optimization, CNS-directed treatment, hematopoietic stem cell transplantation (HSCT), risk stratification, supportive care measures, and novel targeting agents [4]. Following the first reports of disease remission in 1948, pediatric ALL has become a beacon of hope within the oncology world as survival rates skyrocketed from near-zero to over 90% today.

History

In the early 1900s, children with ALL had little hope for survival; however, over the past seventy years, many remarkable researchers have pioneered various treatment strategies resulting in overall survival rates of 90%. Dr. Sidney Farber, an American pediatric pathologist, is considered the "father of modern chemotherapy" for his fight against ALL in the mid-twenieth century [7-9]. In 1948, Farber and his team used a folic acid antagonist to induce a "temporary remission" in 10 out of 16 evaluable children [5]. Farber is also the founder of the Children's Hospital Cancer Research Foundation [6].

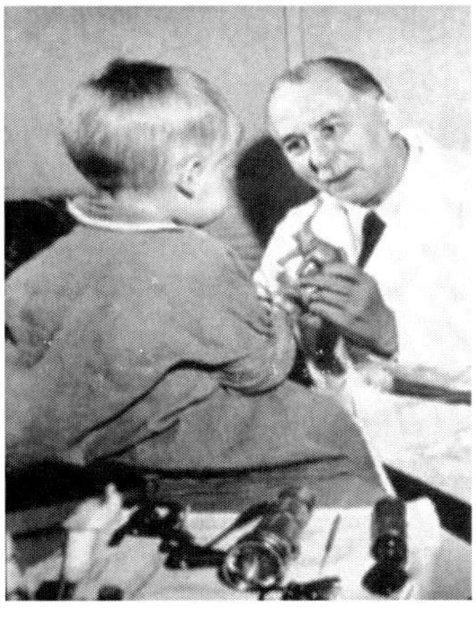

Sidney Farber, M.D. is considered the "father of chemotherapy" due to his work with folic acid antagonists to fight leukemia. Courtesy of the National Institutes of Health.

In 1961, Emil Frei III fortified Farber's breakthrough with a combination of mercaptopurine and methotrexate to achieve a CR rate of 59% and a 2-year survival rate of 20% in patients [7]. Despite these monumental discoveries, ALL continued to be fatal in the majority of patients until 1962 when St. Jude Children's Research Hospital was established and Donald Pinkel commenced "total therapy" for select ALL patients [8]. Total therapy is a curative approach consisting of remission induction, central nervous system (CNS)-directed therapy (including cranial irradiation and intrathecal methotrexate), intensification therapy, and continuation treatment. These four components of therapy continue to be the pillar of ALL treatment today. With this approach, one study found there was an estimated 50% cure rate among their 35 patients [9]. During the 1970s, only ten years after Pinkel's initial trials, two studies found that intensification therapy following remission-induction could advance cure rates to nearly 70% [10, 11]. More recently, ALL pathobiology, the various mechanisms of drug resistance, and the nature of antileukemic drugs are better understood leading to improved individualized care. ALL can now be classified according to specific genetic factors and abnormalities with the use of genome and transcription sequencing. Completion of full genomic sequencing should further elucidate the underlying pathogenesis of leukemia and guide future therapy to push ALL cure rates closer to 100%. An emerging challenge will be to identify patients who may require less intensive treatment, therefore sparing them from untoward short- and long-term chemotherapy complications.

EPIDEMIOLOGY

Acute leukemias, although rare, possess the highest rate of cancer-related mortality in children less than 20 years of age [4]. Acute leukemias account for 97% of all childhood leukemias [4]. In 2018, ALL will represent about 0.3% of all new cancer cases within the United States; however, this equates to 5,960 new cases and 1,470 deaths from ALL [2]. From 2011-2015, over 55% of ALL cases were children less than 20 years of age, while 14.5% of deaths were children <20 years of age. Males are more likely than females to be diagnosis with ALL. Hispanic children appear more likely to develop ALL than African American or Caucasian children [2]. Adult patients with ALL fare significantly worse than their pediatric counterparts in terms of long-term survival (40% versus 90%) [2, 4]. The disparity in long-term survival between adults and children is multifactorial. Adults who acquire acute leukemias tend to be older with complicated comorbidities, and therefore unable to receive intensive chemotherapy required for optimal leukemic eradication. In addition, adult patients also appear to experience significant genetic mutations leading to aggressive and potentially chemotherapy-resistant disease [3].

Etiology

While there is no known cause of ALL, several correlating risk factors are currently being investigated. Most likely, the development of acute leukemia is multifactorial, involving a complex interplay of genetic, environmental, infectious, immunologic, and socioeconomic factors. Genetically, there are several syndromes associated with ALL, including Bloom Syndrome, Down syndrome, Diamond-Blackfan anemia, Fanconi anemia, Noonan syndrome, and Klinefelter syndrome, among others. These cancer predisposition syndromes are increasingly recognized through advances in next-generation sequencing technology, which help identify germline mutations early and facilitate critical discussion and monitoring for those at risk. Siblings of those with leukemia have a four times greater risk of occurrence than those without siblings with leukemia. Known environmental toxins include ionizing radiation, herbicides and pesticides, in utero exposure to contraceptives, cigarettes, drugs, alcohol, coffee, cola, and contaminated water [12]. Exposure to Epstein-Barr virus (EBV) and Human T-lymphocyte virus (HTLV-1 and HTLV-2) also have a strong link to ALL [13]. Alkylating agents, anthracyclines, and epipodophyllotoxins are all commonly used chemotherapy agents showing a propensity to cause secondary cancer, within 5-10 years of exposure [14].

Pathogenesis and Pathologic Features

Normal hematopoiesis is a dynamic and intricate process controlled by various growth factors and nuclear transcription factors that activate specific gene sequences. The development of leukemia results when a series of genetic mutations occur, resulting in alterations of regulatory processes [15]. ALL is characterized by clonal lymphoid cells with genetic defects leading to altered maturation and cessation of hematopoietic differentiation. These alterations in hematopoiesis result in an accumulation of highly proliferative immature lymphoblasts that overtake the bone marrow and stymie normal hematopoiesis [15]. Lymphoblasts can either be of the B-cell or T-cell lineage, with identification occurring early on in the diagnostic process due to the poor prognosis typically identified with T-cell ALL.

Fluorescence in situ hybridization (FISH) commonly reveal chromosomal abnormalities in roughly 80% of ALL patients, including chromosomal additions, deletions, translocations, and inversions [16]. Chromosomal translocations in ALL help identify specific disease subtypes. For instance, nearly 25% of precursor B cell ALL involves the TEL-AML1 (ETV6-RUNX1) fusion gene generated by the reciprocal translocation of t(12;21)(p13;q22) [17]. In adult ALL, the most common chromosomal translocation, occurring in 25% of patients, is the Philadelphia chromosome, otherwise known as t(9;22). Pediatric patients rarely harbor this translocation, with only 3% of patients testing positive [18]. The t(9;22) translocation results in the *BCR-ABL1* fusion gene and a constitutively active tyrosine kinase associated with a poor prognosis. Overall, leukemias commonly harbor genetic alterations that hopefully can be targeted and exploited with future treatment options.

Disease Classification

Pediatric ALL is classified using several different factors, including age, initial white blood cell (WBC) count, immunophenotype, and specific cytogenetic abnormalities. The French-American-British (FAB) classification system was replaced with the World Health Organization's (WHO) system in 2008, which better incorporates chromosomal alterations, immunophenotype, and molecular markers [19, 20]. The original FAB system placed patients into one of three categories, described as L1, L2, or L3 based on cytologic features of the lymphoblastic marrow. The updated WHO system is much more descriptive and better reflects known prognostic features important in risk stratification and treatment selection.

Table 1. FAB classification system [19]

FAB Subtype	Leukemia Cell	Description
L1	Pre-B or T cell	Small and homogenous
L2	Pre-B or T cell	Large and heterogeneous
L3	B cell	Large, mature cells

FAB = French-American-British.

Clinical Presentation

ALL is an invasion of the bone marrow by leukemic blasts resulting in overcrowding and eventual pancytopenia. Clinical onset following leukemic acquisition is rapid. If treatment is delayed, leukemic infiltration of various organ systems ensues, eventually leading to death within weeks to months. The early signs and symptoms of ALL are nonspecific to leukemia: fever, pallor, bone pain, and lethargy [1]. In a meta-analysis, over fifty percent of children presented with at least one of the following characteristics: palpable liver (64%), palpable spleen (61%), pallor (54%), fever (53%), or bruising (52%) [21]. Anemia, neutropenia, and thrombocytopenia are each early complications of leukemic hyperproliferation and their severity reflect the degree of bone marrow suffocation by leukemic cells. Anemia results in pallor, lethargy, tachycardia, shortness of breath, and potential heart failure. Common neutropenic complications include fever and infections. ALL patients may also experience abnormal bruising, purpura, and recurrent mucosal or internal bleeding caused by thrombocytopenia [1, 21]. CNS involvement occurs in less than 5% of children at diagnosis. Increassed intracranial pressure (headache, morning vomiting, papilledema), parenchymal involvement (convulsions, ataxia, hyperreflexia), hypothalamic syndrome (weight gain, hirsutism, behavioral disturbances), diabetes insipidus (pituitary involvement), and rarely, chloromas (blue-green collection of leukemia cells under skin) are complications of CNS leukemia result from leukemic infiltration of the CNS [21]. Even though rare at diagnosis, CNS leukemia is a common complication in patients who do not receive CNS-directed preventative therapy with either intrathecal chemotherapy or cranial irradiation.

Table 2. WHO classification system [20]

Acute leukemias of ambiguous lineage	Acute undifferentiated leukemia
	Mixed phenotype acute leukemia (MPAL)
B cell lymphoblastic leukemia/lymphoma (B-ALL)	B-lymphoblastic leukemia/lymphoma
	B-lymphoblastic leukemia/lymphoma with t(9;22)
	B-lymphoblastic leukemia/lymphoma with TEL-AML1
	B-lymphoblastic leukemia/lymphoma with hyperdiploidy
	B-lymphoblastic leukemia/lymphoma with hypodiploidy
	B-lymphoblastic leukemia/lymphoma with t(5;14)
	B-lymphoblastic leukemia/lymphoma with t(1;19)
	B-lymphoblastic leukemia/lymphoma with recurrent genetic abnormalities
T cell lymphoblastic leukemia/lymphoma (T-ALL)	T cell lymphoblastic leukemia/lymphoma

ALL = acute lymphoblastic leukemia; WHO = World Health Organization.

DIAGNOSIS

Once a patient presents with suspicious signs and symptoms of leukemia, clinicians should order a Complete Blood Count (CBC) with differential. Common findings will include laboratory abnormalities with platelets, hemoglobin, and red blood cells. The WBC count may be low, normal, or elevated [22]. A complete metabolic panel should also be ordered to evaluate for electrolyte derangements possibly indicative of tumor lysis syndrome (TLS). Lactate dehydrogenase may also appear elevated, correlating with the degree of tumor burden. Due to the non-specific nature of ALL presentation and overlapping morphological and immunophenotypical features with other benign and neoplastic entities, the differentiatial diagnosis is important to evaluate.

Table 3. Differential diagnosis of ALL [22]

Non-Malignant	Malignant
Juvenile idiopathic arthritis	Neuroblastoma
Osteomyelitis	Retinoblastoma
Epstein-Barr virus	Rhabdomyosarcoma
Immune thrombocytopenia (ITP)	Ewing sarcoma
Pertussis	Burkitt lymphoma/leukemia
Aplastic anemia	Peripheral T-cell lymphoma
Acute infectious lymphocytosis	
Hypereosinophilic syndrome	
Benign precursor B-cells (hematogones)	

PROGNOSIS AND RISK STRATIFICATION

Long-term survival rates for pediatric ALL has increased dramatically over the last several decades. One reason for this progress is an improved prognostication system utilizing risk stratification algorithms to ensure appropriate treatment. Nearly 75% of adult patients present with high-risk features, leading to disease-free survival rates of only 25% [23]. Pediatric patients, on the other had, frequently present without high-risk features. Age and initial WBC count are two important indicators of treatment failure. Infants under one year of age and children over ten years are considered to have a higher likelihood of relapse and therefore require higher-intensity therapy. Likewise, children with an initial WBC count $\geq$ 50,000/uL are classified as high risk requiring more intensive therapy [23]. Certain cytogenetic abnormalities also portend a higher overall risk of disease relapse and death. These include BCR-ABL positivity, KMT2A (MLL) rearrangement, and iAMP21 amplification [24].

Table 4 shows the original National Cancer Institute criteria for risk stratification based solely on age and initial WBC count [25]. Alternative risk stratifications have emerged utilizing immunophenotype, ploidy, cytogenetic abnormalities, extramedullary involvement, and response to initial therapy [26, 27]. Table 5 provides current risk stratification strategies for several pediatric consortiums.

Table 4. NCI risk stratification [25]

Factors	Standard Risk	High Risk
Age	1 to 9.99 years	<1 year or ≥ 10 years
Initial WBC count	< 50,000 cells/uL	≥ 50,000 cells/uL

Table 5. Current risk stratification concept [26, 27]

Factors	Low Risk	Standard Risk	High Risk (Requires one of the following)	Very High Risk (Requires one of the following)
Age	1 to 9.99 years	1 to 9.99 years	<1 year or ≥ 10 years	-
Initial WBC count	<50,000 cells/uL	<50,000 cells/uL	≥ 50,000 cells/uL	-
Extramedullary Involvement	None	None	CNS3 or testicular	-
Cytogenetics or Lineage	Presence of either double trisomies 4 and 10, or *TEL/AML1* gene	B-cell	T-cell disease	Presence of any of the following: *BCR-ABL1*, KMT2A (MLL) rearrangement, and iAMP21 amplification, hypodiploidy
MRD	<0.01% at day 8	-	MRD > 0.01% following induction	>5% to 25% blasts following induction

MRD = minimal residual disease; MLL = mixed lineage leukemia; WBC = white blood cell.

Treatment Overview for BCR-ABL1 Negative ALL

ALL is a heterogeneous disease with multiple risk stratifications, leading to various treatment approaches based on classification and risk stratification. Identifying ALL as a clinically and biologically diverse disease has helped fundamentally alter treatment and improve long-term outcomes. Historically, all pediatric patients with ALL were treated with the same multi-agent chemotherapy regimen. This approach led to some patients receiving excessive chemotherapy and others too little. As our understanding of ALL improved, treatment and monitoring became more complex and contigent on various prognostic factors. With risk stratification now in effect, clinicians and oncology consortiums can tailor treatment to a specific patient's need based on initial presentation, cytogenetic abnormalities, and response to initial therapy.

Historically, pediatric ALL resulted in appalling survival rates with >90% of children dying prior to Sydney Farber's momentous chemotherapy trials using aminopterin and other nascent chemotherapy regimens. Following the discovery of multiple leukemocidal agents over the last three decades, cure rates in children rose to nearly 90% in standard risk patients.

Treatment for ALL consists of four primary components, highlighting the complexity and intensity of treating this aggressive disease. Multidrug regimens are frequently employed throughout ALL treatment to help avoid the development of chemotherapy resistance and eventual disease recurrence. The four primary components required for treating newly diagnosed ALL include remission induction, consolidation, maintenance, and CNS prophylaxis (Figure 1).

Standard ALL treatment with induction, consolidation, maintenance, and CNS prophylaxis results in 5 year event-free survival rates ranging from 75% to 90% depending on risk stratification. Low-risk patients with favorable cytogenetic features and good, early response to chemotherapy are projected to have an estimated 5 year event-free survival of greater than 95% [29]. With cure rates under 10% just 50 years ago, the advancement of pediatric ALL survival rates is considered one of modern medicine's great triumphs.

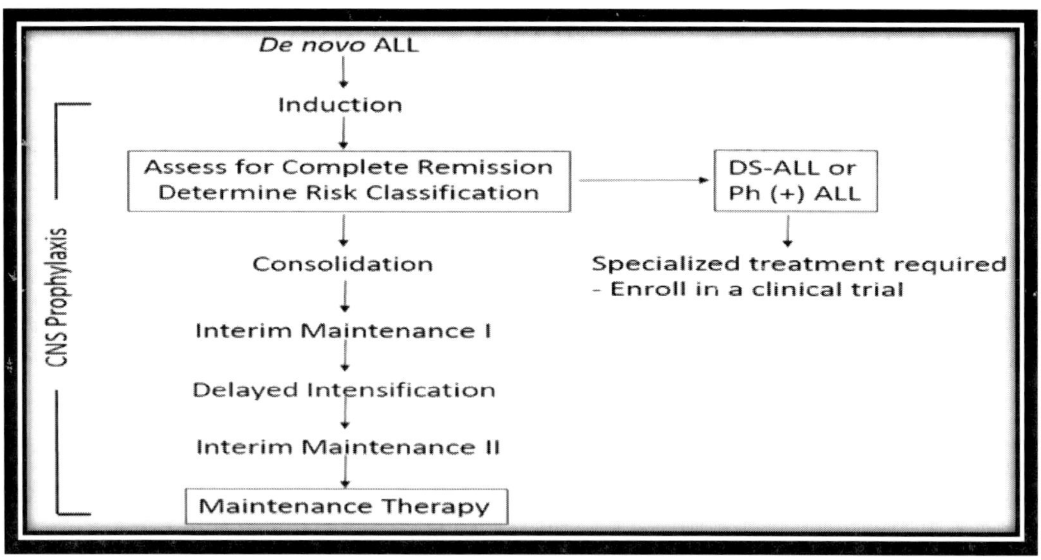

ALL = acute lymphoblastic leukemia; CNS = central nervous system; DS = Down syndrome; Ph+ = Philadelphia chromosome positive.

Figure 1. Example Treatment Schema for Pediatric ALL [28].

Table 6. Selected clinical trials in pediatric ALL [30-36]

Study	Patients (n)	T-cell ALL (%)	Overall Survival (%)	Event Free Survival (%)
AIEOP 95	1,743	11	86	76
BFM-95	2,169	13	87	80
COG-2000	7,153	7	90	90
IC-BFM 2002	5,060	13	82	74
MRC UKALL 2003	3,126	12	92	87
SJCRH XV	498	15	94	87
NOPHO-2000	1,023	11	89	79

Induction

The aim of induction therapy is to obtain a CR, defined as the eradication of all detectable leukemic disease from the marrow with restoration of normal hematopoiesis and no signs or symptoms of extramedullary disease. Induction therapy should reduce the initial leukemic burden from approximately one trillion cells (10^{12}) to less than one billion (10^{9}). Furthemore, induction aims to reduce the bone marrow blast count to <5%. This eradication of more than 99% of leukemic cells allows for restoration of normal hematopoiesis and clinical stability. The remaining leukemia cells make up the minimal residual disease (MRD), which has important prognostic and monitoring implications. MRD evaluation using flow cytometry or PCR allows for detection of one leukemia cell in 10,000 normal cells, which is far more sensitive and reliable than conventional morphological evaluation. Following induction therapy, bone marrow MRD levels <0.01% is a positive predictor of treatment success and is an important component of treatment evaluation [37]. Most protocols call for MRD testing at day 8 of induction and day 29 at the end of induction. MRD evaluation might be the single most powerful predictor of relapse available and is an indispensable tool in the clinician's armamentarium.

Multi-agent chemotherapy remains the primary treatment modality for pediatric patients with ALL. Surgery and radiation have no role in induction therapy. Remission induction is the first step in a long successive line of treatment phases, with the typical induction phase lasting 4 to 6 weeks depending on treatment protocol. Most institutions and protocols require hospital admission for the early stages of induction therapy but discharge is possible once chemotherapy is complete and the patient has clinically stabilized. The goal of induction is to obtain a CR, which 95% of patients achieve following standard induction therapy [30-36]. For those unable to obtain a CR with first induction therapy, half die from treatment-related complications and half experience induction failure and typically require aggressive therapy with allogeneic HSCT.

Table 7. Example induction regimen for high-risk ALL [38][a]

Drug	Dose	Schedule
Vincristine	1.5 mg/m^2/dose IV every 12 hours	Days 1,8,15 and 22
Dexamethasone	5 mg/m^2/dose IV/PO BID	Days 1-14
Pegaspargase (PEG-ASP)	2,500 Internationional Units/m^2/dose IV	Days 4
Daunorubicin	25 mg/m^2/dose IV	Days 1,8,15 and 22

[a] Doses and schedules may vary between treatment protocols. BID = twice daily; IV = intravenous; PO = by mouth.

Common chemotherapeutic agents utilized during induction include vincristine, L-asparaginase, and corticosteroids with certain high-risk populations requiring the addition of an anthracycline. Vincristine and a glucorcorticoid alone induce remission 85% of the time and the addition of L-asparaginase increases remission rates in pediatrics to 95% [39]. The preferred corticosteroid is either dexamethasone or prednisone with dexamethasone showing improved CNS penetration and decreased risk of relapse but with higher rates of complications, including infection, growth delays, and avascular necrosis [40]. Unlike adult leukemias, only daunorubicin and doxorubicin have proven safety and efficacy. Although the inclusion of anthracycline therapy is controversial due to a paucity of efficacy data for induction therapy, most protocols include either daunorubicin or doxorubicin in remission induction for high-risk or slow responders. L-asparaginase products include the native *Escherichia coli* L-asparaginase (Elspar® – no longer commercially available in the United States), Pegylated L-asparagainase (Oncaspar®), and Erwinia asparaginase (Erwinaze®) derived from *Erwinia chrysanthemi* and reserved for patients who experienced a hypersensitivity reaction to one of the E. coli products [41,42].

Table 8. Pharmacology of asparaginase formulations [41, 42]

Formulation	Brand name FDA Approval	Typical Induction Dose (mg)	Elimination half-life
Native L-asparaginase	Elspar 1978	6,000 International Units/m^2 three times weekly	26-30 hours
PEG-aspargase	Oncaspar 1994	2,500 International Units/m^2 every 2-4 weeks	5.5-7 days
Erwinia asparaginase	Erwinaze 2011	25,000 International Units/m^2 6 doses for every PEG-aspargase dose	16 hours

FDA = Food and Drug Administration.

Asparaginase remains one of the most important components for treating pediatric ALL. The clinical efficacy and safety profile have been heavily scrutinized over the last four decades and several improvements have increased the tolerability and efficacy of this chemotherapeutic. L-asparagine is a non-essential amino acid synthesized by the transamination of L-aspartic acid by L-asparagine synthetase. Acute leukemia cells are asparagine-dependent and lack asparagine synthetase activity, therefore requiring exogenous sources of L-asparagine for DNA synthesis and cellular proliferation. The administration of L-asparaginase products prevent leukemic proliferation and leads to apoptosis by catalyzing asparagine into aspartic acid and ammonia (Figure 2) [41, 42]. With insuffcient stores of asparagine, leukemic cells lack the ability to produce proteins or divide and eventually undergo apoptosis. Asparaginase products may result in allergic reactions, including anaphylaxis, in up to 20% of patients. Other complications with both E. coli and Erwinia formulations include pancreatitis, hyperglycemia, thrombosis, hemorrhage, disseminated intravascular coagulopathy, hyperbilirubinemia, nausea, vomiting, and hepatotoxicity. Approximately 2% to 8% of patients receiving L-asparaginase develop neutralizing anti-asparaginase antibodies requiring therapeutic monitoring and product discontinuation [43]. Therapeutic drug monitoring has gained traction with commercially available products now available; however, additional studies are required to fully elucidate appropriate activity levels and treatment algorithms.

Induction failure is an uncommon event, occurring in less than 5% of children, and indicative of a poor overall prognosis with an event-free survival of approximately 15% [44]. Induction therapy should also include intrathecal chemotherapy with methotrexate, cytarabine, and/or hydrocortisone to help reduce and minimize leukemic infiltration of the CNS.

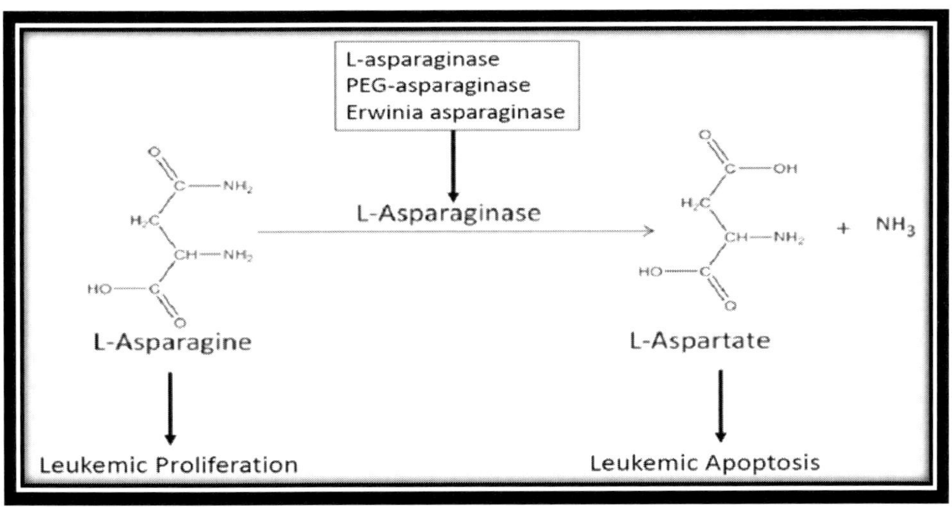

Figure 2. L-asparaginase Mechanism of Action.

Consolidation

Without post-remission consolidation, pediatric patients with ALL eventually succumb to the residual disease not eradicated by induction chemotherapy. Once a CR has been achieved following induction chemotherapy, consolidation is required and involves high-dose, multi-agent chemotherapy. Post-remission consolidation is a period of intense treatment typically lasting between 6 and 9 months. The optimal chemotherapy, dosing, schedule, and duration in post-remission consolidation remains unknown despite decades of clinical trials. The goal of post-induction consolidation is to thwart leukemic growth, eradicate MRD, minimize chemotherapy resistance, and avoid treatment-related complications such as neutropenic fever, hyperglycemia, neuropathy, thrombosis, and anaphylaxis. The goal of post-induction chemotherapy is to eradicate chemotherapy-resistant subclones that escaped induction therapy. In order to eliminate these resistant clones, several different chemotherapy agents are selected.

Within the consolidation phase, several distinct cycles of chemotherapy are required but vary from protocol to protocol. A common progression within consolidation involves the following chemotherapy cycles: "consolidation," "Interim Maintenance I," "Delayed Intensification," and finally "Interim Maintenance II" as the last cycle before starting maintenance therapy. These treatment cycles differ based on overall risk stratification. For instance, a patient with very low risk ALL will receive significantly different post-induction treatment than a patient with high-risk disease. Not only will the various cycles vary between protocols but the doses, schedules, and duration of chemotherapy will differ as well. There are dozens of consolidation regimens in existence with no consensus on the optimal makeup required to achieve post-induction treatment goals.

Intensification of chemotherapy is based on the specific patient and their overall risk classification. Allocating patients to different risk categories allows researchers to reduce or increase intensification appropriately based on the individual patient's prognosis. For patients at low-risk of disease recurrence, less chemotherapy can be incorporated into their treatment plan. This reduced-intensity path may reduce overall treatment-related morbidity and mortality. Conversely, for high-risk patients, chemotherapy intensity should be increased to help overcome leukemic resistance and reduce minimal residual disease.

Consolidation typically involves aggressive chemotherapy and often requires hospital admission and close monitoring for acute and delayed complications. Fortunately, several pediatric institutions afford patients with the opportunity to receive some consolidation therapy in the outpatient setting with close monitoring. Infectious complications are a significant concern during consolidation due to the profound myelosuppression experienced from high-dose chemotherapy and coinciding immunosuppression naturally present in pediatric patients with ALL. Bacteria, viral, and fungal infections are all commonplace and require frequent interrogation during periods of neutropenia, especially in the setting of febrile neutropenia. Neutropenic fever is an oncologic emergency and warrants immediate broad-spectrum antibiotics with antipseudomonal coverage.

Maintenance

Maintenance is the final phase of ALL treatment and typically lasts 2 to 3 years depending on gender and protocol. Boys are treated for an additional 12 months to help eradicate and prevent testicular relapse. Maintenance is less intensive and can be completed on an outpatient basis using a combination of oral and intravenous chemotherapy. Preferred maintenance schedules generally incorporate continuous therapy rather than high-dose, pulse therapy with extended breaks between cycles. It appears continuous therapy is more effective than tradition high-dose chemotherapy used for induction and consolodiation [45]. To help shorten the standard maintenance duration, one clinical trial attempted to intensify earlier treatment and shorten total duration to less than one year [46]. They evaluated 347 previously untreated children and found that early treatment intensification failed to overcome a truncated maintenance phase of only 6 months.

Table 9. Example consolidation cycle [38][a]

Drug	Dose	Schedule
Cyclophosphamide	1000 mg/m^2/dose IV	Days 1 and 29
Cytarabine	75 mg/m^2/dose IV	Days 1-4, 8-11, 29-32, and 36-39
Mercaptopurine	60 mg/m^2/dose	Days 1-14 and 29-42
Vincristine	1.5 mg/m^2/dose IV	Days 15, 22, 43, and 50
Pegaspargase (PEG-ASP)	2,500 Internationional Units/m^2/dose IV	Days 15 and 43

[a] Doses and schedules may vary between treatment protocols. IV = intravenous.

The cornerstone of maintenance therapy includes oral methotrexate and 6-mercaptopurine (6-MP) along with pulses of vincristine and glucocorticoids. Proper medication adherence is especially important for these patients. A randomized, multi-center Children's Oncology Group (COG) clinical trial evaluated medication adherence in 326 pediatric ALL patients undergoing maintenance therapy and found that children who reported taking <95% (non-adherent) of their 6-MP doses exhibited a 2.7 fold increase in disease relapse [47]. Pharmacists and other healthcare professionals must provide in-depth medication education for these patients emphasizing the importance of strict medication adherence. Clinicians should be frequently monitoring complete blood counts in ALL patients on maintenance therapy. These labs help guide dosing decisions for certain chemotherapy agents such as 6-MP and methotrexate. If the absolute neutrophil count does not respond to increasing 6-MP doses, consider medication non-adherence. Obtaining 6-thioguanine and 6-methylmercaptopurine levels can help distinguish medication non-adherence from other possibilities such as thiopurine-S-methyltransferase (TPMT) inactivity, liver dysfunction, or genetic polymorphisms. Most treatment protocols include guidance for managing oral maintenance therapy.

TPMT is responsible for metabolizing thiopurines such as 6-MP. Certain polymorphisms in the TPMT gene may decrease enzyme effectiveness or result in complete loss of function. Pediatric ALL patients with TPMT inactivation or diminished enzyme activity are at higher risk of treatment-related neutropenia and prolonged myelosuppression. Over 24 low-functionioning TPMT variants have been identified, with TPMT*2 and TPMT*3 making up nearly 95% of defective genes. Approximately 10% of pediatric ALL patients witll have TPMT heterozygosity, resulting in intermediate levels of enzyme activity, potentially requiring dose modifications. Only 1 in 300 patients will have TPMT-deficiency as an autosomal recessive trait requiring extreme 6-MP dose modifications [48]. Most ALL protocols do not require TPMT testing prior to 6-MP treatment.

Pulse therapy with glucocorticoids and vincristine are often employed during maintenance therapy but the evidence supporting their use remains controversial. Standard risk patients appear to benefit from pulse therapy compared to patients receiving only oral methotrexate and 6-MP; however, additional research is required to assess the duration of pulse therapy in maintenance [49].

Table 10. Example maintenance cycle (12 week cycle) [47][a]

Drug	Dose	Schedule
Methotrexate	20 mg/m^2/week PO	Once weekly
Dexamethasone	3 mg/m^2/dose PO BID	Days 1-5
Mercaptopurine	75 mg/m^2/dose	Daily
Vincristine	1.5 mg/m^2/dose IV	Day 1

[a] Doses and schedules may vary between treatment protocols.

Prevention of CNS Leukemia

The fourth pillar of ALL treatment is CNS-directed therapy. Up to 95% of newly diagnosed patients will not have leukemic involvement in the CNS [50]. Unfortunately, as researchers discovered in the 1960s and 1970s, without the use of CNS-directed radiation or chemotherapy, 80% or more of patients with a complete bone marrow remission would relapse with leukemic meningitis resulting in treatment failure and death

[51]. In 1962, Donald Pinkel and colleagues at St. Jude's Children Research Hospital conducted groundbreaking research incorporating CNS-directed therapy utilizing cranial irradiation and intrathecal methotrexate into their standard treatment protocol [52]. Results were astonishing and nearly half of the 35 enrolled patients experienced long-term survival. Moreover, the routine use of preventative CNS therapy provided a major therapeutic breakthrough for the treatment of pediatric ALL. Craniospinal radiotherapy remained the standard of care for many years despite significant toxicity, including neuropsychological morbidity [53]. One cancer survivorship study showed a significant increase in secondary brain tumors, leukoencephalopathy, and a decline in verbal functioning and overall intelligence in adults who were treated with cranial radiation as children [54]. The Dana-Farber Cancer Institute conducted a randomized comparison of intensive triple intrathecal chemotherapy (methotrexate, cytarabine, and hydrocortisone) versus cranial radiation in 272 standard risk patients and found intensive intrathecal chemotherapy to be equally effective as cranial radiation in preventing CNS disease [55]. A subsequent trial was conducted in 498 newly diagnosed pediatric ALL patients using triple intrathecal chemotherapy in lieu of crandial radiation [56]. The 5-year cumulative risk for isolated CNS relapse was 2.7% and the 5-year overall survival rate was 94%, demonstrating that intrathecal chemotherapy to be a reliable option for preventing CNS relapse. Given its propensity for intellectual disability and secondary neoplasms, the use of cranial radiation continues to decline in favor of intrathecal chemotherapy. Unfortunately, intrathecal chemotherapy is not without risk and is associated with neurotoxicity, including seizures, leukoencephalopathy, and acute hemiparesis [57]. Typical intrathecal doses for methotrexate, hydrocortisone, and cytarabine can be found in Table 11.

Table 11. Example intrathecal doses for pediatric ALL [55][a]

Drug	Age (years)	Dose (mg)
Methotrexate	1-1.99	8
	2-2.99	10
	3-8.99	12
	≥9	15
Hydrocortisone	1-1.99	8
	2-2.99	10
	3-8.99	12
	≥9	15
Cytarabine	1-1.99	16
	2-2.99	20
	3-8.99	24
	≥9	30

[a] Doses and schedules may vary between treatment protocols.

For patients who relapse with isolated CNS disease, treatment and prognosis are dependent on how long the patient remained in remission following initial induction chemotherapy and if they received cranial irradiation for CNS-directed therapy. If radiation was not administered initially, isolated CNS relapse can be effectively managed with durable remission rates similar to newly diagnosed ALL patients [58].

Treatment Overview for ALL Subgroups

Philadelphia Chromosome Positive ALL

The Philadelphia translocation occurs frequently in patients with chronic myeloid leukemia; however, only 3% of those with pediatric ALL will test positive for this *BCR-ABL1* gene. Philadelphia translocation is a t(9;22)(q34;11) chimeric gene resulting in a contitutively active cytoplasmic tyrosine kinase that induces dysfunctional signaling and abnormal cellular proliferation. ALL patients who are Philadelphia chromosome positive (Ph^+) typically respond poorly to conventional chemotherapy and require the inclusion of tyrosine kinase inihibtors (TKIs) such as imatinib, dasatinib, or nilotinib. Patients with Ph^+ are considered high-risk regardless of other cytogenetic testing or risk stratification criteria. The addition of an active TKI to traditional ALL therapy has increased event-free and overall survival rates [59]. Compared to historical controls, ALL patients taking continuous imatinib obtained a 3-year event free survival rate of 80% compared to 35% of patients on tradition chemotherapy. Patients receiving allogeneic HSCT and imatinib did not benefit compared to allogeneic HSCT alone. Unfortunately, leukemic cells can develop resistance to TKI therapy, requiring patients to switch TKI agents in hopes of experiencing improved efficacy. Ponatinib is a third-generation TKI with proven activity against the native and mutated *BCR-ABL1* tyrosine kinases and remains the only TKI effective against the *BCR-ABL1* T315I mutation [60]. Various studies are ongoing evaluating the different TKIs in up-front therapy for Ph^+ ALL, but regardless of which specific agent is selected, patients must receive TKI therapy throughout induction, consolidation, and maintenance therapy.

T-Cell ALL

T-cell lymphoid leukemia display distinct biochemical and immunologic features compared to B-cell malignancies. Approximately 10% to 15% of pediatric ALL patients will be diagnosed with T-cell ALL, which historically portends a worse overall prognosis compared to precursor B-cell ALL. More recently, however, survival rates in T-cell ALL approach those of B-cell ALL due to aggressive chemotherapy protocols targeting high-risk disease. Even with 5-year event-free survival rates over 85% in recent trials, T-cell ALL continues to be a high-risk factor in newly diagnosed ALL patients. Both age and WBC count at diagnosis are important risk factors in B-cell ALL, but T-cell ALL prognosis is not impacted by either of these factors [61]. Unfortunately, unlike B-ALL, few, if any, genomic alterations affecting T-cell ALL prognosis have been identified. Therefore, risk stratification in T-cell ALL consists of evaluating the CNS status along with MRD following induction chemotherapy. Treatment for T-cell ALL mirrors most pediatric ALL protocols with standard intensive therapy including induction, consolidation, and maintenance phases. The COG initiated a clinical trial evaluating nelarabine, a purine nucleoside analog targeting T-cells, in patients with relapsed disease [62]. Regardless, few options exist to specifically target T-cell ALL.

Infantile ALL

Infants with ALL appear to have a distinct biological and immunological disease compared to standard pediatric ALL. These young children are at particularly high risk for treatment failure and treatment-related complications. Particular worrisome risk factors include diagnosis prior to reaching 6 months of age, *KMT2A* translocation (formerly known as a mixed lineage leukemia gene rearrangement), and elevated initial WBC count. The KMT2A rearrangement is found in approximately 75% to 89% of infant ALL cases. This driver mutation leads to poor results despite highly aggressive chemotherapy. The rate of remission in infants with KMT2A rearrangement is high, but the event-free and overall survival rates remain extremely poor compared to other pediatric ALL subtypes. The COG P9407 and Interfant-99 trials showed 5-year event-free survival rates of 36% and 37%, respectively [63,64]. Novel treatment approaches are needed to help overcome early disease relapse and eventual death in this high-risk population. DNA hypomethylating agents hold some promise, with azacitidine displaying some pre-clinical activity against *KMT2A*-positive blast cells [65].

Adolescent and Young Adult ALL

Adolescent and young adult (AYA) classification will typically involve patients between the ages of 15 and 39 years. The Surveillance, Epidemiology and End Results (SEER) database show 5-year overall survival rates for children to be approximately 90%; however, the overall survival rates for AYA patients were much lower at 42% to 63% depending on age [2]. Lower rates of survival for AYA patients compared to most pediatric cohorts may result from an association between older age and an increased incidence of Ph^+ and T-cell immunophenotypes, which are both high-risk features. Recent clinical evidence suggests AYA patients experience superior outcomes when treated with pediatric-based ALL protocols compared to standard adult regimens [66-68]. A United States intergroup study evaluated 318 AYA patients with ALL using pediatric-based regimens and found an estimated 2-year event-free survival rate of 66%, which was significantly better than the 34% observed in the historic control arm. Pediatric protocols are the preferred option for AYA patients. The main concern involves the inherent toxicity found in these high-intensity regimens.

Patients 40 years and older tend to be rather intolerant to these pediatric regimens and therefore require less intensive therapy. For instance, one clinical trial showed patients older than 40 years had a 10-fold increase in death due to treatment during induction chemotherapy. Researchers at MD Anderson Cancer Center evaluated 106 AYA patients receiving pediatric-like treatment compared to 102 AYA patients treated with standard HYPER-CVAD [69]. The complete remission rate (93% versus 98%), 5-year event-free survival (53% versus 55%) and 5-year overall survival (60% versus 60%) were all statistically similar. The pediatric-like regimen resulted in more hepatotoxicity, pancreatitis, osteonecrosis, and thrombosis compared to HYPER-CVAD; however, it also resulted in fewer cases of myelosuppression-associated complications. AYA patients should be enrolled in clinical trials whenever possible, but only 2% of AYA patients with ALL enroll in a clinical trial compared to 60% of pediatric patients [70]. Furthermore, pediatric patients appear more compliant to treatment regimens, which may help explain some of the outcome disparities [71]. Based on the National Comprehensive Cancer Network (NCCN) guidelines, both pediatric-based regimens and high-dose HYPER-CVAD regimens are acceptable treatment options for AYA patients with B-cell ALL [72].

TREATMENT OF RELAPSED ALL

Pediatric ALL confers excellent long-term survival outcomes in most patients. Unfortunately, 15% to 20% of patients will suffer disease relapse at some point following initial remission [73]. Relapse of childhood ALL is a vexing problem with overall survival remaining ciritically low with little improvement over the past 20 years [32]. Even with intensive treatment that includes allogeneic HSCT, only 40% of relapsed patients will experience a cure. Survival rates vary significantly depending on the location of the relapse (e.g., CNS, bone marrow, testes, etc), when the relapse occurred (e.g., during treatment, within 2.5 year of remission, etc), patient age, cytogenetic abnormalities, and treatment regimen [74]. Nguyen reviewed 1,961 pediatric ALL patients with relapsed disease from a cohort of 9,585 COG-enrolled patients and found that the strongest predictor of survival was the time from initial diagnosis until disease relapse [75]. High-risk patients who relapsed within 18 months of initial diagnosis showed the poorest long-term outcomes, with only 15% of these patients surviving for 5 years. Conversely, 5-year survival rates were highest among those with isolated CNS disease (59%) compared to isolated (24%) or concurrent bone marrow relapse (39%). In addition, initial risk stratification plays a role in prognosis following ALL relapse. Standard risk patients fare better in the relapsed setting than those initially diagnosed with high-risk disease; this is especially true for those with T-cell ALL who exhibit extremely poor long-term survival following relapse [74]. The treatment regimen used following relapse can also make a difference in long-term survival rates. A multicenter, phase III clinical trial evaluated 216 relapsed ALL patients receiving either idarubicin-based or mitoxantrone-based chemotherapy [75]. Mitoxantrone resulted in significantly better rates of overall survival (69% versus 45%) and progression-free survival (65% versus 36%) compared to idarubicin-based therapy.

A second CR following first relapse can be achieved in 65% to 85% of patients receiving re-induction chemotherapy [75]. Current treatment strategies for obtaining a second CR share similarities with first-line therapies for newly diagnosed ALL patients. Various protocols for re-induction are utilized, depending on institution, but most contain vincristine, corticosteroid, L-asparaginase, and an anthracycline. These agents are often given at higher doses or alternative schedules to help overcome chemotherapy resistance. Once a second CR is verified, post-remission treatment is started based on overall risk stratification and cytogenetic findings. Allogeneic HSCT should be considered for most patients unless they experienced late relapsee or had isolated CNS disease. Allogeneic HSCT is usually the best option for achieving long-term survival in those with early relapse, isolated bone marrow disease, high-risk cytogenetic features, and/or T-cell immunophenotype [75].

Due to a dearth of effective alternative treatment options, relapsed patients should be encouraged to enroll in a clinical trial whenever possible. Several emerging therapies have shown promise in improving treatment outcomes in this high-risk population.

Table 12. Children's oncology group risk stratification (IND#117467)

Risk Stratification	Duration of CR and site of relapse
Low	≥ 18 months isolated extramedullary
Intermediate	≥ 36 months with marrow < 18 months isolated extramedullary
High	< 36 months with marrow relapse T-cell ALL

Blinatumomab

Blinatumomab (Blincyto®) is a bispecific T-cell engaging antibody (BiTE) consisting of two antibody domains connected by a non-immunologic marker. The FDA approved blinatumomab in 2014 for the treatment of Philadelphia chromosome negative relapsed or refractory precursor B-cell leukemia. The indication was later expanded in 2017 to include Ph^+ disease in both adults and children, and again in 2018 to include ALL patients in remission but displaying MRD levels ≥0.1%. Derived from a mouse monoclonal antibody, blinatumomab targets CD3-expressing T-cells and CD19 B-cells. Over 90% of B-cells are positive for CD19 cell surface protein antigen, making CD19 an attractive target for immunologic therapy [76]. The rationale behind BiTe therapy is the propensity to form an "immunologic synapse" between cytotoxic T-cells and malignant B-cells, resulting in activation of the immune system and subsequent destruction of the malignant clone [77]. Blinatumomab dosing varies depending on weight, indication, and cycle (Tables 13 and 14) [78].

Table 13. Blinatumomab dosing strategies in relapsed/refractory ALL [78]

Weight	Dose
<45 kg	Cycle 1: 5 mcg/m²/day (maximum: 9 mcg/day) administered as a continuous infusion on days 1 to 7, followed by 15 mcg/m²/day (maximum: 28 mcg/day) as a continuous infusion on days 8 to 28 of a 6-week treatment cycle. Cycles 2 through 5: 15 mcg/m²/day (maximum: 28 mcg/day) administered as a continuous infusion on days 1 to 28 of a 6-week treatment cycle. Cycles 6 through 9: 15 mcg/m²/day (maximum: 28 mcg/day) administered as a continuous infusion on days 1 to 28 of a 12-week treatment cycle.
≥45 kg	Cycle 1: 9 mcg daily administered as a continuous infusion on days 1 to 7, followed by 28 mcg daily as a continuous infusion on days 8 to 28 of a 6-week treatment cycle. Cycles 2 through 5: 28 mcg daily administered as a continuous infusion on days 1 to 28 of a 6-week treatment cycle. Cycles 6 through 9: 28 mcg daily administered as a continuous infusion on days 1 to 28 of a 12-week treatment cycle.

Involves two induction cycles with three consolidation cycles and up to four cycles of continued therapy (up to nine total cycles). ALL = acute lymphoblastic leukemia.

Table 14. Blinatumomab dosing strategies in MRD positive ALL [78]

Weight	Dose
<45 kg	Cycles 1 to 4: 15 mcg/m^2/day (maximum: 28 mcg/day) as a continuous infusion on days 1 to 28 of a 6-week treatment cycle.
≥45 kg	Cycles 1 to 4: 28 mcg daily administered as a continuous infusion on days 1 to 28 of a 6-week treatment cycle

Involves one induction cycle followed by up to three additional consolidation cycles (total of up to four cycles). ALL = acute lymphoblastic leukemia.

An open-label, phase I/II clinical trial was conducted evaluating blinatumomab in pediatric patients with relapsed or refractory precursor B-cell ALL [79]. For patients who received the recommended dose, 39% achieved a CR within the first two cycles and 52% were MRD negative. These patients were followed for 24 months. Of the 27 responders, four were alive and in CR, two were alive in relapse and three had withdrawn consent. The remaining 18 patients consisted of three patients who died in CR following allogeneic HSCT and 15 patients experienced disease relapse and death. The median relapse-free survival was 4.4 months. Common adverse events included anemia, pyrexia, headache, nausea, and thrombocytopenia. Eight patients experienced cytokine release syndrome, a potentially fatal complication resulting from an elevation of inflammatory cytokines and severe immune reaction.

Another report in high-risk pediatric ALL patients showed an event-free survival of 30% in 9 patients who received a total of 18 cycles following post-transplant relapse [80]. These patients were heavily pre-treated and molecularly resistant to previous therapy. Based on these promising results, along with adult data, the COG elected to study blinatumomab in a randomized, phase III clinical trial in first relapse of precursor B-cell ALL. The Children's Oncology Group AALL1331 Risk-Stratified Randomized Phase III Testing of Blinatumomab (IND#117467, NSC#765986) in First Relapse of Childhood B-Lymphocytic Leukemia (B-ALL) trial was activated in 2014 and is currently still ongoing.

Chimeric Antigen Receptor T Cells (CAR-T)

Genetically engineered immunotherapy may have the potential to cure patients with highly-resistant ALL. Chimeric antigen receptor T cells (CAR-T) is a novel therapeutic option for patients with relapsed or refractory precursor B-cell ALL. CAR-T is an example of adoptive cell transfer involving genetically modifying T-cells to express chimeric antigen receptors targeting CD19 positive B-cells. Chimeric antigen receptors are engineered receptors that redirect T-cell activity to a pre-specified target. Following T-cell harvesting via leukapheresis, effector lymphocytes are engineered *ex vivo* to enforce an immune response targeting malignant leukemic cells [81]. Second-generation products contain dual-signaling receptors that effectively expand T cell function and enable T-cell longevity. Once these "living drugs" have been effectively programed to target CD19-positive cells, they are then expanded *ex vivo* and eventually reinfused into the patient to bind to tumor antigens, activating an immune response leading to leukemic apoptosis.

Several clinical trials using CAR-T therapy have provided impressive results in various cancers, including relapsed and refractory non-Hodgkin's lymphoma, chronic lymphocytic leukemia, and lymphoblastic leukemias [82-84]. Over 1,000 patients have been treated in the United States alone since the FDA approved the first CAR-T applications in 2007. Furthermore, the highest response rates reported with CAR-T therapy was in pediatric B-cell ALL. An initial phase I trial evaluating CAR-T therapy was conducted at the Children's Hospital of Philadelphia. They enrolled 25 pediatric patients with relapsed or refractory B-cell ALL and demonstrated impressive results [85]. The overall and event-free survival at 6-months were 78% and 67%, respectively, with 90% of patients experiencing a CR. These patients were heavily pretreated with over 50% failing a previous allogeneic HSCT and two patients also failing blinatumomab therapy. A follow-up phase I/II clinical trial also conducted at the Children's Hospital of Philadelphia evaluated an additional 34 children and young adults with B-cell ALL in at least their second relapse [86]. Of the 59 pediatric patients, 44 had detectable disease before beginning CAR-T therapy. Following one month of treatment with CAR-T therapy, 93% of patients were in a CR. Even more impressive, 88% of patients were MRD negative. With 12 months of follow-up, 58% of patients were still in remission and overall survival was 79%. Unfortunately, CAR-T therapy dose pose significant adverse effects, including cytokine release syndrome, hypogammaglobulinemia, encephalopathy, and seizures.

In Auguts 2017, the FDA approved tisagenlecleucel (Kymriah®) suspension for intravenous infusion for the treatment of patients (under 26 years of age) with relapsed or refractory precursor B-cell ALL. This was the first form of gene-transfer therapy to receive FDA approval. A Risk Evaluation and Mitigation Strategy (REMS) program was mandated by the FDA to help ensure education and training for the management of complications relating to CAR-T treatment, most notably cytokine release syndrome. Several clinical trials evaluating CAR-T therapy for frontline or second-line treatment are ongoing or in the planning phase. ClinicalTrials.gov currently lists 300 CAR-T trials, with potential indications ranging from leukemias and lymphomas to solid tumors (i.e., glioblastomas, melanoma, sarcoma, pancreatic cancer, etc). Several limitation exist, ranging from extreme cost, long manufacturing delays, and severe adverse events.

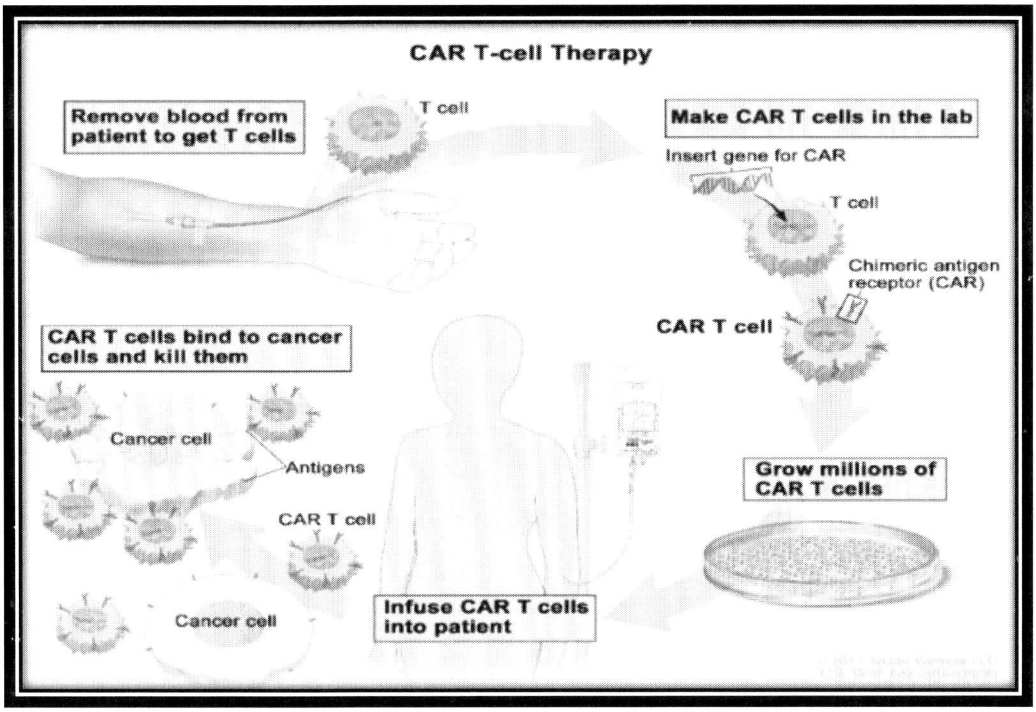

Illustration 1. "CAR T cell Therapy" Publication Year: 2017, Original Graphic: https://visualsonline.cancer.gov/details.cfm?imageid=11776. © 2017 Terese Winslow LLC, U.S. Govt. has certain rights.

Allogeneic HSCT

Allogeneic HSCT or high-intensity chemotherapy following disease relapse has been widely debated. It appears HSCT is superior to chemotherapy, showing long-term disease-free survival rates of 20% to 40%, but success is highly dependent on a number of factors [87]. Donor status, comorbidities, time to relapse, previous treatment, and degree of match all play a role in long-term outcomes. Although a potentially curative option, HSCT is a complicated procedure requiring extensive medical care with potential devastating short- and long-term sequelae. The field of bone marrow transplantation is rapidly advancing, with some ALL patients receiving allogeneic HSCT as front-line therapy for high-risk features. Furthermore, treatment-related mortality continues to decline with HSCT thanks to improved graft-versus-host-disease management and healthcare provider understanind of the disease. Allogeneic HSCT is a powerful tool in a clinician's armamentarium.

Supportive Care of ALL

Pediatric patients with ALL are at an increased risk for several potentially life-threatening disease- and treatment-related complications. Several common chemotherapy agents lead to myelosuppression, mucositis, nausea/vomiting, hepatotoxicity, and nephrotoxicity. See Table 15 for common chemotherapy complications. In addition to these chemotherapy-related concerns, patients with ALL are considered to have high risk for developing TLS, which is a common oncologic emergency requiring early identification and management [88].

Prevention and treatment is similar to adults at risk for TLS. Aggressive hydration initiation followed by TLS prophylactic measures such as allopurinol and, in some cases, rasburicase administration are required. Frequent metabolic derangements resulting from TLS include hyperkalemia, hyperuricemia, hyperphosphatemia, and hypocalcemia. Routine laboratory monitoring is required to catch early TLS and to monitor the resolution of metabolic derangements. ALL patients also frequently require blood product support such as packed red blood cells and platelet transfusions. Myelosuppression may result in neutropenic fever, which remains a significant cause of morbidity and mortality in patients with acute leukemias. Pediatric ALL patients require early identification and rapid administration of appropriate empiric antibiotics with broad-spectrum activity to prevent and treat these life-threatening infections.

Table 15. Common chemotherapy complications [89][a]

Chemotherapy	Adverse Events
Anthracyclines	Myelosuppression, nausea/vomiting, mucositis, cardiotoxicity, red secretions
Corticosteroids	Agitation, insomnia, hyperglycemia, hypertension, psychosis, fluid retention
Cyclophosphamide	Myelosuppression, hemorrhagic cystitis, hyponatremia, nausea/vomiting
Cytarabine	Conjunctivitis, flu-like syndrome
Etoposide	Infusion-related reactions, mucositis
Mercaptopurine	Hepatotoxicity, rash, myelosuppression
Methotrexate	Transaminitis, nephrotoxicity, myelosuppression, mucositis
Peg-Aspargase	Hypersensitivity reactions, coagulopathies, hyperglycemia, pancreatitis
Vincristine	Peripheral neuropathies, constipation

[a]This is not an exhaustive list of all complications; rather, this should highlight a few of the common complications patients may experience from each agent.

Conclusion

ALL is the most common childhood malignancy, resulting from a series of genetic mutations and manifesting with signs and symptoms of anemia, thrombocytopenia, and neutropenia. Substantial progress in the identification, diagnosis, risk stratification, treatment, and overall management of these patients has occurred over the past 50 years. Modern treatment strategies for children with

ALL include remission-induction, consolidation, CNS-directed therapy, and maintenance therapy with or without allogeneic HSCT. Using multi-agent chemotherapy, cure rates for pediatric ALL is 80% to 90%. Unfortunately, 15% to 20% of patients will relapse following their first complete remission and few treatment options provide long-term survival for these high-risk patients. Targeted therapy with blinatumomab or CAR-T therapy may help improve survival rates in high-risk patients and is a cause for cautious optimism. Much progress has been made since the 1950s, but continued research using multi-centered randomized clinical trials are necessary to identify and interrogate emerging therapeutic options.

References

[1] Lanzkowsky P. Leukemias. *Manual of Pediatric Hematology and Oncology.* [Fifth Edition]. Elsevier 2010; 518-566. June 17, 2018.

[2] Noone AM, Howlader N, Krapcho M, et al. *SEER Cancer Statistics Review*, 1975-2015, National Cancer Institute. Bethesda, MD, https://seer.cancer.gov/csr/1975_2015/, based on November 2017 SEER data submission, posted to the SEER web site, April 2018.

[3] Terwilliger T, Abdul-Hay M. Acute lymphoblastic leukemia: a comprehensive review and 2017 update. *Blood Cancer Journal.* 2017;7(577):1.

[4] Pui C-H, Evans WE. A 50-Year Journey to Cure Childhood Acute Lymphoblastic Leukemia. *Seminars in Hematology.* 2013;50(3):185-196.

[5] Farber S, Diamond LK, Mercer RD, et al. Temporary remissions in acute leukemia in children produced by folic acid antagonist, 4-aminopteroyl-glutamic acid 374. *N Engl J Med* 1948; 238:787–93.

[6] Farber, Sydney: Image Details. *NCI Visuals Online*. https://visualsonline.cancer.gov/details.cfm?imageid=1926. Published January 1, 2001. Accessed July 20, 2018.

[7] Frei E, Freireich EJ, Gehan E, et al. Studies of Sequential and Combination Antimetabolite Therapy in Acute Leukemia: 6-Mercaptopurine and Methotrexate. *Blood* 1961; 18:431–54.

[8] Pinkel D. Five-year follow-up of "total therapy" of childhood lymphocytic leukemia. *JAMA* 1971;216:648–52.
[9] Aur RJ, Simone J, Hustu HO, et al. Central nervous system therapy and combination chemotherapy of childhood lymphocytic leukemia. *Blood* 1971; 37:272–81.
[10] Henze G, Langermann HJ, Brämswig J, et al. The BFM 76/79 acute lymphoblastic leukemia therapy study (author's transl). *Klin Padiatr* 1981; 193:145–54.
[11] Sallan SE, Hitchcock-Bryan S, Gelber R, et al. Influence of intensive asparaginase in the treatment of childhood non-T-cell acute lymphoblastic leukemia. *Cancer Res* 1983; 43:5601–7.
[12] Thomopoulos TP, Ntouvelis E, Diamantaras AA, et al. Maternal and childhood consumption of coffee, tea and cola beverages in association with childhood leukemia: A meta-analysis. *Cancer Epidemiol* 2015;39:1047–1059.
[13] Deschler B, Lubbert M. Acute myeloid leukemia: Epidemiology and etiology. *Cancer* 2006;107:2099–2107.
[14] Spector LG, Ross JA, Robison LL, et al. Epidemiology and etiology. Pui CH. *Childhood leukemias.* 2nd ed 2006 Cambridge University Press Cambridge, UK 48-66.
[15] Cline MJ. The molecular basis of leukemia. *N Engl J Med* 1994;330:328-336.
[16] Moorman AV, Chilton L, Wilkinson J, et al. A population-based cytogenetic study of adults with acute lymphoblastic leukemia. *Blood* 2010;115(2):206.
[17] Pui CH, Relling MV, Downing JR. Acute lymphoblastic leukemia. *N Engl J Med* 2004;350:1535-1548.
[18] Arico M, Schrappe M, Hunger SP, et al. Clinical outcome of children with newly diagnosed Philadelphia chromosome-positive acute lymphoblastic leukemia treated between 1995 and 2005. *J Clin Oncol* 2010;28:4755–4761.
[19] Bennett JM, Catovsky D, Daniel MT, et al. Proposals for the classification of the acute leukaemias. French-American-British (FAB) co-operative group. *Br J Haematol* 1976; 33:451.
[20] Arber DA, Orazi A, Hasserjian R, et al. The 2016 revision to the World Health Organization classification of myeloid neoplasms and acute leukemia. *Blood* 2016;127(20):2391.
[21] Clarke RT, Van den Bruel A, Bankhead C, et al. Clinical presentation of childhood leukaemia: a systematic review and meta-analysis. *Arch Dis Child* 2016; 101:894.
[22] Onciu M. Acute lymphoblastic leukemia. *Hematol Oncol Cin N Am* 2009;23:655-674.
[23] Faderl S, Jeha S, Kantarjian HM. The biology and therapy of adult acute lymphoblastic leukemia. *Cancer* 2003;98(7):1337–54.
[24] Harrison CJ. Cytogenetics of paediatric and adolescent acute lymphoblastic leukaemia. *Br J Haematol* 2009;144(2):147.

[25] Smith M, Arthur D, Camitta B et al. Uniform approach to risk classification and treatment assignment for children with acute lymphoblastic leukemia. *J Clin Oncol* 1996; 14(1): 18-24.

[26] Borowitz MJ, Devidas M, Hunger SP et al. Clinical significance of minimal residual disease in childhood acute lymphoblastic leukemia and its relationship to other prognostic factors: A children's oncology group study. *Blood.* 2008; 111(12): 5477-85.

[27] Schultz KR, Pullen DJ, Sather HN et al. Risk- and response-based classification of childhood b-precursor acute lymphoblastic leukemia: A combined analysis of prognostic markers from the pediatric oncology group (pog) and children's cancer group (ccg). *Blood* 2007;109(3):926-35.

[28] Cooper SL and Brown PA. Treatment of pediatric acute lymphoblastic leukemia. *Pediatr Clin North Am* 2015;62(1):61-73.

[29] Borowitz MJ, Devidas M, Hunger SP, et al: Clinical significance of minimal residual disease in childhood acute lymphoblastic leukemia and its relationship to other prognostic factors: a Children's Oncology Group study. *Blood* 2008;111(12):5477-5485.

[30] Conter V, Aricò M, Basso G, et al. Long-term results of the Italian Association of Pediatric Hematology and Oncology (AIEOP) Studies 82, 87, 88, 91 and 95 for childhood acute lymphoblastic leukemia. *Leukemia* 2010;24:255-264.

[31] Möricke A, Zimmermann M, Reiter A, et al. Long-term results of five consecutive trials in childhood acute lymphoblastic leukemia performed by the ALL-BFM study group from 1981 to 2000. *Leukemia* 2010;24:265-284.

[32] Hunger SP, Lu X, Devidas M, et al. Improved survival for children and adolescents with acute lymphoblastic leukemia between 1990 and 2005: A report from the Children’s Oncology Group. *J Clin Oncol* 2012;30:1663-1669.

[33] Stary J, Zimmermann M, Campbell M, et al. Intensive chemotherapy for childhood acute lymphoblastic leukemia: Results of the randomized intercontinental trial ALL IC-BFM 2002. *J Clin Oncol* 2014;32:174-184.

[34] Vora A, Goulden N, Mitchell C, et al. Augmented post-remission therapy for a minimal residual disease-defined high-risk subgroup of children and young people with clinical standard-risk and intermediate-risk acute lymphoblastic leukaemia (UKALL 2003): A randomised controlled trial. *Lancet Oncol* 2014;15:809-818.

[35] Pui CH, Pei D, Campana D, et al: A revised definition for cure of childhood acute lymphoblastic leukemia. *Leukemia* 2014;28:2336-2343.

[36] Schmiegelow K, Forestier E, Hellebostad M, et al. Long-term results of NOPHO ALL-92 and ALL-2000 studies of childhood acute lymphoblastic leukemia. *Leukemia* 2010;24:345-354.

[37] Borowitz MJ, Devidas M, Hunger SP, et al. Clinical significance of minimal residual disease in childhood acute lymphoblastic leukemia and its relationship to other prognostic factors: A Children's Oncology Group Study. *Blood* 2008;111:5477–5485.

[38] Larsen EC, Devidas M, Chen S, et al. Dexamethasone and high-dose methotrexate improve outcome for children and young adults with high-risk B-acute lymphoblastic leukemia: a report from Children's Oncology Group Study AALL0232. *J Clin Oncol* 2016;34(20:2380-2388.

[39] Ortega JA, Nesbit ME Jr, Donaldson MH, et al. L-Asparaginase, vincristine, and prednisone for induction of first remission in acute lymphocytic leukemia. *Cancer Res* 1977;37: 535–540.

[40] Mitchell CD, Richards SM, Kinsey SE, et al. Benefit of dexamethasone compared with prednisolone for childhood acute lymphoblastic leukaemia: results of the UK Medical Research Council ALL97 randomized trial. *Br J Haematol* 2005;129(6):734–45.

[41] Pegaspargase. In: *Lexi-Drugs Online* [Pediatric & Neonatal Lexi-Drugs®] Hudson, Ohio: Lexi-Comp, Inc.; January 29, 2018. Available from http://online.lexi.com. Subscription required to view.

[42] Erwinia chyrsanthemi. In: *Lexi-Drugs Online* [Pediatric & Neonatal Lexi-Drugs®] Hudson, Ohio: Lexi-Comp, Inc.; January 29, 2018. Available from http://online.lexi.com. Subscription required to view.

[43] Strullu M, Corradini N, Audrain M, et al. Silent hypersensitivity to Escherichia coli asparaginase in children with acute lymphoblastic leukemia. *Leuk Lymphoma* 2010;51:1464-1472.

[44] Silverman LB, Gelber RD, Young ML, et al. Induction failure in acute lymphoblastic leukemia of childhood. *Cancer* 1999;85:1395–1404.

[45] Moricke A, Zimmermann M, Reiter A, et al.: Long-term results of five consecutive trials in childhood acute lymphoblastic leukemia performed by the ALL-BFM study group from 1981 to 2000. *Leukemia* 2010*;*24:265-284.

[46] Toyoda Y, Manabe A, Tsuchida M, et al.: Six months of maintenance chemotherapy after intensified treatment for acute lymphoblastic leukemia of childhood. *J Clin Onco 2000;*18:1508-1516.

[47] Bhatia S, Landier W, Shangguan M, et al. Nonadherence to oral mercaptopurine and risk of relapse in Hispanic and non-Hispanic white children with acute lymphoblastic leukemia: a report from the children's oncology group. *J Clin Oncol* 2012;30:2094-2101.

[48] Krynetski EY, Tai HL, Yates CR, et al. Genetic polymorphism of thiopurine S-methyltransferase: clinical importance and molecular mechanisms. *Pharmaco-genetics* 1996 Aug;6(4):279-90.

[49] Childhood ALLCG: Duration and intensity of maintenance chemotherapy in acute lymphoblastic leukaemia: overview of 42 trials involving 12 000 randomised children. Childhood ALL Collaborative Group. *Lancet* 1996;347:1783-1788.

[50] Levinsen M, Taskinen M, Abrahamsson J, et al. Clinical features and early treatment response of central nervous system involvement in childhood acute lymphoblastic leukemia. *Pediatr Blood Cancer* 2014 Aug;61(8):1416-21.

[51] Evans AE, Gilbert ES, Zandstra R. The increasing incidence of central nervous system leukemia in children. (Children's Cancer Study Group A). *Cancer* 1970;26(2):404.

[52] Aur RJ, Simone J, Husto HO, et al. Central nervous system therapy and combination chemotherapy of childhood lymphocytic leukemia. *Blood* 1971;37:272-281.

[53] on der Weid N, Swiss Pediatric Oncology Group (SPOG). Late effects in long-term survivors of ALL in childhood: experiences from the SPOG late effects study. *Swiss Med Wkly* 2001;131(13-14):180.

[54] Krull KR, Zhang N, Santucci A, et al. Long-term decline in intelligence among adult survivors of childhood acute lymphoblastic leukemia treated with cranial radiation. *Blood* 2013;122(4):550-553.

[55] Moghrabi A, Levy DE, Asselin B, et al. Results of the Dana-Farber Cancer Institute ALL Consortium Protocol 95-01 for children with acute lymphoblastic leukemia. *Blood* 2007;109(3):896.

[56] Pui CH, Campana D, Pei D, et al. Treating childhood acute lymphoblastic leukemia without cranial irradiation. *N Engl J Med* 2009;360(26):2730.

[57] Mahoney DH Jr, Shuster JJ, Nitschke R, et al. Acute neurotoxicity in children with B-precursor acute lymphoid leukemia: an association with intermediate-dose intravenous methotrexate and intrathecal triple therapy--a Pediatric Oncology Group study. *J Clin Oncol* 1998;16(5):1712.

[58] Ritchey AK, Pollock BH, Lauer SJ, et al.: Improved survival of children with isolated CNS relapse of acute lymphoblastic leukemia: a pediatric oncology group study. *J Clin Oncol 1999;*17:3745-3752

[59] Schultz KR, Bowman WP, Aledo A, et al. Improved early event-free survival with imatinib in Philadelphia chromosome-positive acute lymphoblastic leukemia: a children's oncology group study. *J Clin Oncol* 2009;27(31):5175–81.

[60] Cortes JE,Kim DW,Pinilla-Ibarz J, et al. A phase 2 trial of ponatinib in Philadelphia chromosome-positive leukemias. *N Engl J Med* 2013;369-371.

[61] Hastings C, Gaynon PS, Nachman JB, et al. Increased post-induction intensification improves outcome in children and adolescents with a markedly elevated white blood cell count with T cell acute lymphoblastic leukaemia but not B cell disease: a report from the Children's Oncology Group. *Br J Haematol* 2015;168:533–546.

[62] Berg SL, Blaney SM, Devidas M, et al. Phase II study of nelarabine (compound 506U78) in children and young adults with refractory T-cell malignancies: A report from the Children's Oncology Group. *J Clin Onco.* 2005;15:3376–82.
[63] Dreyer ZE, Hilden JM, Jones TL, et al: Intensified chemotherapy without SCT in infant ALL: Results from COG P9407 (Cohort 3). *Pediatr Blood Cancer* 2015;62:419-26.
[64] Pieters R, Schrappe M, De Lorenzo P, et al: A treatment protocol for infants younger than 1 year with acute lymphoblastic leukaemia (Interfant-99): an observational study and a multicentre randomised trial. *Lancet* 2007;370:240-50.
[65] Stumpel DJ, Schneider P, van Roon EH, et al: Absence of global hypomethylation in promoter hypermethylated Mixed Lineage Leukaemia-rearranged infant acute lymphoblastic leukaemia. *Eur J Cancer* 2013;49:175-84.
[66] Cancer Group; Cancer and Leukemia Group B studies. What determines the outcomes for adolescents and young adults with acute lymphoblastic leukemia treated on cooperative group protocols? A comparison of Children's Cancer Group and Cancer and Leukemia Group B studies. *Blood* 2008;112(5):1646-1654.
[67] StockW, Luger SM, Advani AS, et al. Favorable outcomes for older adolescents and young adults (AYA) with acute lymphoblastic leukemia (ALL): early results of US Intergroup trial C10403. *Blood* 2014;124(21):abstr 796.
[68] Huguet F, Leguay T, Raffoux E, et al. Pediatric-inspired therapy in adults with Philadelphia chromosome-negative acute lymphoblastic leukemia: the GRAALL-2003 study. *J Clin Oncol* 2009;27(6):911-918.
[69] RyttingME, Jabbour EJ, Jorgensen JL, et al. Final results of a single institution experience with a pediatric-based regimen, the augmented Berlin-Frankfurt-Münster, in adolescents and young adults with acute lymphoblastic leukemia, and comparison to the hyper-CVAD regimen. *Am J Hematol* 2016;91(8):819-823.
[70] Fern LA, Whelan JS. Recruitment of adolescents and young adults to cancer clinical trials – international comparisons, barriers, and implications. *Semin Oncol* 2010;37:e1-8.
[71] Schmiegelow K, Heyman M, Gustafsson G, et al. The degree of myelosuppression during maintenance therapy of adolescents with B-lineage intermediate risk acute lymphoblastic leukemia predicts relapse. *Leukemia* 2010;24:715-720.
[72] *The NCCN Clinical Practice Guidelines in Oncology™ Acute Lymphoblastic Leukemia (Version 1.2018).* National Comprehensive Cancer Network, Inc. Available at: www.NCCN.org. Accessed May 18, 2018.
[73] Teachey DT, Hunger SP. Predicting relapse risk in childhood acute lymphoblastic leukaemia. *Br J Haematol* 2013;162(5):606-20.
[74] Nguyen K, Devidas M, Cheng SC, et al. Factors influencing survival after relapse from acute lymphoblastic leukemia: a Children's Oncology Group study. *Leukemia* 2008;22(12):2142.

[75] Parker C, Waters R, Leighton C, et al. Effect of mitoxantrone on outcome of children with first relapse of acute lymphoblastic leukaemia (ALL R3): an open-label randomised trial. *Lancet* 2010;376(9757):2009.
[76] Ribera JM, Ferrer A, Ribera J, et al. Profile of blinatumomab and its potential in the treatment of relapsed/refractory acute lymphoblastic leukemia. *Onco Targets Ther* 2015;8:1567–1574.
[77] Buie LW, Pecoraro JJ, Horvat TZ, et al. Blinatumomab: A First-in-Class Bispecific T-Cell Engager for Precursor B-Cell Acute Lymphoblastic Leukemia. *Ann Pharmacother* 2015;49(9):1057–1067.
[78] Blinatumomab. Lexi-Drugs. *Lexicomp*. Wolters Kluwer Health, Inc. Riverwoods, IL. Available at: http://online.lexi.com. Accessed June 10, 2018.
[79] von Stackelberg A, Locatelli F, Zugmaier G, et al. Phase I/Phase II Study of Blinatumomab in Pediatric Patients With Relapsed/Refractory Acute Lymphoblastic Leukemia. *J Clin Oncol* 2016;34(36):4381–4389.
[80] Schlegel P, Lang P, Zugmaier G, et al. Pediatric posttransplant relapsed/refractory B-precursor acute lymphoblastic leukemia shows durable remission by therapy with the T-cell engaging bispecific antibody blinatumomab. *Haematologica* 2014;99(7):1212–1219.
[81] Maude SL. Future directions in chimeric antigen receptor T cell therapy. *Curr Opin Pediatr* 2017;29(1):27–33.
[82] Kochenderfer JN, Wilson WH, Janik JE, et al. Eradication of B-lineage cells and regression of lymphoma in a patient treated with autologous T cells genetically engineered to recognize CD19. *Blood* 2010;116:4099-4102.
[83] Porter DL, Levine BL, Kalos M, et al. Chimeric antigen receptor–modified T cells in chronic lymphoid leukemia. *N Engl J Med* 2011;365:725-733.
[84] Brentjens RJ, Davila ML, Riviere I, et al. CD19-targeted T cells rapidly induce molecular remissions in adults with chemotherapy-refractory acute lymphoblastic leukemia. *Sci Transl Med* 2013;5:177.
[85] Maude SL, Frey N, Shaw PA, et al. Chimeric antigen receptor T cells for sustained remissions in leukemia. *N Engl J Med* 2014;371(16):1507–1517.
[86] Maude SL, Teachey DT, Rheingold SR, et al. Sustained remissions with CD19-specific chimeric antigen receptor (CAR)-modified T cells in children with relapsed/refractory ALL. *J Clin Oncol*; 2016 ASCO Annual Meeting; Chicago, IL. 2016.
[87] Gaynon PS, Harris RE, Altman AJ. Bone marrow versus prolonged intensive chemotherapy for children with acute lymphoblastic leukemia and an initial bone marrow relapse within 12 months of the completion of primary therapy. *J Clin Onc* 2006;24(19):3150-3156.

[88] Cairo MS, Coiffier B, Reiter A, et al. Recommendations for the evaluation of risk and prophylaxis of tumour lysis syndrome (tls) in adults and children with malignant diseases: An expert tls panel consensus. *Br J Haematol* 2010;149(4):578-86.

[89] Lexi-Drugs. *Lexicomp*. Wolters Kluwer Health, Inc. Riverwoods, IL. Available at: http://online.lexi.com. Accessed July 24, 2018.

In: Frontiers in Leukemia Pharmacotherapy
Editor: Lunawati L. Bennett

ISBN: 978-1-53614-960-9

Chapter 14

METASTASIS IN LEUKEMIA

Ifeoluwa Babatunde**, PharmD
Case Western Reserve University, Cleveland, Ohio, US

ABSTRACT

Metastasis has been an attribute of concern that has affected the treatment and outcome of most malignancies. High mortality rates and treatment failure make understanding the metastatic process of utmost importance. While most solid cancers undergo similar steps in acquiring the propensity to migrate, hematologic tumors are seen to be inherently capable of seeding successfully in a secondary site. This chapter outlines biological principles in metastasis and the factors responsible for the characteristic migration ability of metastatic leukemia.

Keywords: metastasis, migration, leukemia, leukocyte, microenvironment

ABBREVIATIONS

ADAM12	a disintegrin and metalloproteinase domain
AML	acute myeloid leukemia
ALL	acute lymphoblastic leukemia
CAM	calcium-dependent cell adhesion molecule
CLL	chronic lymphoblastic leukemia
CML	chronic myeloid leukemia
CTCs	circulating tumor cells

* Corresponding Author Email: iob3@case.edu.

CXCL12	chemokine ligand-12
CXCR4	chemokine receptor-4
ECM	extracellular matrix
EMT	epithelial-mesenchymal transition
N-Cadherin	mesenchymal neural-cadherin
MMPs	matrix metalloproteinases
VEGF	vascular endothelial growth factor
VLA-4	very late antigen-4
VCAM-1	vascular cell adhesion molecule-1

INTRODUCTION

Metastasis is an inherent characteristic of most forms of cancer and remains a major cause of mortality [1-2]. Due to cellular features and the mutations that tumor cells undergo, most solid cancer types are prone to tumorigenesis in other sites other than their primary formation place [2].

The cells or "seeds" from the original cancer can migrate towards sites or suitable "soil" to promote growth and proliferation. The invasion of the circulatory system by the primary cancer cells followed by the extravasion and seeding of the cancerous cells at the metastatic sites, is the principles of how metastatic cascade are being activated [1].

Without an exception, hematologic cancer forms such as leukemia and lymphoma are proned to metastasize to secondary sites which contribute to relapse, resistant to treatment, and death in patients with the diseases [1].

PRINCIPLES OF SOLID ORGAN AND BLOOD METASTASIS

For metastasis to occur, cells need to be able to survive and proliferate at rates which are not controlled by biochemical pathways and biological measures at a site foreign to the tumor's primary site [1]. The processes required to prepare cells for transit and survival are 1) dissemination, 2) intravasation, 3) extravasation, and 4) colonization.

Firstly, dissemination/migration. The metastasis cascade of events typically involves the cell acquisition of properties which enable the dissemination and invasion of foreign sites in the body. As shown in *in vitro* model, solid tumor cells are able to migrate through the epithelial-mesenchymal transition (EMT) by which cells exist in trans-differentiation states allowing for the loss of E-cadherin mediated cell-cell adhesion and promoting migration by intravasation through the circulatory system, follow by extravasation into the metastatic microenvironment [3]. A key player in the adhesive nature of cells is the calcium-dependent cell adhesion molecule (CAM) E-cadherin. E-cadherin serves to promote attachment between cells and the basement membrane. It inadvertently further serves as a tumor suppressor gene which makes E-cadherin an important force to overcome cancer and metastatic development [4]. In EMT, E-cadherin is seen to be downregulated and another CAM, mesenchymal neural-cadherin (N-cadherin) is seen to be upregulated which then facilitates the non-adhesive transition of cells.

With this process, cells no longer are adhered to the epithelial layer and they become polarized towards mesenchymal cells. More changes including changes to the adherens junctions and cytoskeletal polarity through genetic modification all go towards preparing the cells to migrate and invade the new tumor site [4, 5]. The extracellular matrix (ECM) which stringently controls cell function also undergoes remodeling for metastatic dissemination [5].

The cancer ECM demonstrates biological changes through genes and chemical differences in the glycation process that contribute to increase the activity of Matrix Metalloproteinase (MMP), a major family of enzymes that play a role in the apoptosis, angiogenesis and metastasis [6, 7]. Two major proteases which are seen to be increasingly expressed include MMP2 and MMP9 [5].

Secondly, intravasation. Cancer cells detached from the primary soon invade the circulatory system as a route to the intended metastatic site. These cells known as circulating tumor cells (CTCs), travel as single or colony which dwell in the vasculature or lymphatic system for short periods of time before clearance occurs [3]. Early research even showed CTCs to exist during early cancer stages and with an advancing technology CTCs can be used as a biomarker in detecting cancer progression and metastasis of solid tumors. An important characteristic of CTCs which have undergone EMT is their lack of cytokeratin proteins that are known to support cytoskeleton in cells [8].

Furthermore, these CTCs also are found to lack most of their epithelial cell-surface markers that link the seeds with the originating cancer and reveal their original identity [3].

Thirdly, extravasation. After all the changes that occur in the vasculature and lymphatic space, the seeds extravasate into the microenvironment of the destination tissue. Through transendothelial migration (TEM), the cells irreversibly cross from the permeable vasculature into the new epithelial environment and adhere to the new parenchymal tissue. The integrity of the vasculature is disrupted due to molecules such as VEGF, MMPs, and ADAM12. Inflammatory monocytes also help aid the extravasation [3, 9].

Lastly, colonization. Once the CTCs are at the new site, normal body processes will try to eliminate these seeds [5]. While some are eventually be eliminated, others either fall into a state of dormancy as a result of a failure to initiate cancer growth and adapt to the new microenvironment, or the CTCs will become disseminated cancer cells or micro-metastatic clusters that lead to the development of new cancers [3, 10].

Leukemia Specific Patterns of Metastasis

Leukemias have shown to be an aggressive and rapidly spreading malignancy. It's prominence in children reveals its very virulent nature. While most cancer take years to develop mutations, leukemia's early presentation indicates short period of time needed to develop mutations [1]. The natural properties of leukocytes allow these cells to carry out immune and inflammatory functions in the body. Hence, these cells are able to migrate to different parts of the body in response to pathogen invasion or due to damage to the tissues [11]. Leukocytes flow through the circulatory system and extravasate to the site of inflammation through chemokine and lipid attractants [11]. This intrinsic property of leukocyte mirrors the steps in the EMT program and hence allows leukemic cells to innately have migratory/metastatic properties [1].

The bone marrow microenvironment has been demonstrated to have an importance in the tumorigenesis and metastasis of leukemia [1]. It fosters the survival and migration of leukemic cells to seed at other sites to form secondary cancers. Stromal cells in the bone marrow promote tumor progression through events that mimic normal wound healing, fibrosis and remodeling [12]. These stromal cells also play a significant role in hematopoiesis, and they contribute to the increased survival of leukemic cells in collaboration with the altered state of the bone marrow architecture [13]. Their survival is increased with more stromal cells in close proximity.

Hematopoietic stem cells (HSC) and hematopoietic progenitor cells (HPCs) are characterized by ligands and molecules at the surface that lead to interactions that aid the proliferation and differentiation and migration of these cells. Some of these ligands and receptors include: VLA-4,VCAM-1, E-selectin, Notch-1/Jagged-1, CXCL12/CXCR4 [13].

VLA-4/VCAM-1

Very late antigen 4 (VLA-4) or $\alpha4\beta1$ integrin (integrin alpha 4, CD 49/integrin beta 1, CD29) is an integrin expressed on the surface of many cell including hematopoietic cells. It's multifunctions have been widely studied and deemed responsible for many inflammatory and autoimmune activities in the body. It is studied for its role in diseases like multiple sclerosis, Crohn's disease, and others [14].

VLA-4 proteins expressed on hematopoietic cells have significant pattern changes during differentiation that lead to mobilization of stem cells in the bone marrow micro environment [15]. VLA-4 binds to its receptor at the vascular cell adhesion molecule (VCAM-1) on the surface of cells which is expressed after cytokine stimulation. VCAM-1 is usually upregulated by cytokines which increase the adhesiveness of cells to vascular endothelium.

The VLA-1/VCAM-1 complex serve many functions; however, it's important to metastasis and migrate is ability of this integrin to integrate a cell to it's environment. While the functions of VLA-1 has somewhat been well defined in chronic leukemia, conflicting results show an inconclusive function of the VLA-1 integrin in acute leukemia [14].

CXCL12/CXCR4

CXCL12 is a chemokine which is also known as stromal-derived factor 1(SDF-1) which plays important role in the activation of VLA-1. SDF-1 initiates a conformational change in the integrin's components that leads to an increase in adhesion of the endothelium.

CXCL12 is highly involved in hematopoiesis and was first identified to stimulate the proliferation of B cells in the bone marrow. By interacting with it's receptor CXCR4, an elicited response as indicated is the retention of hemopoeitic cells in the bone marrow [13, 16]. This prevents apoptosis and allows the cells to acquire mutations necessary for migration to secondary sites.

Although common in all leukemia, the acute forms seem to express CXCR4/CXCR12 the most. In AML, the CXCR4/CXCR12 complex is said to promote what appears to be an "emperipolesis-like" activity, blast cells containing normal hematopoietic cells which promotes survival, but cause problem of gingival and skin tissue [13, 16].

E-Selectin

E-selectin is also an adhesion molecule similar to VLA-1 and VCAM [17]. This molecule mediates tissue infiltration and found abundantly in the circulatory system during periods of inflammation which can be used as biomarker of cancer progression. Together with it's receptor CD44, E-selectin enhances migration of leukocyte cells [17]. In the bone marrow microenvironment, E-selectin contributes to the survival of leukemic cells but cause chemoresistance [18]. This molecule is being explored as a target for drug development in cancer treatment.

Notch-1/Jagged-1

Notch signaling has been reported to be involved in EMT and metastasis and plays a significant, but not exclusive role in breast cancer metastasis. Notch1 on progenitor cells interact with Jagged1 ligands on stromal cells [19]. These promote growth and proliferation [13].

In other solid cancers such as breast, colon, and cervical cancer, this interaction often leads to the induction and expression of metastatic and migratory markers such as MMP2 and MMP9 [19]. Less understood is its role in leukemia. However, it is hypothesized that the interaction between Notch-1 and Jagged-1 results in an excessive self-renewal and abnormal proliferation in acute leukemia [20].

METASTATIC SITES OF LEUKEMIA

Similar to other cancers, leukemic cells like to disseminate to a number of sites in the body. Although it is originating from the bone marrow, leukemic cells usually spread to liver, spleen, breast and other organs. Due to the leukemia's inherent migratory properties, the lymph nodes serve as condusive environments for leukemic cells [21]. Although leukemic cells usually metastasize to the same sites like solid cancers, the central nervous system (CNS) involvement is different than other cancers [22]. An estimated 40% of patients develop cancer that metastases to the CNS which is seeded from other primary sites [22-23]. Although leukemias and lymphomas metastasize to the CNS, they rarely involve the brain tissue. If leukemia or lymphomas metastasize to the brain, it is usually affecting the layer surrounding the brain and spinal cord, leptomeninges, thus this is known as Leptomeningeal (LM) tumors [21]. About 10-30% of ALL patients are found to have leptomeningeal dissemination at early time during the diagnosis, but it is rarely seen in patients with chronic leukemias like CLL or CML [24].

LM was historically diagnosed during autopsy. Current gold standard for diagnosis of LM is through lumbar puncture (LP) of CSF (cerebro spinal fluid) accompany with neuro imaging using MRI to compliment the findings from the LP. Signs and symptoms of LM include headaches, nausea, vomiting, neuropathic pain, weakness in extremities, nuchal rigidity and other neurologic abnormalities such as photophobia [23].

CONCLUSION

Metastasis to distant organs remains an interesting phenomenon and although complex, it still remains common among all cancers. It is also interesting to note the strategic format in which cells are fortified to thrive at "foreign" soil.

Due to their innate function, leukocytes are naturally equipped to migrates and survives in foreign sites. It is no surprise that leukemic cells can proliferate to almost any sites in the body.

REFERENCES

[1] Trendowski, M. The inherent metastasis of leukemia and its exploitation by sonodynamic therapy. *Critical Reviews in Oncology/Hematology,* http//dx.doi.org/ 10.1016/j.critrevonc.2014.12.013.

[2] Zubair, H., Ahmad, A. Cancer Metastasis: An Introduction. In: Ahmad, A. (eds) *Introduction to Cancer Metastasis.* Elsevier Inc, San Diego, CA.

[3] Lambert, A., Pattabiraman, D. R., Weinberg, R. A. Emerging Biological Principles of Metastasis. *Cell, 168.* http://dx.doi.org/10.1016/j.cell.2016.11.037.

[4] Pecina-Slaus, N. Tumor suppressor gene E-cadherin and its role in normal and malignant cells. *Cancer Cell International,* 2003, 3:17.

[5] Lamouille, S., Xu, J., Derynck, R. Molecular mechanisms of epithelial-mesenchymal transition. *Nat. Rev. Mol. Cell Biol.*, 2014 March; 15(3):178 - 196. Doi:10.1038/nrm3758.

[6] Cox, T. R., Erler, J. T. Remodeling and homeostasis of the extracellular matrix: implications for fibrotic diseases and cancer. *Disease Models and Mechanisms,* 2011; 4:165 - 178. doi:10.1242/dmm.004077.

[7] Jabłońska-Trypuć, A., Matejczyk, M., Rosochacki, S. Matrix metalloproteinases (MMPs), the main extracellular matrix (ECM) enzymes in collagen degradation, as a target for anticancer drugs. *Journal of Enzyme Inhibition and Medicinal Chemistry,* 2016; 31:177 - 183.

[8] Marrinucci, D., Bethel, K., Kolatkar, A., et al. Fluid Biopsy in Patients with Metastatic Prostate, Pancreatic and Breast Cancers. *Phys. Biol.*, 2012 9(1): 016003. doi:10.1088/1478-3975/9/1/016003.

[9] Muller, W. A. Mechanisms of Leukocyte Transendothelial Migration. *Annu. Rev. Pathol.,* 2011; 6:323 - 344. Doi:10.1146/annurev-pathol-011110-130224.

[10] Dasgupta, A., Lim, A. R., Ghajar, C. M. Circulating and disseminated tumor cells: harbingers or initiators of metastasis. *Molecular Oncology*, 2017;11(1):40 - 61. doi:10.1002/1878-0261.12022.

[11] Nourshargh, S., Alon, R. Leukocyte Migration into Inflamed Tissues. *Immunity, 41.* 2014. http://dx.doi.org/10.1016/j.immuni.2014.10.008.

[12] Bussard, K. M., Mutkus, L., Stumpf, K., et al. Tumor-associated stromal cells as key contributors to the tumor microenvironment. *Breast Cancer Research,* 2016; 18:84. DOI 10.1186/s13058-016-0740-2.

[13] Sison, E. A., Brown, P. The bone marrow microenvironment and leukemia: biology and therapeutic targeting. *Expert Rev. Hematol.*, 2011; 4(3): 271 - 283. Doi:10.1586/ehm.11.30.

[14] Becker, P., Appelbaum, F. VLA-4 Function and Prognosis in AML. In: Andreeff, M. (eds) Targeted Therapy of Acute Myeloid Leukemia. *Current Cancer Research,* Springer, 2015; New York, NY.

[15] Bönig, H., Kim, Y. M. VLA4 in Acute Lymphoblastic Leukemia. In: Andreeff, M. (eds) Targeted Therapy of Acute Myeloid Leukemia. *Current Cancer Research,* Springer, New York, NY.

[16] Rastogi, V., Sharma, R., Misra, S. R., et al. Emperipolesis – A Review. *Journal of Clinical and Diagnostic Research,* 2014; 8(12): ZM0 1-ZM02. DOI:10.7860/ JCDR/2014.

[17] Kang, S. A., Blache, C. A., Bajana, S., et al. The effect of soluble E-selectin on tumor progression and metastasis. *BMC Cancer,* 2016; 16:331. DOI 10.1186/ s12885-016-2366-2362.

[18] Chien, S., Haq, S. U., Pawlus, M., et al. Adhesion Of Acute Myeloid Leukemia Blasts To E Selectin In The Vascular Niche Enhances Their Survival By Mechanisms Such As Wnt Activation. *Blood,* 2013; 122 (21) 61.

[19] Li, D., Masiero, M., Banham, A. H., et al. The Notch ligand Jagged1 as a target for anti-tumor therapy. *Frontiers in Oncology,* 2014: 4: 254.

[20] Shuji Tohda, Nobuo Nara. Expression of Notchl and Jaggedl Proteins in Acute Myeloid Leukemia Cells. *Leukemia and Lymphoma*, 2001; 42:3, 467 - 472, DOI: 10.3109/10428190109064603.

[21] DeAngelis, L. M.: Leukemia and lymphoma metastases. In *Cancer in the Nervous System.* Edited by Levin, V. A. New York: Oxford University Press; 2002:362 – 373.

[22] Aragon-Ching, J. B., Zujewski, J. A. CNS metastasis: An old problem in a new guise. *Clin. Cancer Res.*, 2007; 13:1644 - 1647. DOI: 10.1158/1078 0432.CCR-07-0096.

[23] Pekmezci, M., Perry, A. Neuropathology of brain metastases. *Surg. Neurol.,* Int. 2013; 4(Suppl. 4): S245–S255. Doi: 10.4103/2152-7806.111302.

[24] Enting, R. H. Leptomeningeal Neoplasia: Epidemiology, Clinical Presentation, CSF Analysis and Diagnostic Imaging. In: Abrey, L. E., Chamberlain, M. C., Engelhard, H. H. (eds) *Leptomeningeal Metastases. Cancer Treatment and Research*, 2005. vol 125. Springer, Boston, MA.

In: Frontiers in Leukemia Pharmacotherapy
Editor: Lunawati L. Bennett
ISBN: 978-1-53614-960-9

Chapter 15

REDOX HOMEOSTASIS IN LEUKEMIA

Lunawati L. Bennett**, PhD, PharmD
Union University, School of Pharmacy, Jackson, Tennessee, US

ABSTRACT

Exogenous and endogenous antioxidants work by eliminating oxidizing free radicals also known as ROS (reactive oxygen species), thus preventing cellular damage to the normal cells. Many anti-cancer drugs such as alkylating agents and anthracylines work by generating free radicals causing cellular damage and necrosis to the cancer cells, but also causing damage to the normal cells. Since there are many cancer patients taking antioxidants as supplementation during their chemotherapeutic regimens, concern has logically developed as to taking antioxidants concurrently during the chemotherapy. Can antioxidants be beneficial or detrimental? This chapter highlights our understanding on how free radicals are formed, antioxidants mechanism of action, redox homeostasis, and potential ROS-producing therapeutic agents for leukemia treatment.

Keywords: ROS, RNS, free radicals, chemo-prevention, vitamins, natural products, antioxidants, redox homeostasis

ABBREVIATIONS

ROS	reactive oxygen species
RNS	reactive nitrogen species
SOD	superoxide dismutase

* Corresponding Author Email: llbennett@uu.edu.

HO-1	heme oxygenase
GSH	glutathione sulfhydryl
TRx	thioredoxin
Prx	peroxiredoxin
AML	acute myeloid leukemia
ALL	acute lymphocytic leukemia
CML	chronic myeloid leukemia
CLL	chronic lymphocytic leukemia
APL	acute promyelocytic leukemia
ATO	arsenic trioxide
AA	ascorbic acid

INTRODUCTION

Antioxidants in cancer treatment and prevention remains an area of rapid growth and evolution. Antioxidants have been extensively studied for their abilities to prevent cancer in humans [1-2]. The therapeutic implications of antioxidant therapy has gained substantial traction and attention, especially since several chemotherapeutic agents deplete the body's endogenous antioxidant supplies, potentially leading to inflammation and infectious complications.

While many believe antioxidants diminish toxicity and enhance efficacy, legitimate concerns exist surrounding antioxidants interference with the oxidative mechanisms of some chemotherapeutic agents such as alkylating agents and anthracyclines. This disruption may lead to a diminished free radical formation, ultimately increasing cancer cell survivability.

Understanding the redox environment of leukemia cells will improve our understanding of the benefits and detrimental effects of antioxidants. In addition, learning redox biochemistry that occurs between normal and cancer cells is essential for the design and development strategies to overcome oxidative damage and chemotherapy resistance.

Enhancing the capacity of antioxidants to protect cells from redox-related changes or environmental toxins are the aim of antioxidants cytoprotective strategies against cancer. On the contrary, the strategy to deplete antioxidants or to create prooxidants aiming to sensitize cancer cells are another strategy in our fight against cancer.

Free Radicals and Oxidative/Nitrosative Stress

Free radicals are generally known as ROS (reactive oxygen species) or reactive nitrogen species (RNS). Constant generation of ROS/RNS is a natural biochemical event in all aerobic organisms. ROS/RNS are oxidants natural products formed during cell vital metabolism activity which play important role in proliferation, migration, defense, vasorelaxation, autophagy and apoptosis signals that act as second messengers, as an integral part of the signal transduction network [3-5]. RNS are produced by endothelium inducing vascular relaxation when vascular smooth muscle cells are stimulated by vasodilators [4-5]. ROS are heterogeneous group diatomic oxygen derived from free and non-free radicals species with a wide range of reactivity [6-7].

The free radical formation begins with the univalent reduction of oxygen to produce superoxide radical anions ($O2^{\cdot-}$), that give rise to many highly reactive species such as peroxyl radicals (ROO·), hydroxyl radical (·OH), and nitric oxide (NO·), hypochlorous acid (HOCl), hydrogen peroxide (H_2O_2), peroxynitrite (ONOO−), and singlet oxygen (1O2) [8]. ROS/RNS formation involves enzymes of the mitochondria respiratory chain, NADPH oxidase, xanthine oxidase, and cytochrome P450 system. Dysfunctional endothelial nitric oxide synthase (eNOS) and free redox-active metals such as iron and copper via their catalytic decomposition of H_2O_2 (Fenton reaction) also play important role in free radical formation [8-10].

Antioxidants

In order to maintain appropriate ROS/RNS and to regulate their functions, the body has natural defenses against oxidative stress by using endogenous antioxidatives. The endogenous antioxidative system includes: a) enzymes such as superoxide dismutase (SOD), catalase, Peroxiredoxins (PRx); b) glutathione sulfhydryl-linked system (GSH), such as glutathione peroxidase, glutathione S-transferase, glutathione reductase; c) non-enzymes such as cysteine, thioredoxin (Trx), and d) metal-binding proteins such as ferritin, metallothionein, and ceruloplasmin [3, 11]. Components of the endogenous antioxidant defense system work together in concert with exogenous antioxidants from dietary or supplementation such as ascorbic acid, vitamin E, carotenoids, and polyphenols (flavonols, isoflavones) to prevent or to reduce oxidative stress and to maintain redox homeostasis [12]. Antioxidants activity of these enzymes and compounds are reliant upon trace elements such as selenium, copper, manganese, and zinc [13].

Based on animal, cell line, and preclinical experiments, antioxidants supplements are beneficial for patients undergoing chemotherapy because they alleviate toxic effects of chemotherapeutic agents allowing patients to tolerate the full course of treatment [14-15].

In the clinical trials; however, the data suggested a lack of benefit and possibly harmful [16-17]. The discrepancy of the studies might be due to the fact that depending on the drug class being used, many chemotherapeutic agents such as alkylating agents (cyclophosphamide, ifosfamide), anthracycline antibiotics (doxorubicin, idarubicin), or mitotic inhibitors (vincristine, vinorelbine) works by creating cellular damage to the cancer cells by increasing their ROS/RNS productions [8, 18]. While not all anti-cancer drugs causing increased in ROS/RNS production, patients with cancer who take large amounts of antioxidants during the chemotherapy may actually block ROS/RNS-induced apoptosis of the cancer cells [3].

REDOX HOMEOSTASIS

Maintaining the balance between the generation of ROS/RNS and the activity of endogenous or exogenous antioxidants enzymes are very intricate. From decades of redox biology studies, a paradigm has emerged our understanding on redox homeostasis. In general, cancer cells have relatively high levels of ROS due to alterations in pro- and antioxidants pathways. Low levels of ROS; however, plays an important role as secondary messengers, facilitating a number of signaling pathways involving kinases, phosphatases and other transcription factor. Low level of ROS also can cause drug resistance [19-20]. When the ROS level is very high, this promotes genomic instability, reduce survival and growth signaling of cancer cells, and promote oxidative damage of cancer cells through lipid peroxidation, amino acid oxidation, and DNA damage [19-21]. Figure 1. depicts ROS levels in leukemic versus normal cells and the difference in biological outcomes [19].

Leukemic cells frequently alter the expression and the activity of antioxidant pathways by neutralizing free radicals to less-reactive molecular components, preventing catastrophic redox imbalance [19]. Irwin et al. compiled a study on different effects of six antioxidants such as SOD, catalase, HO-1, GSH, Trx and Prx that are dysregulated in leukemic cells from the patients with ALL, AML, CLL, and CML. Endogenous antioxidants are reported to be both up- and down-regulated in leukemia models and primary human leukemia cells [19]. Up regulation and protein expression and activity of SOD, GSH, Trx, Prx, HO-1 and catalase enzymes observed in these samples maybe due to the imbalance in the redox status of leukemic cells leading to oxidative stress allowing survival of cancer cells. While most of the antioxidant proteins are up regulated, down regulation of antioxidant activity and expression are also noticed which maybe transient in response to therapy or permanent in response to genetic inhibition. Specifically, SOD and catalase activity are reduced in lymphocytes from ALL and CLL patients [19, 22-23].

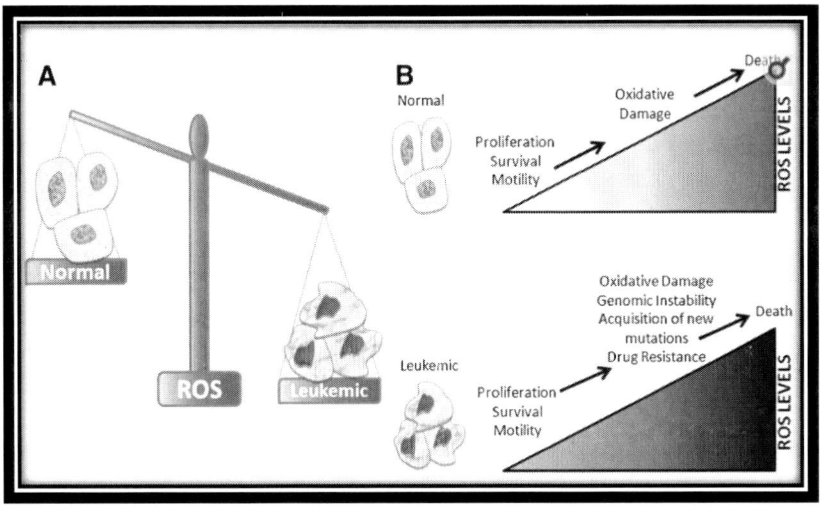

Figure 1. ROS are elevated in leukemic cells compared with normal cells, leading to differing biological outcomes. (**A**) The balance of ROS levels is tipped to denote that leukemic cells have higher basal levels of ROS than normal cells (B) Within normal cells (top panel), low levels of ROS are constitutively produced (light shading in the *triangle*), which contributes to cell proliferation, survival, and motility. As these levels increase (darker shading), oxidative damage can occur to cells that ultimately results in cell death. Leukemic cells (*bottom panel*) have constitutively elevated levels of ROS (darker shading in the *triangle*) due to alterations in redox control. However, due to this altered redox status, elevated ROS is beneficial rather than detrimental to leukemic cells. Elevated ROS in leukemic cells not only provides the same benefits as low levels of ROS in normal cells but also promotes genomic instability and drug resistance due to oxidative damage. Ultimately, further elevations in ROS, such as those produced by therapeutic agents, can lead to the death of leukemia cells. ROS, reactive oxygen species [19].

Besides antioxidants, oncogenes such as BCR/ABL, Flt3-ITD, Ras, and c-kit directly manipulate leukemia cell signaling, but these oncogenes can also alter the redox homeostasis of cancer cells [24]. ROS levels was elevated in blast crisis samples of CML that have mutations in BCR/ABL. BCR/ABL is also capable of influencing ROS production through manipulation of the NADPH oxidase (NOX) complex leading to tyrosine kinase inhibitors resistant in CML patients [25]. FLt3-ITD causes increased levels of ROS in AML cell lines, while c-kit and Ras can also regulate NOX activity causing production of ROS [26]. The major endogenous source of ROS in any cell types of leukemia are mitochondrial electron transport chain (ETC) and NOX complexes [19, 25-26]. Mitochondrial ETC generates about 90% of ROS in most leukemic cells [27-28]. Mitochondrial ETC is the principal contributor of the production of adenosine triphosphate (ATP) within cells, viable for both normal and cancer cells. Almost all oxygen consumed during respiration is converted to water; however, 1-2% is partially reduced for generation of superoxide anion [27-28].

Mutation in mitochondrial DNA (mtDNA) appears in leukemia resulting in alterations of mitochondrial ETC and potentially elevated ROS production [29-30]. Paradoxically, mitochondrial ROS also induce apoptosis, rather than survival of AML cells [28]. MtETC in the leukemic cells can also promote growth, survival, and drug resistance, but also sensitizing leukemic cells to death by some chemotherapeutics agents [19]. Leukemic cells show an increased expression of NOX components as well as the production of the rate limiting substrate, NADPH, by transferring an electron from NADPH through NOX complex to oxygen [24, 31]. Additionally, metabolic and detoxification pathways such as xanthine oxidoreductase (XO/XDO) complex and cytochrome P450 may contribute to leukemic cells ROS production [32-33]. Elevations of XO activity are found in relapsed AML contribute to increase in ROS level [32]. Figure 2 depicts endogenous routes of leukemic induction of ROS.

Therefore, as with many other cancers, it was observed that ROS/RNS levels are up regulated in leukemia. Elevated production of ROS can occur due to the use of certain chemotherapeutic agents, activation of leukemic oncogenes, mutations within mitochondria or cytochrome P450 systems independent of oncogene activity, or down regulation of antioxidants. Increased in total ROS level or decreased in clearance of ROS can also be used as therapeutic approach to treat refractory AML, ALL, CML, CLL, and other hematologic malignancies.

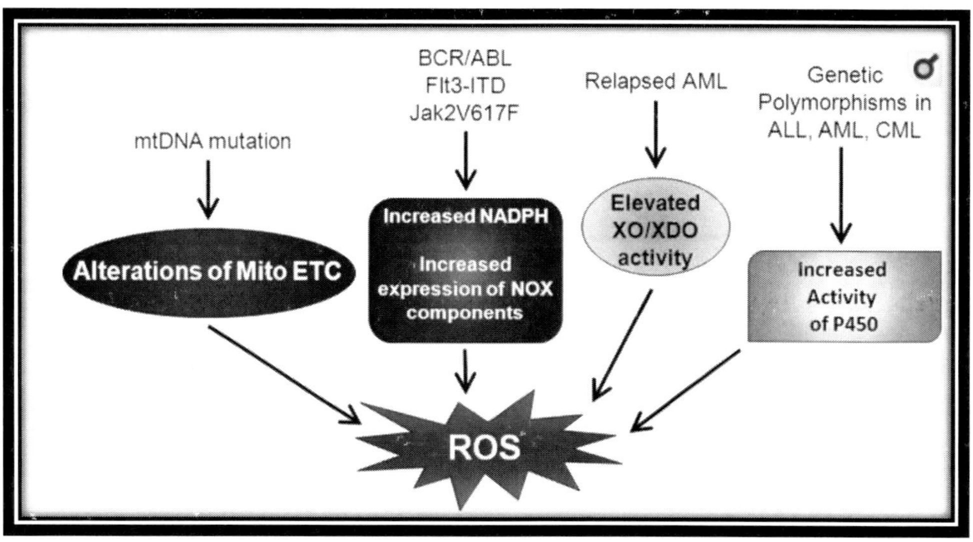

Figure 2. Highlighted endogenous routes of leukemic induction of ROS. A myriad of pathways can result in elevated ROS production in leukemic cells. Mutations in the mitochondrial DNA (mtDNA) can lead to alterations of the ETC, resulting in ROS production. Activation of the BCR/ABL, and Flt3-ITD pathways and mutation of Jak can lead to alterations in the NADPH oxidase (NOX) system and ultimately increase ROS levels. In AML, xanthine oxidoreductase activity (XO/XDO) is elevated, which can induce up regulation of ROS. Activating polymorphisms of cytochrome P450, which results in elevated ROS levels, can be found in ALL, AML, and CML. ALL, acute lymphocytic leukemia; AML, acute myeloid leukemia; BCR/ABL, breakpoint cluster region–Abelson leukemia virus; CML, chronic myeloid leukemia; ETC, electron transport chain; Flt3, fms-like receptor tyrosine kinase 3; ITD, internal tandem duplication; XO, xanthine oxidase; XDO, xanthine dehydrogenase [19].

ROS-PRODUCING CHEMOTHERAPEUTIC AGENTS

Because ROS levels are elevated in leukemic cells, the use of drugs that promote further production of ROS to tip the scales toward cell death have been explored. Although a number of cytotoxic chemotherapeutic drugs such as purine analogs, mitotic inhibitors and antibiotic antracyclines have been used as frontline standard of care in leukemia; unfortunately, relapse and resistance remain critical issues. For example, pyrimidine analogs such as cytarabine, an antimetabolite drugs that when phosphorylated incorporated unto DNA poisoning the DNA replicating leukemic cells. Induction of ROS appears early in the apoptosis cascade, which could be reversed by antioxidant N-acetyl cysteine (NAC) causing a large decrease in endogenous GSH [19]. This explain why cytarabine use for remission of AML is short live, with 5 year event free survival and overall survival rates of only 35% and 40%, respectively [34]. Another example is anthracyclines such as doxorubicin, idarubicin, mitoxantrone. These drugs work by interfering macromolecular biosynthesis causing DNA adduct formation, by interfering with topoisomerase II, and by causing free radical formation [35]. Anthracyclines are substrates for XO and Trx. Bioactivation of theses enzymes cause anthracyclines to produce free radicals [36-37]. The free radicals induce direct damage to DNA and may interact with oxygen to promote ROS formation [35]. Anthracyclines may also complex with free iron in cells, leading to chemical reaction known as Fenton reaction which generates further ROS through combination of iron and H_2O_2 [35]. Although the accumulation of ROS and free radical damage within leukemic cells lead to cytotoxic oxidative stress, antracyclines are susceptible to resistance due to cancer cells ability to repair their DNA and evade apoptosis [38-39]. Antracyclines cause myelosuppression, mucosititis and cardiotoxicity showing as arrhythmias, dilated cardiomyopathy with heart failure that can occur even 24 hours after a single dose or can happen years later due to the generation of ROS within myocardium [38-41]. Therefore, there is a need to develop chemotherapeutic drugs that can prolonged or cause increased in the production of ROS.

A recently approved ROS producing chemotherapeutic drug is arsenic trioxide (ATO, $As_2 O_3$, Trisenox ®), which is a traditional Chinese medicine that is used for the treatment of various cancers and acute promyelocytic leukemia (APL). A number of suggested mechanisms through which ATO exerts its cytotoxic effect are: a) causing degradation of chimeric PML/RAR-α protein (fusion gene on chromosome 15 and 17, [t (15; 170(q24; q21) which disrupts the gene for nuclear receptor for retinoic acid that fuses with PML gene), b) inducing apoptosis through a mitochondrial dependent process resulting increased in ROS production, and c) activating caspases cell signaling responsible for apoptosis [19, 42-46]. By manipulation of intracellular redox control, ATO induce NOX components and mitochondrial ETC. Figure 3. depicts mechanism of ATO-induced death of leukemic cells.

Besides ATO, potential therapeutic avenues to modulate redox homeostasis include drugs that potentiate ROS production or inhibit ROS. Histone deacetylase (HDACs) inhibitors or HO-1 inhibitors can increase the production of ROS pushing the oxidative balance resulting in leukemic cell death, while drugs such as NOX inhibitors, XO/XDO inhibitors, SOD and catalase delivery system are aimed to cause genomic instability and increased drug sensitivity by inhibiting ROS production. For instance, there are several HDAC inhibitors that have been developed, such as vorinostat, romidepsin, and benzamides that affect production of ROS and control the transcription of endogenous antioxidants [47]. HDAC inhibitors were shown to elevate the expression of NOX2, inhibit Trx enzymes, promoting proapoptotic BCl2 family leading to alteration of mitochondrial and potentiation of apoptosis. Using samples from ALL and CML patients, HDAC inhibitors showed to cause a significant increase in ROS level alone or in combination with tyrosine kinase inhibitors, leading to enhanced DNA damage and cell death [47]. There are several clinical trials combining HDAC inhibitors with other standard care chemotherapy to treat refractory ALL, AML, CML, or CLL.

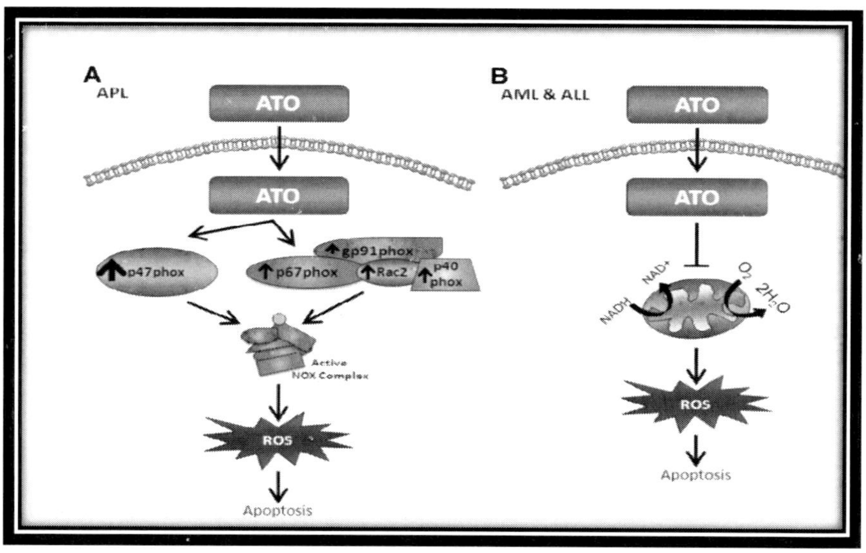

Figure 3. Mechanisms of ATO-induced death of leukemia cells. ATO passes through the plasma membrane into the cytosol. Once inside the cell, ATO either (**A**) directly induces elevations of NOX subunits (p47phox: 400-fold induction; p67phox, Rac2, p40phox, and gp91phox: 2-fold induction), leading to induction of the active NOX complex (in APL) or (**B**) inhibits the mitochondrial respiratory chain (in AML and ALL). Both scenarios lead to increased ROS generation and subsequent apoptosis of leukemic cells. APL, acute promyelocytic leukemia [19].

VITAMIN C

Ascorbic acid (AA, vitamin C, ascorbate) has a controversial history in cancer treatment [48]. It was first reported that when AA was given by intravenous (i.v.) for 10 days and then orally in pharmacologic doses of 10 g daily, it was effective in treating some cancers and in improving patients' survivals [49-50]. However, the same dose had no effect in patient well-being and survival in 2 subsequent double-blind placebo-controlled trials when given orally [51-52]. Interestingly, another study showed AA has a significant effect in cancer treatment [53].The differences between the studies are due to the route used i.e., intravenous followed by oral versus oral only. The pharmacokinetics studies in men and women showed that 10 g AA when given intravenously produced 70 times higher plasma concentration than oral administration [54]. In lymphoma and human leukemic cell lines, several studies found that when these cell lines were incubated with buffered neutralize AA for 1 hr. to mimic clinical i.v. use, it caused 50% cancer cell death using AA at 2 mM and 2.8mM, respectively [53-54].

It was postulated that high dose AA mediated cell death due to the generation of protein-dependent extracellular H_2O_2 via ascorbate radical formation from AA as the electron donor. High dose AA can only be achieved with i.v. resulting in pharmacological concentration distribution to the extracellular water space [55]. No detectable H_2O_2 was accumulated in the blood. H_2O_2 generation is outside cells at the pharmacological concentrations. AA acts as prodrug generating H_2O_2 extracellular induces apoptosis or necrosis to the cancer cells but not to the normal cells [56]. In leukemic cell lines, high dose AA also down regulate HIH-1α which regulate BCl_2 family such as MCl-1, $BCl\text{-}_{xL}$ essential for the growth and survival of leukemic cells by preventing the induction of apoptosis by ROS [57-59]. Inhibition of HIH-1α along with high AA causing generation of H_2O_2 suggests an alternative option for cancer therapy. Complementary and alternative medicine practitioners worldwide have used i.v. AA in some patients since there is no apparent harm with high dose of this antioxidant. Currently, there are 13 clinical trials examine the use of i.v. AA as monotherapy, or in combination with ATO, dexamethasone and thalidomide in AML, ALL, APL, myelodysplastic syndrome (MDS). See ClincalTrials.gov for more detail.

CONCLUSION

Despite a significance interest in the role of redox homeostasis in leukemia cell survival, growth, progression, relapse and drug resistance, direct inhibitors of antioxidants or prooxidants are still fairly young in the development. Targeting the dysregulated redox environment within the leukemic cells could provide treatment selectivity, allowing less overall toxicity than traditional chemotherapy. Further study is needed to quantify the levels of oxidative stress *in vitro* and *in vivo* and to learn how to control redox system to balance between ROS and the antioxidants.

Patients with advanced disease and poor prognosis have dysregulated expression of certain ROS/RNS-metabolizing enzymes. These patients may not benefit and, in fact, may experience deleterious effects from taking antioxidants. These ill effects may result from the advanced cancer cells utilizing antioxidants to scavenge high ROS/RNS levels. Because cancer cells are able to adapt to the altered redox homeostasis due to their rapid growth and their ability to alternate metabolic pathways, making them less sensitive to exogenous stressors, an effective modulation of oxidative stress may provide a promising strategy in cancer treatment. Although a "universal" antioxidant may not be developed due to the complex system of redox homeostasis, antioxidant that should be absorbed readily, able to chelate donor oxygen or nitrogen atoms, inhibit cell proliferation, behaving as prooxidant, suppressing the metabolic activation of carcinogens, and possess low toxicity will be ideal options treatment for leukemia pharmacotherapy.

REFERENCES

[1] Lamson DW, Brignall MS. Antioxidants in cancer therapy: their actions and interactions with oncologic therapies. *Alternative Med Ev* 1999;4:5-304-329.

[2] Sing DK, Lippman SM. Cancer chemoprevention part 1: retinoids and carotenoids and other classic antioxidants. *Oncology* 1998;12:1643-1660.

[3] Kwee JK. A paradoxical chemoresistance and tumor suppressive role of antioxidant in solid cancer cells: a strange case of Dr. Jekyll and Mr. Hyde. *BioMed Res International*. 2014. http://dx.doi.org/10.1155/2014/209845.

[4] McCormick WJ. Cancer: the preconditioning factor in pathogenesis: a new etiologic approach. *Arch Pediatr* 1954;71:313-322.

[5] Chen Q, Espey MG, Sun AY, et al. Pharmacologic doses of ascorbate act as a prooxidant and decrease growth of aggressive tumor xenographs in mice. *Proc Natl Acad Sci USA* 2008;105 (32):11105-11109.

[6] Takemura Y, Satoh M, Satoh K, et al. High dose of ascorbic acid induces cell death in mesothelioma cells. *Biochem Biophys Res Commun* 2010; 394:249-253.

[7] Levine M, Padayatty SJ, Espey MG. Vitamin C: a concentration-function approach yields pharmacology and therapeutic discoveries. *Adv Nutr* 2011;2:78-88.

[8] Poprac P, Jomova K, Simunkova M, et al. Targeting free radicals in oxidative stress-related human diseases. *Trends in Pharmacological Sciences*. 2017. http;//dx.doi.org/10.1016/j.tips.2017.04.005.

[9] Siegel BV, Moton JI. Vitamin C and immunity: natural killer cell factor. *Int J Vitam Nutr Res* 1983;53 92): 179-183.

[10] Valko M. Free radicals and antioxidants in normal physiological functions and human disease. *Int J Biochem Cell Biol* 2007;39:44-84.

[11] Zalewska M, Trefon J, Milnorowicz H. The role of metallothionein interaction with other proteins. *Proteomics* 2014.

[12] Rio DD, Mateos AR, Spencer JPE, et al. Dietary (poly) phenolics in human health: structures, bioavailability, and evidence of protective effects against chronic diseases. *Antioxidants and Redox Signaling* 2013;18:1818-1892.
[13] Romero-Canelon I, Sadler PJ. Next generation metal anticancer complexes: multitargeting via redox modulation. *Inorganic Chemistry* 2013;52:12276-12291.
[14] Fuchs-Torlovsky V. Role of antioxidants in cancer therapy. *Nutrition* 2012;29:15-29.
[15] Vincent DT, Ibrahim YF, Espey MG, et al. The role of antioxidant in the era of cardiooncology. *Cancer Chemotherapy and Pharmacol* 2013;72:1157-1168.
[16] Goodman M, Bostick RM, Kucuk O, Jones DP. Clinical trials of antioxidants as cancer prevention agents: past, present, and future. *Free Rad Biol Med* 2011;51:1068-1084.
[17] Bjelakovic G, Nikolova D, Gluud C. Antioxidant supplement and mortality. *Current Opion in Clinical Nutrition and Metabolic care*. 2014; 17:40-44.
[18] Halliwell B. Oxidative stress and cancer: have we moved forward? *Biochem J* 2007;401:1-11.
[19] Irwin ME, Valle NR-Del, Chandra J. Redox control of leukemia: from molecular mechanisms to therapeutic opportunities. *Antioxidants & Redox Signaling* 2013;18 (11): 1349-1383.
[20] Finkel T. Signal transduction by reactive oxygen species. *J Cell Biol* 2011;194: 7-15.
[21] Teachootham D, Lu W, Ogasawara MA, et al. Redox regulation of cell survival. *Antioxid Redox Signal* 2008;10:1343-1374.
[22] Senturker S, Karahalil B, Inal M, et al. Oxidative DNA base damage and antioxidant enzyme levels in childhood ALL. *FEBS Lett* 1997;416:286-290.
[23] Oltra AM, Carbonell F, Tormos C, et al. Antioxidant enzyme activities and the production of MDA and 8-oxopdG in CLL. *Free Radic Biol Med* 2001;30:1286-1292.
[24] Reddy MM, Fernandes MS, Salgia R, et al. NADPH oxidases regulate cell growth and migration in myeloid cells transformed by oncogenic tyrosine kinase. *Leukemia* 2011; 25:281-289.
[25] Mayerhofer M, Florian S, Krauth MT, et al. Identification of heme oxygenase-1 as a novel BCR/ABL dependent survival factor in CML. *Cancer Res* 2004; 64:3148-3154.
[26] Maraldi T, prata C, Vieceli DSF, et al. NADPH oxidase isoform Nox2 plays a prosurvival role in human leukemia cells. *Free Radic Res* 2009;43:1111-1121.
[27] Silva A, Girio A, Cebola I et al. Intracellular reactive oxygen species are essential for P13k/Akt/mTOR-dependent IL-7 mediated viability of T cell ALL cells. *Leukemia* 2011;25:960-967.

[28] Quillet-Mary A, Jaffezou JP, Mansat V et al. Implication of mitochondrial hydrogen peroxide generation in ceramide-induced apoptosis. *J Biol Chem* 1997;272:21388-21395.

[29] Carew JS, Huang P. Mithochondrial defects in cancer. *Mol Cancer* 2002; 1:9.

[30] Carew JS, Zhou Y, Albitar M et al. Mitochondrial DNA mutations in primary leukemia cells after chemotherapy: clinical significance and therapeutic implications. *Leukemia* 2003;17:1437-1447.

[31] Naughton R, Quiney C, Turner SD, Cotter TG. BCR-ABL mediated redox regulation of the P1`3k/Akt pathway. *Leukemia* 2009; 23;1432-1440.

[32] Zhang Z, Blake DR, Stevens CR, et al. A reappraisal of xanthine dehydrogenase and oxidase in hypoxic reperfusion injury: the role of NADH as an electron donor. *Free Radic Res* 1998;28:151-164.

[33] Xu W, Zhang XA, Wang DW. The roles of CYP450 epoxygenases and metabolites, epoxy eicosatrienoic acids in cardiovascular and malignant diseases. *Adv Drug Deliv Rev* 2011;63:597-609.

[34] Lowenberg B, Pabst T, Vellenga E, et al. Cytarabine dose for AML. *N Engl J Med* 2011;364:1027-1036.

[35] Gewirtz DA. A critical evaluation of the mechanisms of action proposed for the antitumor effects of anthracnycline antibiotics adriamycin and daunorubicin. *Biochem Pharmacol* 1999; 57:727-741.

[36] Celik H, Arinc E. Bioreduction if idarubicin and formation of ROS responsible for DNA cleavage by NADPH cytochrome P450 reductase and its potential role in the antitumor effect. *J Pharm Sci* 2008;11:68-82.

[37] Ravi D, Das KC. Redox-cycling of anthracyclines by thioredoxin system: increased superoxide generation and DNA damage. *Cancer Chemother Pharmacol* 2004;54:449-458.

[38] Nielsen D, Maare C, Skovsgaard T. Cellular resistance to anthracyclines. *General Pharmacology The Vascular System*. 1996: 27(2); 251–255.

[39] Pendleton MJ, Linsdsey RH, Felix CA, et al. Topoisomerase II and leukemia. *Ann NY Acad Sci* 2014;1310:98-110.

[40] DenBoer ML, Pieters R, Veerman AJP. Mechanisms of cellular anthracycline resistance in childhood acute leukemia. *Leukemia*. 1998;12(11):1657–1670.

[41] Cutts SM, Swift LP, Rephaeli A, Nudelman A, Phillips DR. Recent advances in understanding and exploiting the activation of anthracyclines by formaldehyde. *Current Med Chem Anti Cancer Agents*. 2005;5(5):431– 447.

[42] McCulloch D, Brown C, Illand H. Retinoic acid and arsenix trioxide in the treatment of acute promyelocytic leukemia: current perspective. *Onco Tarets Ther.* 2017;10:1585-1601. doi: 10.2147/OTT.S100513.

[43] Rowley JD, Golomb HM, Dougherty C. 15/17 translocation, a consistent chromosomal change in APL. *Lancet*. 1977;1(8010):549–550.

[44] Zhang X, Yu D, Geng H, et al. Dual effects of arsenic trioxide on tumor cells and the potential underlying mechanisms. *Oncol Lett* 2018;16(3): 3812-3820.
[45] Chen GQ, Shi XG, Tang W, et al. Use of arsenic trioxide (As2O3) in the treatment of acute promyelocytic leukemia (APL): I. As2O3 exerts dose-dependent dual effects on APL cells. *Blood.* 1997;89:3345–3353.
[46] Pelicano H, Feng L, Zhou Y, et al. Inhibition of mithocndrial respiration: a novel strategy to enhance drug-induced apoptosis in human leukemia cells by a reactive oxygen species-mediated mechanism. *J Biol Chem* 2003;278:37832-37839.
[47] Nguyen T, Dai Y, Attkisson E et al. HDAC inhibitors potentiate the activity of the BCR/ABL kinase inhibitor KW-2449 in imatinib sensitive or resistant BCR/ABL $^+$ leukemia cells in vitro and in vivo. *Clin Cancer Res* 2011; 17:3219-3232.
[48] Padayatty SJ, Levine M. Reevaluation of ascorbate in cancer treatment: emerging evidence, open minds and serendipity. *J Am Coll Nutr* 2000;19:423-425.
[49] Cameron E, Pauling L. Supplemental ascorbate in the supportive treatment of cancer: prolongation of survival times in terminal human cancer. *Proc Natl Acad Sci USA* 1976;73:3685-3689.
[50] Cameron E, Pauling L. Supplemental ascorbate in the supportive treatment of cancer : reevaluation of prolongation of survival times in terminal human cancer. *Proc natl Acad Sci* USA 1978;75: 4538-4542.
[51] Creagan ET, Moertel CG, O'fallon JR, et al. Failure of high-dose ascorbic acid therapy to benefit patients with advanced cancer. A control trial. *N Engl J Med* 1979;301:687-690.
[52] Moertel CG, Fleming TR, Creagen ET, et al. High dose vitamin C versus placebo in the treatment of patients with advanced cancer who have had no prior chemotherapy. A randomized double-blind comparison. *N Engl J Med* 312:137-141.
[53] Chen Q, Espey MG, Krishna MC, et al. Pharmacologic ascorbic acid concentrations selectively kill cancer cells: action as a pro-drug to deliver hydrogen peroxide to tissues.P*NAS* 2005; 102 (38): 13604-13609.
[54] Kawada H, Kanek M, Sawanobori M, et al. High concentrations of L-ascorbic acid specifically inhibit the growth of human leukemic cells via downregulation of HIF-1α transcription. *Plos One* 2013;8:4-e62717.
[55] Semen GL. Targeting HIF-1 for cancer therapy. *Nat Rev Cancer* 2003;3:721-732.
[56] Du J, Cullen JJ, Buettner GR. Ascorbic acid: chemistry, biology and the treatment of cancer. *Biochim Biophys Acta* 2012;1826:443-457.
[57] Glaser SP, Le EF, Trounson E, et al. Anti-apoptotic MCl-1 is essential for the development and sustained growth of acute myeloid leukemia. *Genes Dev* 2012;26:120-125.
[58] Del Principe MI, Del Poeta G, Venditti A, et al. Apoptosis and immaturity in AML. *Hematology* 2005;10:25-34.

[59] Gonzalez MS, DeBrasi CD, Bianchini M, et al. BAX/BCL-XL gene expression ratio inversely correlates with disease progression in CML. *Blood Cells Mol Dis* 2010;45:192-196.

In: Frontiers in Leukemia Pharmacotherapy
Editor: Lunawati L. Bennett
ISBN: 978-1-53614-960-9

Chapter 16

Supportive Care in Leukemia

Lunawati L. Bennett*, PhD, PharmD

Union University, College of Pharmacy, Jackson, Tennessee, US

Abstract

Cancer patients are at increased risk of serious adverse events due to the cancer or the drug therapy or both; therefore, the management of these complications by supportive care or symptoms management are important to be addressed. Common adverse events encountered by the patients includes suppression of the immune system (myelosuppression), venous thromboembolism (VTE), tumor lysis syndrome (TLS), nausea/vomiting, fatigue and pain. Specific drugs also produce specific toxicities require treatment with antidotes. For example, cyclophosphamide can cause hemorrhagic cystitis require treatment with Mesna. This chapter highlights common adverse events and their supportive cares.

Keywords: tumor lysis syndrome, supportive care, myelosuppression, nausea, vomiting, fatigue, filgrastim, cytokine release syndrome

Abbreviations

AML	acute myeloid leukemia
ALL	acute lymphoblastic leukemia
CML	chronic myeloid leukemia
CLL	chronic lymphocytic leukemia

* Corresponding Author Email: llbennett@uu.edu.

CRF	cancer related fatigue
CRP	cancer related pain
TLS	tumor lysis syndrome
MDS	myelodysplastic syndrome
NSAIDs	non-steroidal anti-inflammmatory drugs
VTE	venous thromboembolism
EPO	erythropoietin
ESA	erythropoiesis stimulating agent
MGF	myeloid growth factors
N/V	nausea, vomiting

INTRODUCTION

Standard care for leukemia involves supportive care measures that include observation, psychosocial support, routine quality of life assessment, and clinical monitoring of drug efficacy to prevent toxicity and undesirable adverse events. AML and patients with different types of leukemia are often extremely ill requiring comprehensive management of bone marrow support with red blood cells and platelet transfusions, prevention of infections, correction of coagulopathies (deep vein thrombosis or venous thromboembolism), and prevention of tumor lysis syndrome (TLS) occurances.

Common chemotherapy adverse events and toxicities due to: 1) anthracyclines are myelosuppression, nausea/vomiting (N/V), mucositis, and cardiotoxicity; 2) cyclophosphamide are myelosuppression, hemorrhagic cystitis, hyponatremia, and N/V; 3) cytarabine are conjunctivitis and flu-like syndrome; 4) etoposide are infusion-related reactions and mucositis; 5) mercaptopurine are hepatotoxicity, rash, and myelosuppression; 6) methotrexate are nephrotoxicity, myelosuppression, and mucositis; 7) Peg-Asparaginase are hypersensitivity reactions, coagulopathies, hyperglycemia, and pancreatitis; 8) vincristine are peripheral neuropathies and constipation; and 9) corticosteroids are agitation, insomnia, hyperglycemia, hypertension, psychosis and fluid retention, respectively [1]. This chapter highlights common adverse events of chemotherapeutic drugs.

DISORDERS OF BLOOD CELL

Disorder of blood cell production usually manifested as anemia, leukopenia, or thrombocytopenia. Under ordinary condition, blood cells production ranged from 2 x 10^{11} erythrocytes (red blood cells, RBC), 5 x 10^{10} neutrophils, and 2.5 x 10^{11} platelets along with other component of blood such as lymphocytes, macrophages, antigen processing cells, eosinophils, and basophils [2]. Cancer and chemotherapeutic agents are often associated with profound perturbation of blood cells production.

Incidence of anemia in cancer is common, and it contributes to bleeding, malnutrition, iron, folate and B12 deficiencies, hemolysis, myelosuppresion, endogenous erythropoietin (EPO) deficiency and chronic illness [2]. Deficiency in EPO has been associated with increased production of hepcidin, an iron regulatory peptide in the liver [3-4]. Hepcidin binds to inactivates iron transporter ferroportin causing impaired absorption of dietary iron and depleted storage of iron pools [3-4]. Anemia is usually treated with erythropoiesis stimulating agents (ESAs). Although ESAs are generally well tolerated, but due to recent safety concerns regarding increased formation of red blood cells aplasia (PRCA), development of venous thromboembolism (VTE), and potential effect on cancer progression and survival, ESAs should not be used routinely to treat anemia associated with cancer. Other option include transfusion with RBC, but RBC transfusion is usually limited to patients with severe anemia (hemoglobin level of 8 g/dL or lower) [2].

White blood cells (WBC) disorder such as neutropenia is also important to manage. Neutropenia not only causes life threatening infections, but also can cause reduction in the chemotherapy dose, which makes the patients receive less than optimal chemotherapy dosage. To prevent infection during chemotherapy using drugs that cause myelosuppression, prophylactic antibiotics and myeloid growth factors (MGFs) have been used and shown to be beneficial. Prior to chemotherapy, prophylactic use of antibiotics has advantage of being less costly, but the disadvantage of causing microbial resistance need to be considered as well. There are 3 MGFs recombinant currently available: G-CSF (filgrastim), pegylated recombinant G-CSF (pegfilgrastim), and recombinant GM-CSF (sargramostim). MGFs therapy is associated with an increase in neutrophil numbers and enhanced function of mature neutrophils [5]. Because use of pegfilgrastim is more convenient for the patients, it has become the most frequently used MGFs for the reduction of infection risk during chemotherapy. Pegfilgrastim is both safe and effective when used with chemotherapy regimens that are administered every 2 weeks [6]. When chemotherapy and MGFs are administered on the same day, it is possible that myeloid progenitors will be recruited into cell cycle while cytotoxic chemotherapy is still in their environment. MGFs have paradoxical effect of causing myelosuppression; therefore, it is better to administer MGFs the day after the completion of chemotherapy [7].

The primary regulator of platelets is thrombopoietin (TPO), a glycoprotein that is produced in the liver and is cleared by platelets and their precursors [8-9]. Thrombocytopenia most often occurs with drugs such as bortezomib, gemcitabine, carboplatin, or ifosfamide after multiple cycles of treatment or in cancer patients with liver diseases (due to the decreased TPO production). In general, out-patients with thrombocytopenia who are not bleeding, do not require platelet transfusions unless their platelet count is less than 20,000/μL. Recombinant IL-11, oprelvekin, has been shown to accelerate platelet recovery after chemotherapy. However, adverse events of this drug for causing cardiac arrhythmias, optic neuropathy, and potential anaphylaxis, have limited the usefulness of this drug in oncology practice. Other drugs such as romiplostim, and eltrombopag were approved for minimization of granulocytopenia and for speedy recovery of neutropenic fever after chemotherapy.

VENOUS THROMBOEMBOLISM

Leukemia is associated with an increased frequency of venous thromboembolism (VTE). The incidence of thromboembolic events in patients with leukemia maybe six-fold higher than in general population. Patients with leukemia also have the highest risk of developing VTE more than patients with different kind of cancers [10-11]. Multiple factors contribute to the hypercoagulable state associated with cancer such as: intrinsic characteristics of the cancer, patients characteristics, and environmental factors. Cancer is characterized by uncontrolled growth, metastasis, and aberrant coagulation cascade activation.

Cancer cells can disrupt the blood hemostatic balance *via* several pathways such as production of procoagulant, profibrinolytic, proproteolytic, and proaggregating mediators, and expression of adhesion molecules that mediate direct interactions with the host cells causing secretion of proinflammatory and proangiogenic cytokines [12-13]. Patient-specific factors include older age, African American, having other comorbid conditions such as obesity, prior VTE incidence and genetic thrombophilic states (having factor V Leiden or prothrombin gene mutations) [10]. Environmental factors include recurrence of hospitalization, immobilization, indwelling venous caterer, and transfusion of blood products.

Chemotherapeutic agents such as platinum, bevacizumab, lenalidomide, and L asparaginase have been associated with increased incidence of VTE. Cancer patient commonly get thromboprophylaxis with unfractionated heparin, deltaparin, enoxaparin, rivaroxaban, or fondaparinux [10]. Management of VTE in the cancer patients is complex due to persistent coagulable state, tendency toward heparin resistant with the development of thrombocytopenia, high risk of bleeding, anticoagulant interactions with chemotherapy, nutrition status of the patients, and possible development of secondary malignancy.

TUMOR LYSIS SYNDROME

Tumor lysis syndrome (TLS) is a fatal metabolic derangements that occur when malignant cells are rapidly killed, causing a massive release of intracellular metabolites into the bloodstream [14]. Sign of TLS includes fever, shortness of breath, peripheral edema, weakness, sweating and tachycardia. Symptoms of TLS are hyperuricemia, hyperkalemia, hyperphosphatemia, hypocalcemia, cardiac arrhythmia, and renal dysfunction which may lead to acute renal failure.

Appropriate management includes risk stratification of all patients prior to getting chemotherapy drugs that more likely causing TLS. Often patients required hospitalized and require intravenous (i.v.) hydration to promote urinary excretion of uric acid and phosphate. Hyperurecimia and hyperphosphatemia should be treated promptly to prevent acute renal failure. Allopurinol or rasburicase are usually given to prevent xanthine and hypoxanthine conversion back into uric acid [15]. Rasbirucase is contraindicated in patients with glucose-6-phosphate dehydrogenase deficiency because of the high risk development of methemoglobinemia and hemolytic anemia after receving rasbirucase [16].

NAUSEA AND VOMITING

Nausea and vomiting (N/V) are common adverse events associated with chemotherapy that are most feared by the patients. Several distinct sites in the brainstem believed to be critical for the control of emesis. These sites include: a) "vomiting center" which is not anatomically discrete, but cause initiation of the vomiting reflex which is controlled by the complex system located in the brainstem, b) chemoreceptor trigger zone (CTZ) located outside blood-brain barrier, c) vesticular system initiating the vomiting reflex, and d) cerebral cortex involve in anticipatory emesis in the patients who previously experienced chemotherapy-induced N/V [17].

Based on their frequency of causing N/V, cancer drugs can be divided into: 1) high risk, greater than 90% frequency of emesis (cisplatin, cyclophosphamide, dacarbazine), 2) moderate risk, 30-90% frequency of emesis (arsenic trioxide, doxorubicin, methotrexate), 3) low risk, 10-30% frequency of emesis (cytarabine, gemcitabine, temsirolimus), and 4) minimal risk, less than 10% frequency (asparaginase, fludarabine, gemtuzumab ozogamicin, rituximab, vincristine), respectively [18].

There are 3 kinds of emesis: acute, anticipatory, and delayed; each of this N/V has different treatment. Anti-emetic to treat acute N/V includes 5HT3 antagonist (ondansetron, granisetron, dolasetron, and palonosetron), neurokinin 1 antagonist (aprepitant), dopamine antagonists (metoclopramide, prochlorperazine), cannabinoids (dronabinol), benzodiazepines (lorazepam), and corticosteroids [17]. Anticipatory N/V can be effectively treated with benzodiazepines [18]. Controlling delayed N/V remained problematic. High rates delayed N/V continues to occur in the patients receiving moderately or highly emetogenic chemotherapy. In addition, some patients with complete control of emesis during the acute phase, may experience delayed N/V a few days later [19-20]. Because none of the antiemetic agents is ideal when used alone, a variety combination regimens has been developed to improve efficacy and to cause less or non-overlapping toxicities. Corticosteroids have been used as the "second antiemetic drugs" in combination with other antiemetic drugs, because of their ease of administration and minimal toxicity. Although there is no clear understanding on how corticosteroids work, dexamethasone has been used routinely for moderate N/V [17].

Cancer Related Fatigue

Cancer related fatigue (CRF) is experienced by most patients during diagnosis, treatment, survivorship, and disease progression. Fatigue is almost always multifactorial. Chemotherapy can increase fatigue by causing anemia, poor sleep, suppression of endogenous corticosteroids, release of pro-inflammatory cytokines, poor nutrition from reduced appetite and constant N/V. Therapy for CRF includes use of psychostimulants such as methylphenidate, antidepressant such as paroxetine, progesterone such as megestrol acetate, and erythropoietin. Erythropoietin and methylphenidate reduce fatigue severity in patients with cancer; however, the magnitude of the benefit is still questionable to produce significant clinical data. Use of those agents is potentially further limited by concerns about their safety. Base on a few studies, pharmacologic interventions should not be routinely done to reduce CRF severity. Future meta-analyses should be obtained from clinical trials to better understand how pharmacologic interventions affect fatigue with minimal adverse events [21]. Studies found moderate exercise not only can decrease CRF, but can increase the reserve capacity of entire body system by forming muscle adenosine triphosphate (ATP) as energy source [22].

Cancer Related Pain

Cancer related pain (CRP) is one of the most common and dreaded symptoms associated with cancer. CRP occurs in 25-50% of patients newly diagnosed with cancer, in more than 30% patients undergoing treatment, and in more than 75% patient with advanced disease, respectively [23]. Common pain are due to the direct leukemic cells causing invasion of bone, compression of neural structures, obstruction of hallow visceral, vascular obstruction, or ulceration of mucus membrane (about 70% of the cases). Less than 10% pain are associated with bedsores, constipation, rectal or bladder spasm, postherpetic neuralgia, and more than 20% are related to diagnostic or therapeutic procedures such as bone marrow aspiration, biopsy or lumbar puncture, post amputation or pain after radiation causing injury to plexus, spinal cord, mucosa or peripheral neuropathy [23]. Pain can be classified as a) somatic (constant aching, gnawing, well-localized pain); b) visceral (constant, aching, often associated with nausea); c) neuropathic (paroxysmal shock-like pain on top of a burning, constricting sensation); and d) sympathetic (severe burning, squeezing or constricting with local edema) [23].

Drugs for the treatment of CRP are usually classified as non-opioids, opioids, and adjuvant analgesics. The World Health organizations (WHO) analgesic ladder was introduced as a framework for physicians as they prescribe analgesics. Aspirin, acetaminophen, or non-steroidal anti-inflammatory drugs (NSAIDs) are preferred for mild to moderate pain [24]. If these drugs do not provide adequate analgesia, then codeine, oxycodone, or hydrocodone would be prescribed to provide better relief. For persistent or severe pain, more potent opioids such as morphine are usually used [23]. Drug rotation should be tried also since patients sometimes tolerate one NSAIDs or opioids better than other. Patients with severe pain might need a strong opioid as an initial therapy to ensure rapid pain relief [25]. Moderate to severe pain can be managed with oral opioids "around the clock" to keep pain under control. If tolerance occurs due to cancer progression, opioid doses need to be increased. Addiction is rare in patients with cancer who are taking opioids for pain relief. Adverse events of opioids include withdrawal symptoms, myoclonus, pruritis, sedation, N/V, and constipation. Constipation should be anticipated and treated prophylactically with stool softeners, lubricants, enemas or laxatives [26].

Common adjuvant analgesics such as antidepressants, anticonvulsants, stimulants, corticosteroids, muscle relaxants, benzodiazepines, anti-spasmodic, neuroleptics, and bisphosphonates can be added to opioid or non-opioids regimen to improve pain control [23].

OTHER COMPLICATIONS

The incidence of hemorrhagic cystitis (bladder infection), due to cyclophosphamide or ifosphamide can be decreased from 40-60% to 5% with proper hydration and use of Mesna (2-mercaptoethane sulfonate) that can be given by i.v. or oral [27].

Mucositis, in particular oral mucositis (OM) cause inflammation, atrophy and breakdown of the mucosa or lining of the oral cavity. Several drugs cause mucositis such as etoposide, anthracyclines, and methotrexate. Patients with OM have decreased oral intake and increased risk of systemic infections. Palifermin, a recombinant keratinocyte growth factor is approved to reduce the incidence and duration of severe OM in leukemia and other hematological malignancies [28]. Besides OM, patients taking methotrexate at a dose higher than 500 mg/m^2 can also develop acute kidney injury. Nephrotoxicity is the results of methotrexate crystallization in the renal tubular lumen leading to tubular toxicity and impaired its clearance. Prolonged exposure to toxic concentrations of methotrexate further exacerbates non-renal adverse events such as myelosuppression and hepatoxicity. Increased hydration, use of high dose leucovorin, and glucarpidase are usually sufficient to allow renal recovery without the need for dialysis [29].

Cytokine release syndrome (CRS) is a major adverse event noticed with chimeric antigen receptor T cell immunotherapy (CART). CART also causes neurotoxicities CAR-related encephalopathy syndrome (CRES). CRES clinical presentations include high fever, hypotension, hypoxia and respiratory distress; while early onset is confusion, hallucination, aphasia, and seizure [30].

CRS and CRES are thought due to the release of cytokines such as interleukin (IL)-1 and IL-6. Besides steroids, tocilizumab, an IL 6 blocking agent, and anakinra, an IL 1 blocker, have been studied for prophylaxis of CRS and CRES complications [31].

Conclusion

Patients with leukemia are at an increased risk of several potentially life-threatening complications from their disease and intensive chemotherapy. Intensive chemotherapy often results in the development of tumor lysis syndrome, venous thromboembolism, infectious complications, nausea and vomiting, pain and fatigue. Hyper-vigilant surveillance is required to identify chemotherapy complications and adverse events as soon as possible.

References

[1] *Lexi-Drugs.* Lexicomp. Wolters Kluwer Health, Inc. Riverwoods, IL. Available at: http://online.lexi.com. Accessed October, 2018.

[2] Glaspy J. A Hematologic Problems and Infections: Disorders of Blood cell Production in Clinical Oncology. In: Niederhuber JE et al, eds. *Abeloff's Clinical Oncology*. 5th ed. Philadelphia, PA: Elsevier; 2014: 532-541.

[3] Andrews NC: Anemia of inflammation: the cytokine-hepcidin link. *J Clin Invest.* 113:1251-1253 2004.

[4] Nemeth E, Valore EV, Territo M, et al.: Hepcidin, a putative mediator of anemia of inflammation, is a type II acute-phase protein. *Blood.* 101:2461-2463 2003.

[5] Glaspy JA, Baldwin GC, Robertson PA, et al. Therapy for neutropenia in hairy cell leukemia with recombinant human granulocyte colony-stimulating factor. *Ann Intern Med.* 1988; 109:789-795.

[6] Burstein HJ, Parker LM, Keshaviah A, et al. Efficacy of pegfilgrastim and darbepoetin alfa as hematopoietic support for dose-dense every-2-week adjuvant breast cancer chemotherapy. *J Clin Oncol.*2005; 23:8340-8347.

[7] Meropol NJ, Miller LL, Korn EL, et al. Severe myelosuppression resulting from concurrent administration of granulocyte colony-stimulating factor and cytotoxic chemotherapy. *J Natl Cancer Inst.* 1992; 84:1201-1203.

[8] Kaushansky K. Thrombopoietin. *N Engl J Med.* 1998; 339:746-754.

[9] Kuter DJ, Begley CG. Recombinant human thrombopoietin: basic biology and evaluation of clinical studies. *Blood.* 2002; 100:3457-3469.

[10] Zeidan AM, Forde PM, Streiff MB. Diagnosis, treatment, and prevention of cancer-associated venous thromboembolism. In: Niederhuber JE et al, eds. *Abeloff's Clinical Oncology.* 5th ed. Philadelphia, PA: Elsevier; 2014:542-561.

[11] Chew HK, Wun T, Harvey D et al. Incidence of venous thromboembolism and its effect on survival among patients with common cancers. *Archives of Internal Medicine* 2006;15(66):458-464.

[12] Noble S, pasi J. Epidemiology and pathophysiology of cancer-associated thrombosis. *British J of Cancer* 2010;102 (suppl 1):S2-S9.

[13] Falanga A, Marchetti M. venous thromboembolism in the hematologic malignancies. *J of Clinical Oncology* 2009; 27:4848-4857.

[14] Coiffer B, Altman A, Pui C et al. Guidelines for the management of pediatric and adult tumor lysis syndrome: an evidence-based review. *J Clin Oncol.* 2008;26(16):2767-2778.

[15] Blumel S, Broadway-Duren J. Approaches to managing safety with lenalidomide in hematologic malignancies. *J Adv Pract Oncol* 2014;5:269-279.

[16] Howard SC. Tumor lysis syndrome. In: Niederhuber JE et al, eds. *Abeloff'sClinical Oncology.* 5th ed. Philadelphia, PA: Elsevier; 2014; 591-596.

[17] Hainsworth JD. Nausea and vomiting. In: Niederhuber JE et al, eds. *Abeloff's Clinical Oncology.* 5th ed. Philadelphia, PA: Elsevier; 2014; 626-634.

[18] Morrow GR, Morrell C. Behavioral treatment for the anticipatory nausea and vomiting induced by cancer chemotherapy. *N Engl J Med* 1982; 307: 1476-1480.

[19] Bloechl-Daum B, Deuson RR, Mavros P et al. Delayed nausea and vomiting continue to reduce patients' quslity of life after highly and moderately emetogenic chemotherapy despite antiemetic treatment. *J Clin Oncol* 2006; 24: 4472-4478.

[20] Roila F, herrstedt J, Aaporo M et al. Guideline update for MASCC and ESMO in the prevention of chemotherapy and radiotherapy-induce nausea and vomiting: results of the Perugia consensus conference. *Annal Oncol* 2010;21: v232-v243.

[21] Tomlinson D, Robinson PD, Oberoi S et al. Pharmacologic intervention for fatigue in cancer and transplantation: a meta analysis. *Curr Oncol* 2018; 25(2):e152-e167.

[22] Brown JC, Huedo-Medina TB, Pescatello LS et al. Efficacy of exercise interventions in modulating cancer-related fatigueamong adult cancer survivors: a meta-analysis. *Cancer Epidemiol Biomarkers Prev* 2011; 20:123-133.

[23] Grossman SA, Nesbit S. Cancer Related Pain. In: Niederhuber JE et al, eds. *Abeloff's Clinical Oncology.* 5th ed. Philadelphia, PA: Elsevier; 2014; 608-619.

[24] Nabal M, Librada S, Redondo MJ et al. The role of paracetamol and and non steroidal anti inflammatory in addition to WHO steps III opioids in the control of pain in advanced cancer. A systemic review of literature. *Palliat Med* 2012; 26(4): 305-312.

[25] MacPherson RD. The pharmacological basis of contemporary pain management. *Pharmacol Ther* 2000; 88(2):163-185.

[26] McNicol E, Horowicz-Mehler N, Fisk RA et al. Management of opioid side effects in cancer-related and chronic non cancer pain: A systematic review. *J Pain* 2003; 4(5):231-256.

[27] West NJ. Prevention and treatment of hemorrhagic cystitis. *J of Human Pharmacology and Drug Therapy* 1997. DOIs: 10.1002/j.1875-9114.1997.tb03745.x.

[28] Oronsky B, Goyal S, Kim MM. A review of clinical radioprotection and chemoprotection for oral Mucositis. *Trans Oncol* 2018; 11 (3): 771-778.

[29] Howard SC, McCormick J, Pui CH et al. Preventing and managing toxicities of high dose methotrexate. *Oncologist* 2016;21:1471-1482.

[30] Wang Z, Han W. Biomarkers of cytokine release syndrome and neurotoxicity related to CAR-T cell therapy. *Biomarker Research.* 2018;6(1):4. doi: 10.1186/s40364-018-0116-0.

[31] Liu D, Zhao J. Cytokine release syndrome: grading, modeling, and new therapy. *J Hematol Oncol* 2019; 11:121. doi: 10.1186/s13045-018-0653.

In: Frontiers in Leukemia Pharmacotherapy
Editor: Lunawati L. Bennett
ISBN: 978-1-53614-960-9

Chapter 17

Palliative Care in Leukemia

Emily P. Brandl**, *PharmD
Union University College of Pharmacy, Jackson, Tennessee, US

Abstract

The term *palliative care* often has a negative connotation with both patients and health care providers, likely due to the fact that this term is often used synonomously with hospice. However, palliative care is much more than just end-of-life care. At its core, palliative care is intensive and comprehensive physical and emotional symptom management. Patients who receive palliative care services that are integrated early in the disease course alongside disease-directed therapies routinely report higher quality of life and more satisfaction with symptom control than those who do not receive palliative care. Provision of palliative care services does not necessarily warrant a consult to a palliative care specialist. In fact, the bulk of services can be offered by primary care providers and oncologists. Ensuring primary providers feel competent and confident providing palliative care services can improve quality of life in patients with hematologic malignancies.

Keywords: palliative care, comfort care, end-of-life, hospice, symptom management, hematologic malignancies, leukemia

* Corresponding Author Email: ebrandl@uu.edu.

Abbreviations

ICU	intensive care unit
NCCN	National Comprehensive Cancer Network
NQF	National Quality Forum

Introduction

Based on findings from multiple studies, patients with hematologic malignancies such as leukemia are less likely to utilize palliative care services when compared to patients with solid tumors [1, 2]. However, patients with leukemia that are not offered palliative care services are not receiving the specialized symptom management or psychosocial and spiritual care that comes when palliative care is integrated early in the disease course. Additionally, patients with leukemia are more likely to receive aggressive care, such as powerful chemotherapy or intensive care services, at the end-of-life when compared to patients with solid tumors [1, 2]. With aggressive therapy comes physical and emotional distress for both the patient and the caregiver. When patients with leukemia do utilize palliative care services, it is often within the final stages of life, forgoing much of the support available from diagnosis to death through the provision of palliative care. In a commentary on palliative care for leukemia, hematologic oncologist Thomas LeBlanc cites several potential reasons for low palliative care usage amongst patients with leukemia [3, 4].

First, aggressive treatments are the standard of care for leukemia. In patients with leukemia, aggressive treatments often result in a cure, even in advanced disease or poor prognosis. Therefore, it is difficult to determine when it is appropriate to stop treatment, especially given the fact that prognostication can be quite difficult in hematologic malignancies.

Additionally, quality measures are not applicable to leukemia. Current NQF quality measures for all patients with cancer suggest that intensive care should not be utilized in the last 30 days of life, chemotherapy should not be given in the last 14 days of life, hospice utilization should increase, and hospice should not be utilized for patients with less than 3 days to live. However, the applicability of these measures to leukemia and other hematologic malignancies is debatable. This is due to the aforementioned facts that guideline-directed therapy for patients with leukemia can include aggressive, high-risk treatment with anticancer therapy to achieve cure, and prognostication is difficult in patients with blood cancers.

Another perceived barrier to the provision of palliative care to patients with leukemia is the fact that home-based palliative care may not be appropriate for patients with leukemia. Palliative care services in a home-based setting, such as traditional home hospice, often are not able to meet the needs of patients with hematologic malignancies. For example, patients with blood cancers may derive symptomatic benefit from blood transfusions, which is not feasible to be done in a home-based setting.

Lastly, symptoms often start suddenly in patients with acute leukemias. Unlike these patients, those with solid tumors often have a gradual onset of symptoms. Patients with acute leukemia have acute onset of distressing symptoms, which necessitates quick decision making regarding therapy and treatment goals. The natural tendency of patients with sudden onset of symptoms and a new diagnosis of blood cancer would be to pursue aggressive treatment, especially since cure rates can be high, even in advanced disease. This tendency is also understandably shared by oncologists, as aggressive therapy is the standard of care in most leukemias [3].

Many of the reasons listed above show that the connotation of the term *palliative care* typically means end-of-life care to hematologic oncologists. Ensuring providers and patients understanding that palliative care is more than just hospice or end-of life care, and that it can be provided alongside disease-directed or life-prolonging therapy, is essential to enhance patient quality of life and reducing suffering in patients with leukemia.

PALLIATIVE CARE, COMFORT CARE AND HOSPICE

Palliative care, comfort care, and hospice are all terms that tend to be used interchangeably, but they each have distinct definitions. The relationship between palliative care, comfort care, and hospice is demonstrated in Figure 1 below.

Palliative care is a broad term that can be loosely defined as specialized medical care that focuses on improving the quality of life for patients with serious illness and their families. Palliative care is focused on providing relief from symptoms as well as psychological stresses related to the illness. It can be provided alongside disease-directed or life-prolonging therapies [5, 6]. For example, palliative care for a patient with cancer should include ensuring the patient's symptoms, such as pain and nausea, are well-controlled while she undergoes chemotherapy and radiation.

It may also include ensuring the patient has access to a counselor to address any psychosocial burden the disease may be putting on the patient. Per the NCCN guidelines, palliative care should be initiated by the primary oncology team at diagnosis and should be delivered alongside disease-directed therapies. If additional support is needed, a palliative care specialty team may be consulted [7]. Through the provision of palliative care, patients and families receive an added layer of support during the disease course.

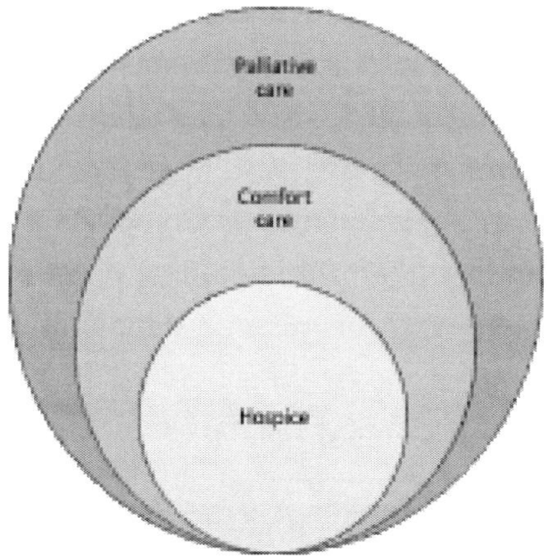

Figure 1. The relationship between palliative care, comfort care and hospice.

Once the focus shifts from aggressive, disease-directed therapy to comfort and symptom management, more specific terminology can be used to describe the care provided. The term *comfort care* refers to symptom management that is provided without curative, aggressive interventions. In other words, comfort care is palliative care provided to patients who have decided to end or forgo disease-directed or life-prolonging therapy. *Hospice* is an even more specific term, referring to a formal care program in which patients with limited life expectancy can enroll. Hospice care is provided by an interdisciplinary team of healthcare providers to patients with a life expectancy of six months or less [6].

The common goal of palliative care, comfort care, and hospice is to ensure patients and caregivers do not suffer, physically or emotionally, during the patients' disease course.

However, the terms should not be used interchangeably as there are distinct differences between the three terms. Comfort care and hospice are specific types of palliative care. For simplicity, this chapter will utilize the broadest term *palliative care*, but the reader should be aware that palliative care encompasses the three types of care described above.

THE ONCOLOGIST'S ROLE IN PALLIATIVE CARE

Screening

The oncologist and oncology team can play a significant role in the early integration of palliative care into the treatment of patients with leukemia. Oncologists should ensure the patient and family are informed about palliative care services, even at the time of diagnosis.

This includes open and honest discussion regarding anticipation and prevention of symptoms as well as advance care planning. In fact, the NCCN guidelines state that oncologists should screen patients at every visit to determine if they are candidates for palliative care.

The guidelines recommend a comprehensive palliative care assessment for patients who meet one or more palliative care screening criteria. These criteria can be found in Table 1 [7].

Table 1. Palliative care screening criteria (from NCCN Palliative Care Guidelines) [7]

Criteria for Full Palliative Care Assessment By Oncologist
Unmanaged symptoms
Moderate to severe distress related to cancer diagnosis or therapy
Serious comorbid physical, psychiatric, and psychosocial conditions
Life expectancy of 6 months or less
Metastatic solid tumors
Patient or family concerns about the course of disease and decision making
Patient or family requests for palliative care

Table 2. Patient circumstances that may warrant palliative care specialist consultation (from NCCN Palliative Care Guidelines) [7]

Physical Circumstances	
Limited anticancer options	Severe comorbid conditions
High symptom burden	Palliative stenting/gastrostomy
Multiple allergies/adverse effects	Rapidly progressing decline
Frequent emergency department visits	High risk for poor pain control
Frequent hospital admissions	Request for hastened death
Complicated ICU admissions	Cognitive impairment
Communication barriers	Goals of care clarification
Resistant to engage in planning	Inadequate social support
Social Circumstances	
Financial limitations	Family conflict
Spiritual or existential distress	Family or caregiver limitations

A comprehensive palliative care assessment, should one be required, includes an evaluation of the benefits versus the burdens of anticancer therapy; personal goals, values, and expectations; physical symptoms; psychosocial distress; educational and informational needs; and cultural values affecting care [7].

Referring to a Palliative Care Specialist

Oncologists are well-respected and well-trusted by their patients due to the nature of their relationship. However, oncologists may feel unequipped to handle some physical or emotional symptoms and social situations that may arise with their patients. Consultation with a palliative care specialist may offer additional support and guidance in these circumstances. Examples of situations that may warrant palliative care consultation can be found below in Table 2.

Management of Distressing Symptoms

Solid tumor cancer symptom burdens have been extensively studied in the literature, but there have been significantly fewer studies assessing the needs of patients with leukemia. However, a recent study by Hochman et al. found that blood cancer patients face a symptom burden that is comparable to or exceeding that of patients with solid tumors. In this study, the authors identified that patients with hematologic malignancies had a higher rate of clinically-significant fatigue and had similar rates of pain, dyspnea, nausea, and anorexia when compared to their counterparts with solid tumors [8].

Cancer Related Fatigue (CRF)

Across several studies, fatigue seems to be one of the most troubling symptoms in patients with hematologic malignancies [8]. Cancer-related fatigue is often described by patients as an overwhelming feeling of exhaustion that cannot be overcome with rest or a good night's sleep [9].

Fatigue can be attributed to many problems, so it is important to thoroughly assess patients in order to assess potential causes.

Commonly seen in leukemia, anemia is a frequent cause of fatigue in this population. Anemia should be treated according to the NCCN guidelines, but the most common treatments include encouraging the patient to eat iron-rich foods, recommending supplements, delaying or modifying chemotherapy or radiation therapy, or providing the patient with red blood cell transfusions. Many patients with advanced anemia due to cancer derive symptomatic benefit from frequent transfusions.

Other interventions for fatigue in the absence of anemia include ensuring patients are getting exercise, practicing good sleep hygeine to improve sleep quality, and ensuring patients are receiving adequate nutrition and calories. Furthermore, adequate treatment of pain and depression or anxiety is crucial, as fatigue may be a manifestation that these symptoms are not adequately controlled.

If none of the above interventions are effective, there are some pharmacologic agents that may be considered to treat fatigue. Most commonly, psychostimulants such as methylphenidate can be considered to improve the feeling of fatigue. Methylphenidate also can be helpful if the patient is having any daytime sedation or drowsiness. There have also been some studies to suggest that corticosteroids may be beneficial in treating symptomatic fatigue [9, 10].

Other Symptoms

Pain is one of the most common symptoms experienced by patients with cancer. This pain can be due to the malignancy itself, diagnostic tests, or treatments related to the cancer. Pain management is essential to improve quality of life of patients suffering with any malignancy, including hematologic malignancies. The NCCN offers comprehensive guidelines on pain management in cancer. They also offer guidance on specific assessments, treatment algorithms, medication dosing, and follow up for cancer patients with pain.

Dyspnea, nausea, and anorexia are also common symptoms seen in patients with cancer. The NCCN offers several supportive care guidelines, including a palliative care guideline, that provide detailed information on management of these symptoms.

End-of-Life Care

Despite the best efforts by an oncology team, some patients will not be cured from their disease. Therefore, it is important that healthcare providers who care for patients with hematologic malignancies are familiar with delivering end-of-life care. Caring for a patient within hours of death can be challenging for the patient as well as the patient's caregivers and family. It is essential to ensure that patients, caregivers, and family members are cared for physically and psychosocially.

The focus of care for an imminently dying patient should be ensuring adequacy of symptom management to provide the maximum amount of comfort for the patient. This includes ensuring the patient has appropriate medications and doses ordered, discontinuing unnecessary interventions and medications, determining alternative medication routes if oral administration becomes difficult or impractical, and ensuring appropriate interventions, such as eye drops or moist mouth swabs, to maintain eye and mouth comfort.

The psychosocial needs of the patient should also be considered. This includes ensuring that any interventions follow the patient's wishes and preferences, religious beliefs, and cultural values. This is an important time to involve chaplains and social workers to ensure that any spiritual or social needs are met. In addition to the patient, it is important to assess any psychosocial needs of caregivers and family members. For example, if a patient has young children, it may be prudent to involve a child life specialist, if available. Ensuring that the family is provided with resources for healthy grieving is also important. Based on family and patient preference, visitors should be allowed to spend uninterrupted time with the patient.

The healthcare provider should ensure that the patient's advance directive is documented and implemented. The provider should also document a "Do Not Resuscitate" or "Allow Natural Death" order in the medical record as appropriate. The patient should be transferred to a private room if available.

After the patient dies, it is important to inform the family if they are not present, offer condolences, and provide family time with the body. Chaplain involvement at this time may be helpful. Additional responsibilities for the healthcare team may include facilitating funeral arrangements, informing insurance companies of the patient's death, and preparing the body for organ donation or autopsy, if appropriate. Bereavement support should also be offered, including a visit or telephone call from the primary providers, followed by a condolence letter or card. Direct bereavement support should be provided by a trained hospice team or a skilled mental health professional [7].

According to most patients and healthcare workers, a good, peaceful death is one that ensures the patient has freedom from pain, spiritual peace, and family presence in the final hours. However, these values may not be shared with every patient. Therefore, it is important to ensure that end-of-life care is flexible enough to accommodate all views of a "good death" [11].

CONCLUSION

Patients with leukemia can benefit from palliative care throughout their entire disease course, not just at the end of their lives. While they may experience distressing symptoms throughout the course of their disease, integration of palliative care early in the disease course may reduce this burden by anticipation, prevention, and treatment of distressing symptoms. Furthermore, if a patient reaches the terminal stages of their disease, palliative care services, in the form of hospice, can provide physical and psychosocial care to the patient as well as their family.

REFERENCES

[1] Howell, D. A., Shellens, R., Roman, E., et al. Hematological malignancy: Are patients appropriately referred for specialist palliative and hospice care? A systematic review and meta-analysis of published data. *Palliat. Med.,* 2011; 25(6): 630 - 641.

[2] Hui, D., Didwaniya, N., Vidal, M., et al. Quality of end-of-life care in patients with hematologic malignancies: A retrospective cohort study. *Cancer,* 2014; 120(10): 1572 - 1578.

[3] LeBlanc, T. W. Palliative care and hematologic malignancies: old dog, new tricks? *J. Oncol. Pract.,* 2014; 10(6):e404-e407.

[4] Odejide, O. O., Salas Coronado, D. Y., Watts, C. D., et al. End-of-life care for blood cancers: a series of focus groups with hematologic oncologists. *J. Oncol. Pract.*, 2014; 10(6):e396-e403.

[5] LeBlanc, T. W., El-Jawahri, A. When and why should patients with hematologic malignancies see a palliative care specialist? *Hematology*, 2015; 2015:471 - 478.

[6] Kelley, A. S., Morrison, R. S. Palliative care for the seriously ill. *NEJM,* 2015; 373(8):747 - 755.

[7] National Comprehensive Cancer Network. *Palliative Care (Version 1.2018).* http:// www.nccn.org/professionals/physician_gls/pdf/palliative.pdf. Accessed August 13, 2018.

[8] Hochman, M. J., Yu, Y., Wolf, S. P., et al. Comparing the palliative care needs of patients with hematologic and solid malignancies. *J. Pain Symptom Manage*, 2018; 55(1):82 - 88.

[9] Leukemia and Lymphoma Society. *Cancer-Related Fatigue.* https://www.lls.org/ treatment/managing-side-effects/cancer-related-fatigue. Accessed August 13, 2018.

[10] National Comprehensive Cancer Network. *Cancer-Related Fatigue* (Version 2.2018). http://www.nccn.org/professionals/physician_gls/pdf/fatigue.pdf. Accessed August 13, 2018.

[11] Steinhauser, K. E., Christakis, N. A., Clipp, E. C. et al. Factors considered important at the end of life by patients, family, physicians, and other care providers. *JAMA,* 2000; 284(19):2476 - 2482.

In: Frontiers in Leukemia Pharmacotherapy
Editor: Lunawati L. Bennett
ISBN: 978-1-53614-960-9

Chapter 18

PHARMACOMETRICS IN LEUKEMIA

Mitali Gaura[1,*], PharmD, Joel S. Owen[1,2], PhD and Andrew Castleman[1], PharmD

[1]Union University School of Pharmacy, Jackson, Tennessee, US
[2]Cognigen Corporation, Buffalo, New York, US

ABSTRACT

Pharmacometrics is a flourishing field that incorporates principles of pharmacokinetics, pharmacodynamics, statistics, and computational modeling to support model based drug development and optimize drug therapy in a given patient population [1]. Pharmacometrics seeks to determine causes of variability among patients and can be used to estimate the dose needed to keep concentrations in an optimum range to produce maximum therapeutic efficacy with minimum toxicities. This chapter introduces the concepts of pharmacometrics and how these tools have been used in the development of drugs for leukemia and in the individualized dosing for patients diagnosed with leukemia.

Keywords: leukemia, pharmacodynamic, pharmacokinetic, pharmacometrics, population pharmacokinetics, therapeutic drug monitoring

ABBREVIATIONS

ADR	adverse drug response
AUC	area under the curve
CL	clearance

* Corresponding Author Email: mgaurav@uu.edu.

IIV	inter-individual variability
IOV	inter-occasion variability
IV	intravenous
mAbs	monoclonal antibodies
MTD	maximum tolerated dose
NCA	non-compartmental analysis
NLME	non-linear mixed effect modeling
PBPK	physiologically based pharmacokinetics
PD	pharmacodynamic
PK	pharmacokinetic
RV	residual variability
TDM	therapeutic drug monitoring
TGN	thioguanine nucleotides
TMDD	target mediated drug disposition
V	volume of distribution
VOD	veno-occlusive disease

INTRODUCTION

The administration of toxic medications to treat life-threatening diseases requires a balance of potential risks and rewards. A thorough understanding of the exposure-response relationships for efficacy and adverse events is necessary to manage dosing of drugs most effectively. Considerable progress has been made in understanding pharmacokinetic (PK) and pharmacodynamic (PD) relationships to identify an appropriate dosing regimen of drugs for leukemia. Strategies to optimize dosing regimens (i.e., route, dose, and frequency) to improve the probability of achieving target exposures and attain clinical success are a major area of current translational research [2].

Chemotherapeutic agents used to treat cancers have often been dosed at the highest tolerated rate to maximize the impact on the cancer with hope that the patient will survive both the cancer and exposure to the drug. The maximum tolerated dose (MTD) regimen has been an acceptable and effective approach for many patients, though it has produced untold individual suffering of patients due to the adverse effects that result from such high exposure. When patient factors can be identified to target more effective and tolerable doses, the patient benefits. For instance, 6-MP used in acute lymphoblastic leukemia (ALL) can be a very effective therapy, but the clinical outcomes can range from life threatening hematologic and hepatotoxic effects to a lack of efficacy in patients, due to partially predictable inter-patient differences in pharmacokinetics that result in various optimal doses for particular individuals [3, 4].

Pharmacometric modeling uses clinical, bioanalytical and other available data to efficiently identify relationships between selected dosing regimens, drug exposure, and drug effects for individuals or the entire patient population. Pharmacometric models can be constructed to describe drug disposition, pharmacodynamic response, biomarkers of response, drug-drug interactions, drug-disease interactions, covariate predictors of effects, and uncertainty of the estimates of each of these. Pharmacometric models can be used to develop and support product labels for individualized dosing and provide guidance for adjustments in treatment as new products or new label indications are developed. This chapter will illustrate some examples of the use of pharmacometrics to support the dosing of drugs for leukemia.

PHARMACOMETRICS

Patients respond to treatments differently even when the disease status and treatment administered are the same. Such differences are primarily due to differences in the physiological characteristics of patients, and result in inter-individual variability (IIV). Pharmacometric models are often constructed with a mathematical relation between covariates and model parameters to explain and quantify the sources and magnitude of variability in patient responses [5].

Covariates are observable and measurable intrinsic or extrinsic characteristics of patients that may be correlated with the individual's parameters of the PK, PD or disease models to explain systematic differences between individuals (e.g., patients that weigh more have a larger clearance value). Examples of intrinsic covariates are age, gender, weight, race, disease status, organ function tests and other laboratory results. Examples of extrinsic covariates are administration of a drug with food or with other concomitant medications. Such population models are often "mixed effect models," which contain both fixed and random effect terms.

Fixed effects are what we often think of as the variables in an equation that take on single numerical values. Together with their mathematical structure, fixed effects represent parameters that describe the consistent trends observed in a population, including systematic differences between individuals explained by covariates, whereas random effects account for the remaining unexplained variability between patients (IIV) or between occasions (IOV) in the same patient.

A second level random effect, residual variability (RV) accounts for differences between predicted and observed concentrations or effects within an individual. Thus, random effects address inter-individual variability and inter-occasion variability at one level, and nested within that, the residual variability within individuals.

Sparse Data

Traditionally, pharmacokinetic studies have included extensive sample collection from patients to provide enough data to describe the PK of a particular drug in each patient. Now, in clinical settings and in large clinical trials, it is common that sparse data are collected due to ethical and resource concerns. Data is referred to as sparse when there is an insufficient number of samples from an individual to conduct the PK analysis with data from only that individual. The desire to analyze sparse data was a primary motivation in the development of the nonlinear, mixed effect modeling approach. Analyzing sparse data gives a significant clinical advantage since populations from which it is most difficult to acquire extensive individual data are often the populations that most require an optimized dosing regimen; for example, critically ill patient groups, neonates, pediatric patients, and in pregnancy [6-8].

We often encounter sparse data in clinical settings where samples are collected in a patient for therapeutic drug monitoring (TDM). TDM approaches have long been practiced for drugs with narrow therapeutic indices, meaning that the difference between an effective dose and a toxic dose is small. The application of TDM involves collection of a single or a few drug concentration samples in a patient and using a previously established understanding of the kinetics of the drug, whether from a developed model or algorithm, to make adjustments to the dosing regimen to achieve target concentrations correlated with safety and efficacy endpoints. Models made for this purpose may be as simple as associations between trough concentrations and an outcome measure, or they may be thoroughly developed PK/PD models that predict a response from a given dose [9].

To carry out model-based approaches of TDM, prior knowledge of the model structure and parameter variances is required. TDM approaches that use a model often apply Bayesian analysis methods to associate sparse observed concentrations in a patient with the likelihood of a certain value of model parameters such as clearance, given a prior understanding of the population's distribution of clearance values. A patient specific model is thus created using the patient's data and the prior model. This patient specific model is useful in predicting drug concentrations at different times, even for untried dosing regimens, and can be utilized to optimize the treatment plan for this patient. By informing these individual estimates of model parameters, TDM is used to confirm or adjust the dosing regimen in the patient. Even though model based, TDM guided therapy adjustments can be very beneficial in a clinical scenario, such methods are not utilized to their full potential because of the complexity and training required for such approaches. However, certain software tools are available that can be used by physicians and clinical pharmacists to accomplish these goals [10].

PHARMACOKINETICS

Where does a drug go in the body after administration to a patient, what concentrations does it reach in the blood and tissues, how long are those concentrations maintained, and how does the body eliminate the drug? These are questions which are studied using pharmacokinetics. Pharmacokinetics explores the characteristics of a drug by attempting to account for processes of absorption, distribution, and elimination (metabolism and excretion). This information is part of what is needed to design appropriate dosing regimens in patients. Pharmacokinetic studies involve the collection of biological samples from the blood, urine, feces, and/or tissues of patients or study subjects, which are analyzed via bioanalytical or imaging methods to determine the concentration of drug in the sample. These data are analyzed mathematically to characterize the pharmacokinetic properties of the drug. There are two main approaches that are used to analyze PK data: non-compartmental analysis (NCA) and model based methods. The NCA method of analysis makes fewer assumptions than the compartmental modeling approach, which makes it convenient to use. The simpler NCA approach can be used as an alternative to or supplement of compartmental modeling approaches that are more sophisticated in explaining a drug's behavior. The primary model based method involves compartmental analysis through nonlinear regression analysis, but the development of physiological based PK methods and quantitative systems pharmacology models are growing areas of pharmacokinetic study.

The PK analysis method one selects depends on the questions that need to be answered, the nature of the data collected, and prior knowledge of the drug's properties. Access to appropriate software, the time available to perform the analysis, and the technical skill of the analyst may also contribute to decisions regarding the selection of the analysis approach.

Because the analysis is performed on a subject-by-subject basis, NCA requires a series of PK observations (e.g., blood concentration measures) within a dosing interval in a single subject. The NCA approach yields metrics of the data that can be computed from simple algebraic approaches (e.g., log-linear regression used to estimate the terminal half-life). NCA provides metrics of drug exposure (area under the curve; AUC), time-course and distribution (the maximum observed concentration, C_{max}; time of the maximum observed drug concentration, T_{max}; elimination half-life, $T_{1/2}$; drug clearance, CL; and the volume of distribution, V). However, there are limitations to the NCA approach. This approach lacks any mechanistic description of the physiological processes or patient factors that might affect the PK of the drug, is not appropriate in cases of nonlinear pharmacokinetics, and requires sufficient data in each subject to perform the analysis. Additionally, the ability to make predictions about the concentration-versus-time profile resulting from an untested dosing regimen is not possible with NCA.

Compartmental model based analysis assumes the body is divided into one or more hypothetical compartments. The compartmental structure provides for an empirical, mathematical description of the observed concentration-versus-time data and does not typically have a physiological interpretation. The amount of drug present in a compartment at a given time is considered to be instantaneously and uniformly distributed in the volume of the compartment. The structural arrangement of the compartments attempts to account for the processes of drug absorption, distribution, metabolism and elimination. Modeled compartments are roughly differentiated based on how well the collection of tissues they represent are perfused or how quickly or slowly drug enters or leaves the tissues. Well-perfused organs with nonrestrictive membranes are represented by the central compartment and is where the systemic drug concentrations in the blood are assumed to be measured. Peripheral compartments are spaces or collections of tissues that are less well perfused or have restricted distribution. Often, peripheral compartments depict distribution behavior to extravascular parts of the body. A general model assumption is that drug transfer between compartments and elimination processes follow linear, first order processes, meaning that the amount of drug transferred in a period of time depends upon the amount of drug present at that time. Although often adequate, the assumptions of linearity are not required. Nonlinear transfer processes can account for nonlinear behavior, such as when metabolic or transport processes are saturated.

Though compartmental pharmacokinetic models are based on assumptions that greatly simplify the complex underlying processes of biology, the approach is largely able to characterize the observed behavior of a drug and support the selection of an appropriate dosing regimen. Unlike a NCA, compartmental models allow the use of simulations (model-based) to predict concentrations of drug with different dosing regimens without administering them to patients. Compartmental models can be relatively simple in structure, or they can be more elaborate, such as target mediated drug disposition (TMDD) models, which account for the limited capacity binding of a drug to receptors and lead to nonlinearity in certain concentration ranges. Compartmental models used for parameter estimation in experimental data generally have a small number of compartments.

Physiologically based pharmacokinetic (PBPK) models attempt to give physiological meaning to their compartmental structure and interpretation and often have many compartments. PBPK models require the collection and integration of biological system parameter values and measures of drug properties from many sources, since they require many more parameters to be estimated than can be accomplished in a single experiment. PBPK models incorporate in vitro and in vivo data regarding biologic and drug related factors. These models have increased in accuracy and utility in recent years due to the growing body of knowledge and development regarding the biology and system parameters in the models. PBPK models have contributed to the information included in drug product labels, especially in applications of drug-drug interactions. Yamazaki S et al. using PBPK modeling were able to demonstrate a reasonable, model based drug-drug interaction prediction of bosutinib with ketoconazole and rifampin (P-glycoprotein inhibitor and inductor respectively) [11]. PBPK models allow the prediction of drug concentrations or amounts in target tissues or organs by taking into account mechanisms of formulation performance, drug absorption, distribution among many organs and tissues, and complex models of metabolism and excretion. PBPK models may describe the effects of intrinsic (e.g., organ function, gender, age, or genetics) and extrinsic (e.g., drug-drug interactions, environment, or diet) patient factors on drug exposure and response in more mechanistic model systems than do traditional compartmental models [12].

In recent years, monoclonal antibodies (mAbs) have become an integral part of chemotherapy. These mAbs have different PK characteristics from small molecule drugs due to the dramatic differences in physical size, chemical composition, and biological and immunological interactions. Developing models to describe the PK properties of mAbs can be a complex process. Typical metabolic and renal excretion pathways of small molecules are frequently not relevant to the PK properties of mAbs, which may be eliminated by proteolytic, endocytotic, or immunologic pathways. Some PBPK models have been developed to describe the PK of mAbs. Additionally, TMDD models may be useful to describe the PK/PD properties of a biologic drug and to give insight into target suppression time and concentration at the target site [13]. In certain concentration ranges, when fixed capacity binding has been saturated, traditional compartmental models may adequately describe the PK of mAbs as well.

Variability in Pharmacokinetics in Cancer Patients

In addition to accounting for the typical behavior of a drug, the assessment of the magnitude and sources of PK variability is also important. When the sources are understood, some variability in a patient's exposure to the drug can be controlled by proper dosing regimen selection. Pharmacometric models reported for drugs used to treat leukemia have evaluated sources of variability in PK and PD.

One source of variability is the drug assay. The selection of which molecular species to assay may contribute to minimizing variability. Studies may evaluate concentrations of the parent drug, active metabolite, or other metabolites dependent upon available assay methodology, the ability of the assay to detect low concentrations, and which species is associated with PD effects. When measured concentrations are low, relative to the limits of the assay, the variability in concentrations is often elevated and the assay measurement may be a significant source of variability.

Additional variability may result from the decision about what exposure measurement to use in the PD analysis. Drug exposure measurements used for correlation with pharmacodynamic effects most commonly include the maximum (C_{max}) or minimum (C_{min}) concentration of the drug during a dosing interval, the area under the concentration-time profile of the drug (AUC), or the time that the drug concentration remains above a threshold concentration. Single-point measures (e.g., C_{max} and C_{min}), have greater inherent variability than aggregate measures (e.g., AUC).

The route of administration may also contribute to variability. Oral and intravenous (bolus or infusion) drug administration are the two most common routes for administration of chemotherapeutic drugs. Intravenous administration minimizes variability in systemic exposure compared to oral administration since it bypasses the variable processes involved in drug product disintegration, in vivo drug stability, drug dissolution, absorption, and first-pass metabolism.

In addition, pharmacokinetic variability may occur due to any of the intrinsic or extrinsic patient physiological factors, pathologic disease conditions, or even the dosing regimen of the drug product.

1. Physiologic Conditions

Patient physiological conditions can represent important intrinsic factors that contribute to IIV. Pharmacokinetic variability among elderly patients appears to be significant for some drugs. Literature reports of clinical studies demonstrate that considering biological age rather than chronological age as a covariate of PK parameters may account for a significant portion of PK heterogeneity in elderly patients [14]. Chemotherapy in elderly patients can be more toxic when compared to young patients. Hence, physicians may often make empirical decisions to give lower doses of chemotherapy drugs to this population. Where the relationship between intrinsic factors and drug exposure are known, adjusting the treatment regimen according to physiological criteria may help in targeting the most appropriate dose for safety and efficacy in a particular patient [15, 16]. In pediatric patients, variation in PK parameters are often associated with age. Methotrexate, busulfan, vancomycin (used in malignant hematological disease) are a few drugs with these documented variations [17-20]. Changes in body composition and maturation of enzyme systems may also lead to variation in drug exposure and PK parameters [21]. To understand the effect of intrinsic and extrinsic factors on the exposure to a drug, appropriate inclusion criteria should be used in clinical trial protocols so relevant patients are included the study of cancer treatments

2. Pathological Conditions

Disease condition may change how the body handles a drug. If any of the major organs is dysfunctional, its altered effectiveness may be seen on the PK or PD properties of a drug. Renal impairment may lead to drug accumulation and drug toxicity requiring adjustment of the dosing regimen or the selection of an alternate drug treatment. When the glomerular filtration rate is less than 70% of the normal value, dose adjustments may be useful for those drugs that themselves or their active metabolite are primarily excreted by the kidneys. Hepatic impairment can also alter the PK and PD properties of a drug. Such impairment may lead to accumulation of the drug, failure to convert a drug into its active or inactive metabolite, alteration in bioavailability, or changes in drug-protein binding. Many drugs bind to plasma proteins, some with greater affinity or capacity than others. The free drug, which is not bound to plasma proteins, is most able to reach the target site and therefore the cellular effects are often more closely related to free drug concentration than to the total drug concentration. Hypoproteinemia that may occur due to renal or hepatic impairment, malnutrition or other disease states may result in unpredicted chemotherapy-induced toxicity as the free drug concentration is altered by the lower amount of protein. The addition of extra compartments can change the PK of a drug (e.g., in ascites, edema, and plural effusion) as this alters distribution space and perhaps the time course of elimination of the drug from the body. Additionally, variation in pH and constitution of the gastrointestinal tract and alterations in visceral motility may drastically affect the characteristics of a drug especially when taken orally [16].

3. Drug Dose Calculations

Another source of IIV can be the algorithms and adjustment methods used to dose chemotherapy agents. The use of body surface area to calculate the dose of a drug for patients in oncology settings is a routine practice. In many cases, this may be appropriate, but in others, this may lead to increased variability and inappropriate dosing. There should be evidence-based support for the selection of dosing algorithms. In a study conducted by Tatsuya Kawaguchi et al. the authors concluded that the imatinib dose in CML is affected by age, gender, and BSA and should be reduced from 400 mg/day to 300 mg/day in older patients and patients with lower BSA values [22]. In contrast, another study conducted by Cahu et al. assessed the relationship of BSA and patient characteristics, dose adjustment, physician strategy and clinical outcomes in younger adults diagnosed with AML and treated with anthracyclines and cytarabine [23]. Patients who had high (>2.15 m^2) BSA values had their doses reduced, which was associated with poor clinical outcomes. The authors suggested these patients would benefit from the full dose calculated using their actual BSA value.

4. Drug Interactions

Chemotherapy is by nature toxic and can cause serious adverse events if not administered in correct doses. Combinations of cytotoxic drugs are often used in the treatment of leukemia. Anthracyclines and cytarabine have remained the first line of treatment for AML. Combining additional drugs with these in an attempt to improve outcomes has led to adverse drug interactions. For example, bortezomib (a CYP3A4 substrate and CYP3A4 inhibitor) when combined with cytarabine and doxorubicin (a CYP3A4 inhibitor) may have its metabolism drastically reduced and result in serious clinical outcomes [24].

PHARMACODYNAMICS

Pharmacodynamics describes what effects a drug has on the body. According to Derendorf et al. PD includes all of the "pharmacological actions, pathophysiological effects, and therapeutic responses, both beneficial and adverse, of the drug ingredient, therapeutic moiety and/or its metabolite(s) on various systems of the body from subcellular effects to clinical outcomes." [25]. PD models help in bridging the gap between drug concentrations and observed responses. Together, PK and PD models help to explain the time-course and magnitude of pharmacological effects of a drug. PD models in oncology seek to assess the effects of a drug on tumors as well as on normal cells and to assess the clinical outcome measures of both efficacy and safety. In oncology, PD response endpoints may include biomarkers, clinical outcomes, or surrogate endpoints. These responses can be continuous values (e.g., tumor size), graded categorical responses (e.g., pain ratings), or dichotomous responses (e.g., progressed or not progressed).

Pharmacodynamic Endpoints and Models

Pharmacodynamics of antineoplastic drugs were not well studied until the 1980s. Data on PD was historically limited since the studies conducted placed little emphasis on understanding the relationship between drug concentrations and clinical efficacy or safety. It was after the development of a better understanding that dose intensity was related with response rate in drug sensitive cancers and studying the relationship between the concentration and drug effect became important to researchers [26]. As interest in modeling pharmacodynamics has developed, a variety of data types and modeling endpoints have emerged as important to the understanding of drug effects in leukemia.

1. Biomarker Model

The NIH defines a biomarker as "a characteristic that is objectively measured and evaluated as an indicator of normal biologic processes, pathogenic processes or pharmacologic responses to a therapeutic intervention" [27]. Identifying a biomarker as a predictor of clinical outcomes can be an important process for the development of understanding of drug effects. Biomarkers can contribute to earlier understanding of patient response to a treatment, and thus improve predictions of disease progression and facilitate the incorporation of individualized disease and drug monitoring. In depth study of disease progression in PK/PD models is carried out by associating clinical outcomes with several candidate biomarker targets before deciding if a particular biomarker is a valid reflection of an outcome. Almufti et al. suggests using nonlinear mixed effect modeling (NLME) to "standardize biomarker kinetics analysis methodologies to ensure the optimized development of novel serum biomarkers and avoid pitfalls of traditional markers" [28]. The NLME approach has been used in cancers like small cell lung cancer, gestational neoplasia, and gastrointestinal stromal tumor [1].

2. Tumor Size Model

Tumor size is one of the most commonly used biomarkers in oncology because it serves as a measure of several PD endpoints, e.g., progression rate of the disease, time to failure of the treatment, disease free survival, and overall treatment response. There are numerous challenges and opportunities that researchers face while analyzing the predictive abilities of a tumor growth model, including analysis of the time course of the individual lesions stratified by the affected organ compared with the pooled analysis of all tumor lesions, maintaining a proper account of new lesions and generating useful information from the preclinical data for its utilization in clinical settings [1]. These authors suggest using tumor size along with the RECIST score to assess clinical outcomes. Continuous monitoring of disease progression via tumor size and the modeling of concentration-effect relationships may lead to a greater understanding of drug effects and lead to improvements in dosing regimen design.

3. Adverse Event Model

Drugs used to treat cancer not only exert their pharmacological effects on the cancer cells, but also on healthy cells and tissues of the body. Since antineoplastic drugs are often highly toxic in nature, significant adverse drug responses (ADR) are common in treated patients. Toxicities range from nausea and vomiting to hematological toxicities and organ failure caused either by the drug, its metabolite, or by drug-drug interactions. Drug doses are often delayed or reduced to mitigate adverse effects, which may lead to a reduction in efficacy. Since cancer treatment includes polypharmacy, clinicians may opt for a reduction in doses of one or more of the drugs a patient receives. This effort to control ADRs may lead to diminished drug effects or disease relapse, since optimum concentrations may not be maintained. Well-defined PK/PD strategies can substantially refine the clinical management of patients by informing evidence-based decisions regarding the dosing regimen in the attempt to balance ADRs and treatment benefits. Various adverse event models have been developed. For example the Friberg et al, adverse event model gives a description of drug-induced myelosuppression [29]. This model has been widely used to describe neutropenia, thrombocytopenia, and leukopenia toxicities [1].

4. Clinical End Point Model

Time-to-event (i.e., survival) analysis is commonly used in pharmacometrics to characterize when events such as disease progression occur and the relationship of that progression with predictors such as drug treatment or intrinsic or extrinsic patients' factors. Survival models identify a hazard function (i.e., the instantaneous event rate). Understanding the hazard with respect to time can help define the survival function (i.e., the probability of not progressing in disease and thus remaining in the study). Identification of the hazard distribution not only allows calculating a hazard ratio between two groups but also helps in simulating different scenarios and calculating hazard ratios between scenarios. Since these models may utilize both constant and time-varying covariates, these models also help to address the sources variability in overall survival across subjects. These models may be predictive of events like time of disease progression, time to an adverse event, progression free survival, and time to complete response along with overall survival [1, 30].

APPLICATION OF PHARMACOMETRICS IN LEUKEMIA

PK Dose Adaptation Strategy

Individualized dosing in chemotherapy for leukemia is of special interest because of the potential toxicities these drugs can cause, the need to have adequate exposure for beneficial effect, and the narrow therapeutic window between these levels of exposure. When exposure targets for safety and efficacy are known and measurable sources of variability of drug exposure are understood, it essential to utilize individualized dosing to attain maximum opportunity for efficacy with minimum toxicity. Designing dosing regimens without considering the sources of IIV in exposure may lead to unanticipated exposures in a patient. This may lead to under dosing which compromises the therapeutic efficacy of the drug or over dosing which can cause an increased risk of ADRs. Hence, the development and application of pharmacometric models is essential to enhance optimal individualized dosing, reduce clinical variability, reduce toxicities, and achieve maximum efficacy.

Mercaptopurine is one of the most commonly used drugs to treat childhood ALL. This drug shows a considerable amount of pharmacokinetic variability in plasma concentration and intracellular accumulation of the active metabolite. Erythrocytes have been considered a surrogate marker to analyze the accumulation of 6-thioguanine nucleotides (TGN) as a PD parameter. Strong correlation between TGN concentrations and therapeutic efficacy and toxicity have been demonstrated. An optimum level of TGN accumulation within erythrocytes has to be maintained so that neutropenia (high level of TGN accumulation) and relapse (low TGN accumulation) can be avoided. Since treatment of ALL includes a complex treatment regimen with a number of drugs, it is difficult to associate observed adverse events with a particular drug. Oncology regimens consist of drugs that can cause serious toxicities and have narrow therapeutic window, this makes dosing a drug such as mercaptopurine a challenge. Routine testing of the polymorphic enzyme thiopurine methyl transferase (TPMT), which is responsible for mercaptopurine metabolism, can be utilized to identify subjects who are TPMT-heterozygous or TMPT-deficient. Understanding the metabolic capability of the individual patient may help identify subjects that are at greater risk of toxicities or relapse. Monitoring TGN levels in erythrocytes along with WBC counts is suggested as an approach to individualized mercaptopurine dosing regimen in pediatric patients suffering from ALL [26].

Informing Product Labels

When pharmacometric approaches are applied well and with sufficient data, they can contribute to optimized product label guidance for dose selection for particular populations. This was accomplished for busulfan treatment of pediatric patients with chronic myelogenous leukemia (CML) when in 2002 a 2-step dosing regimen was added to the product label of busulfan after the FDA approved its addition to the special population section for pediatrics [31].

Busulfan is used along with cyclophosphamide prior to hematopoietic stem cell transplantation as a preparative regimen for CML. Busulfan absorption following oral administration is highly variable, and the drug has a narrow therapeutic index, which requires TDM to keep drug concentrations at an optimum level [32, 33]. An AUC lower than 900 μM·min (3.7 $\mu g \cdot h \cdot mL^{-1}$) has been associated with engraftment failure, whereas an AUC higher than 1500 μM·min (5.5 $\mu g \cdot h \cdot mL^{-1}$) has been associated with veno-occlusive disease (VOD) [34]. To achieve the optimum exposure levels following oral dosing requires dosing patients with a large number of 2 mg busulfan tablets that leads to nausea and vomiting, loss of busulfan dose(s) and contributes to pharmacokinetic variability in patients.

Booth et al. [31] conducted a trial to study the pharmacokinetics of IV busulfan in a pediatric population to establish the dosing regimen for IV busulfan. Twenty-four pediatric patients diagnosed with malignant or nonmalignant CML disease that required hematopoietic stem cell transplantation were enrolled in this particular study. VOD was clinically diagnosed in these patients. Intravenous busulfan was infused for over 2 hours at 1.0 mg/kg in patients of 4 years of age or younger, and in patients older than 4 years, 0.8 mg/kg of IV, busulfan was administered every 6 hours for 16 doses. Some patients had their dose adjusted depending on their AUCs after the first dose administration. Cyclophosphamide (50 mg/kg) was administered to the patients for 4 days following the completion of the busulfan cycle. Hematopoietic stem cells were infused after a 1-day rest period. Blood samples were collected following doses 1, 9, and 13. Dense sampling (6-8 samples) was conducted after administration of doses 1 and 9. After dose 13, sparse sample collection (2-3 samples) occurred. The pharmacokinetic properties of busulfan were described using a 1-compartment open model with intravenous infusion and first-order elimination. The addition of weight on clearance and volume of distribution as covariates significantly reduced the minimum objective function along with inter-occasion variability. CL and VD were found to be 4.04 L/h/20kg and 12.8 L/20kg, respectively. Monte Carlo simulations were carried out to determine the appropriate dosing regimen. Simulation demonstrated that mg/kg and mg/m^2 dosing algorithms were identical and 60% of the population under the study was able to attain the desired target exposure. This study suggests a dosing regimen for pediatric patients with CML where children weighing less than 12 kg receive a dose of 1.1 mg/kg and children weighing less than 12 kg receive a dose of 0.8 mg/kg. This study also recommended carrying out TDM for subjects who fall out of the therapeutic range to improve clinical outcome and efficacy by reducing the toxicity and adverse events. From this work, the therapeutic window for busulfan was changed to 900-1350 μM·min for the pediatric population.

Pharmacometric models describing PK/PD relationships in a clinically relevant manner are available for some of the key drugs used in the treatment of leukemia. However, the application of such models in a clinical setting is not a trivial accomplishment. Oncologists and clinical pharmacy specialists in oncology must appreciate the benefits of these models and be trained in the use of a software tool for the individualization of dosing regimen for their patients.

One such tool, optimized to use pharmacometric models for the individualized dosing of patients is BestDose™ [35]. This software is designed for use by clinicians, to improve dosing accuracy through Bayesian approaches. Other tools are available that require more in-depth knowledge by the user regarding the structure and methods of modeling, as well as the analytical methods and technical details of the software used. Recent introductory texts have been published to assist the orientation of the clinician to certain analytical methods that can be useful for the individualization of dosing [10, 36].

CONCLUSION

Oncology in general and leukemia in particular are therapeutic areas with significant unmet medical needs. Much research is being conducted to find ways to treat leukemia in a more effective manner, and to maximize the benefits and reduce the toxicities of drug therapy. Pharmacometrics is an important tool to accomplish these goals. Pharmacometrics combines population PK, PD, and disease progression data, with pharmacological knowledge, to build models that can be used predict the right dose for the right patient. With the ability to analyze sparse data and to combine data from different studies and experimental conditions, the application of pharmacometrics is critically important in drug development and could be used to a greater extent in the clinical setting. Maximizing the clinical use of pharmacometric approaches to optimize the treatment of patients will require increased availability of clinically focused tools, and an increased level of training for clinicians.

REFERENCES

[1] Buil-Bruna N, López-Picazo J-M, Martín-Algarra S, Trocóniz IF. Bringing Model-Based Prediction to Oncology Clinical Practice: A Review of Pharmacometrics Principles and Applications. *The Oncologist*. 2016; 21(2):220-232. doi:10.1634/theoncologist. 2015-0322.

[2] Theuretzbacher U. Pharmacokinetic and Pharmacodynamic Issues for Antimicrobial Therapy in Patients With Cancer. *Clinical Infectious Diseases*, 2012; 54 (12): 1785-1792, https://doi.org/10.1093/cid/cis210.

[3] Ogungbenro K, Aarons L. *The CRESim & Epi-CRESim Project Groups J Pharmacokinet Pharmacodyn* 2014; 41: 173. https://doi.org/10.1007/s10928-014-9355-3.

[4] Yang JJ, Landier W, Yang Liu, et al. Inherited NUDT15 variant is a genetic determinant of mercaptopurine intolerance in children with acute lymphoblastic leukemia. *Journal of Clinical Oncology*, 2015;*33*(11):1235-1242. http://ascopubs.org/doi/10.1200/JCO.2014.59.4671.

[5] Food and Drug Administration, Guidance for Industry, *Population Pharmacokinetics*. February 1999. https://www.fda.gov/downloads/drugs/guidances/UCM072137.pdf.

[6] Sheiner LB, Beal SL. Evaluation of methods for estimating population pharmacokinetic parameters. I. Michaelis-Menten model: routine clinical pharmacokinetic data. *Journal of Pharmacokinetics and Biopharmaceutics*, 1980; *8*(6), 553-571.

[7] Sheiner LB, Beal SL. Evaluation of methods for estimating population pharmacokinetic parameters II. Biexponential model and experimental pharmacokinetic data. *Journal of Pharmacokinetics and Biopharmaceutics*, 1981; *9*(5),635-651. https://doi.org/10.1007/BF01061030.

[8] Sheiner LB, Beal SL. Evaluation of methods for estimating population pharmacokinetic parameters. III. Monoexponential model: routine clinical pharmacokinetic data. *Journal of Pharmacokinetics and Biopharmaceutics*, 1983; *11*(3),303-319. https://doi.org/10.1007/BF01061870.

[9] Teng JF, Mabasa VH, Ensom MH. The role of therapeutic drug monitoring of imatinib in patients with chronic myeloid leukemia and metastatic or unresectable gastrointestinal stromal tumors. *Therapeutic drug monitoring*, 2012; *34*(1), 85-97. DOI:10.1097/FTD.0b013e31823cdec9.

[10] Owen JS, Fiedler-Kelly. J. *Introduction to population pharmacokinetic/ pharmacodynamic analysis with nonlinear mixed effects models*. 2014. Wiley.

[11] Yamazaki S, Loi CM, Kimoto E, Costales C et al. Application of Physiologically Based Pharmacokinetic Modeling in Understanding Bosutinib Drug-Drug Interactions: Importance of Intestinal P-Glycoprotein. *Drug Metabolism and Disposition* 2018, DOI:10.1124/dmd.118.080424.

[12] Zhao P, Zhang L, Grillo J. et al. Applications of physiologically based pharmacokinetic (PBPK) modeling and simulation during regulatory review. *Clinical Pharmacology & Therapeutics*, 2011; *89*(2), 259-267. DOI:10.1038/ clpt.2010.298.

[13] Zhao L, Shang EY, Sahajwalla CG. Application of pharmacokinetics–pharmacodynamics/clinical response modeling and simulation for biologics drug development. *Journal of pharmaceutical sciences*, 2012; *101*(12): 4367-4382. DOI: 10.1002/jps.23330.

[14] Monfardini S, Chabner B. Joint NCI-EORTC Consensus Meeting on Neoplasia in the Elderly. *European Journal of Cancer,* 1991; 27(5):553-554.

[15] Freyer G, Maire P, Ardiet C et al. Cytotoxic chemotherapy in elderly patients: present and future. *Bulletin du cancer*, 1995; *82*(7): 531-540.

[16] Freyer G, Ligneau B, Tranchand B, et al. Pharmacokinetic studies in cancer chemotherapy: usefulness in clinical practice. *Cancer Treatment Reviews*, 1997; *23*(3): 153-169. https://doi.org/10.1016/S0305-7372(97)90036-0.

[17] Zhao W, Zhang D, Fakhoury M, et al. Population pharmacokinetics and dosing optimization of vancomycin in children with malignant hematological disease. *Antimicrob Agents Chemother*. 2014; 58(6):3191-3199.

[18] Borsi JD, Revesz T, Schuler D. Prognostic importance of systemic clearance of methotrexate in childhood acute lymphoblastic leukemia. *Cancer Chemotherapy and Pharmacology*. 1987;*19*(3):261-264. https://doi.org/10.1007/BF00252984.

[19] Lind, MJ, Margison JM, Cerny T et al. Prolongation of ifosfamide elimination half-life in obese patients due to altered drug distribution. *Cancer Chemotherapy and Pharmacology*. 1989; *25*(2): 139-142. https://doi.org/10.1007/BF00692355.

[20] Nakamura E, Moritani T, Kanetaka A. Biological age versus physical fitness age. *Eur J Appl Physiol Occupational Physiology*, 1989; *58*(7):778-785. https://doi.org/10.1007/BF00637391.

[21] Peyrade F, Frenay M, Etienne MC, et al. Age-related difference in tamoxifen disposition. *Clinical Pharmacology & Therapeutics*, 1996;*59*(4), 401-410.

[22] Kawaguchi T, Hamada A, Hirayama C, et al. Relationship between an effective dose of imatinib, body surface area, and trough drug levels in patients with chronic myeloid leukemia. *International J of Hematology*. 2009; *89*(5): 642-648. doi: 10.1007/s12185-009-0315-4.

[23] Cahu X, Carré M, Recher C, et al. Impact of body-surface area on patients' outcome in younger adults with acute myeloid leukemia. *Eur J Haematol*. 2017; 98:443–449. https://doi.org/10.1111/ejh.12850.

[24] Calcabrini C, Turrini E, Carulli G et al. Pharmacokinetic Interactions in Combination Therapies for Acute Myeloid Leukemia. *SM Journal Human Leukemias*.

[25] Derendorf H, Lesko L, Chaikin P, et al. Pharmacokinetic/pharmacodynamic modeling in drug research and development. *Journal of Clinical Pharmacology*, 2000; *40*(12): 1399-1418.

[26] Evans, W. E. Pharmacodynamics of cancer chemotherapy: childhood ALL as a model. In *International Congress Series*, 2001; (Vol. 1220, pp. 203-222). Elsevier. https://doi.org/10.1016/S0531-5131(01)00298-9.

[27] Atkinson AJ, Colburn WA, DeGruttola et al. Biomarkers and surrogate endpoints: Preferred definitions and conceptual framework. *Clinical Pharmacol Ther*. 2001; 69:89-95. https://doi.org/10.1067/mcp.2001.113989.

[28] Almufti R, Wilbaux A, Oza A, et al. A critical review of the analytical approaches for circulating tumor biomarker kinetics during treatment, *Annals of Oncology*, 2014; 25: 41-56. https://doi.org/10.1093/annonc/mdt382.

[29] Friberg LE, Henningsson A, Maas H. et al. Model of Chemotherapy-Induced Myelosuppression With Parameter Consistency Across Drugs. *Journal of Clinical Oncology* 2002; 20(24): 4713–4721. https://doi.org/10.1200/JCO.2002.02.140.

[30] Holford N. A Time to Event Tutorial for Pharmacometricians. *CPT: Pharmacometrics & Systems Pharmacology*. 2013;2(5):e43 doi:10.1038/psp.2013.18.

[31] Booth, BP, Rahman A, Dagher R et al. Population Pharmacokinetic–Based Dosing of Intravenous Busulfan in Pediatric Patients. *The Journal of Clinical Pharmacology*, 2007; *47*(1): 101. https://doi.org/10.1177/0091270006295789.

[32] Czerwinski M, Gibbs JP, Slattery JT. Busulfan conjugation by glutathione S-transferases alpha, mu, and pi. *Drug Metabolism and Disposition*, 1996; *24*(9): 1015-1019.

[33] Gibbs JP, Murray G, Risler L et al. Age-dependent tetrahydrothiophenium ion formation in young children and adults receiving high-dose busulfan. *Cancer Research,* 1997; 57(24): 5509-5516.

[34] Slattery J, Clift R, Buckner C et al. Marrow Transplantation for Chronic Myeloid Leukemia: The Influence of Plasma Busulfan Levels on the Outcome of Transplantation. *Blood* 1997; 89(8): 3055-3060.

[35] Best Dose, *Laboratory of Applied Pharmacokinetics*. 2000-2013. Laboratory of Applied Pharmacokinetics.

[36] Lavielle M. Mixed effects models for the population approach: models, tasks, methods and tools. *Biostatistics Series*. 2014. Chapman and Hall/CRC.

In: Frontiers in Leukemia Pharmacotherapy
Editor: Lunawati L. Bennett
ISBN: 978-1-53614-960-9

Chapter 19

FUTURE CHEMOTHERAPY

Lunawati L. Bennett**, *PhD, PharmD
Union University, College of Pharmacy, Jackson, Tennessee, US

ABSTRACT

Responses to current protocols for the treatment of leukemia (acute or chronic) are quite variable. While some frontline intensive chemotherapies for acute myeloid leukemia (AML), acute lymphoid leukemia (ALL), or chronic lymphocytic leukemia (CLL) are still in protocols, newer therapies follow a paradigm for the importance of "personal medicine" instead of "the one-size-fits-all" approach. Several clinical trials are ongoing for new entities mimicking previously successful monoclonal antibodies (mAbs) directed against CD19, CD33, or others. Some newer mAbs are conjugated to toxins to increase cytotoxicity and to prevent relapse. Novel therapy includes use of cancer vaccination, gene therapy and others. In recent time, there is a trend to investigate drugs that have been used for other diseases and repurposing them to use for cancer treatment with chemotherapy regimens to achieve synergistic effect.

Keywords: CAR-T, clinical trials leukemia, cancer vaccination, cancer repurposing, monoclonal antibody, refractory leukemia, gene therapy, conjugates mAbs

ABBREVIATIONS

CD	cluster differentiation
FDA	Food and Drug Administration
ADCC	antibody-dependent cell-mediated cytotoxicity

* Corresponding Author Email: llbennett@uu.edu.

MAbs	monoclonal antibodies
ALL	acute lymphoblastic leukemia
AML	acute myeloid leukemia
CML	chronic myeloid leukemia
CLL	chronic lymphocytic leukemia
APL	acute promyelocytic leukemia
MDS	myelodysplastic syndrome
VA	valproic acid
mTOR	mammalian target of rapamycin

INTRODUCTION

Over the past 10 - 20 years, therapy for AML, ALL, and CLL has improved. The notable improvement is primarily attributed to the increase in the number and activity of therapeutic agents currently made available to treat these diseases. As Dr. Kenneth Anderson, the president of the American Society of Hematology stated, " The reason that we've had so many novel therapies approved is the incredible, heartfelt commitment of the Food and Drug Administration (FDA) to look carefully at these many novel agents that we bring forward together to show efficacy and safety. Honestly, the number of agents that have been approved for the last 10 to 15 years, but particularly in the last year, has been phenomenal" [1].

In addition, improved our understanding of the genetic and the epigenetic alteration underlying leukemia development has refined prognostic algorithms and generate better treatment options for patients [2]. Individualized approaches to treat different kinds of leukemia with combinations of chemotherapy, kinase inhibitors, cell cycle inhibitors, conjugate monoclonal antibodies (mAbs), and epigenetic-targeted therapies have been very encouraging with some treatment providing longer remission and improved overall survival.

This chapter is divided into 3 parts: drugs that are in clinical trials, novel drugs, and drugs that being repurposing. There are many drugs in clinical trials; this chapter highlights only a few drugs.

DRUGS IN CLINICAL TRIALS

Relapsed or refractory leukemia is difficult to treat. There are several clinical trials combining new drugs with conventional therapy. Since conventional therapy such as methotrexate, vincristine, cyclophosphamide usually are directed at stopping the growth of cancer by either killing the cells, stopping the cells from dividing, or stopping them from spreading; they are usually toxic to the normal cells. Adding new drugs such as dasatinib or other mAbs, which are usually, less toxic, may be treatment options that are pursued by researchers and oncologists. There are currently several multi-center clinical trials combining new drugs such as blinatumomab, dasatinib, and others with prednisone for older ALL patients to study adverse events and to investigate how well blinatumomab works with other traditional chemotherapy.

Another clinical trial is using temsirolimus (Torisel®), an mTOR inhibitor, with etoposide and cyclophosphamide in relapsed ALL and everolimus or temsirolimus in combination with Hyper-CVAD (cyclophosphamide, vincristine, adriamycin, dexamethasone). Preclinical data indicate the combination of mTOR inhibitors with chemotherapy is beneficial to reduce adverse events in refractory T lymphocyte-ALL. mTOR (mammalian target of rapamycin or mechanistic target of rapamycin) is one of the key effectors of the signaling pathway in leukemia pathophysiology; therefore, inhibiting mTOR and its complex involvement in P13K/Akt signaling provides promising treatment options. Three classes of mTOR inhibitors are in several preclinical studies such as 1) allosteric mTOR inhibitor (rapamycin and its derivative RAD001/everolimus, CCI-779/temsirolimus), 2) ATP-competitive dual P13k/mTOR inhibitors targeting P13K, mTORC1 and mTORC2, and 3) ATP-competitive mTOR kinase inhibitors (TORKIs) that target mTORC1 and mTORC2, but not P13K [3-6]. Allosteric mTOR inhibitor blocked IL7-dependent proliferation and cell cycle progression, causing apoptosis by up regulating TP53, a tumor suppressor gene, and decreasing total DNA methytransferase in T-ALL [7-8]. Co-treatment of allosteric mTOR inhibitor with doxorubicin, idarubicin, cyclophosphamide and methotrexate has also been studied in animal and cell lines [9-11]. Dual P13K/mTOR inhibitors (P1-103, NVP-BEZ235) had been shown to have more pro-apoptotic activity than rapamycin alone when combined with Calcineurin or c-Myc inhibitor in animal models [12-13]. TORK1s were developed to reduce toxicity of dual P13K/mTOR inhibitor [3-4]. Two TORKIs cause inhibition of oncogenic proteins such as MCL-1, survivin, and CDK-2 and caused up regulation of TP53 in different cell lines [14]. TORKI (TAK-228, rapalog (Sapanisertib ®), an ATP-competitive mTOR kinase inhibitor, in combination with a variety of drugs is also ongoing clinical trials. For detail information, see www.clinicaltrials.gov. Identifier NCT01614197, NCT03328104, NCT02484430.

There are a number of antibody therapeutics that is in several stages of clinical trials including ublituximab, coltuximab ravtansine, moxetumomab pasudotox, CSL36, and others [15-23]. Ublituximab (LFB-R603, TGT-1101, TGTX-1101) is a type I glycoengineered anti-CD20 mAb that binds to a specific epitope. This mAb has low fucose content that can improve FcγRIIIa binding and enhanced antibody-dependent cell-mediated cytotoxicity (ADCC) as compared to rituximab [15]. A recent phase 3 trial known as GENUINE evaluated the safety and efficacy of ublituximab alone or in combination with ibrutinib in 126 patients with relapse or refractory CLL. Based on the result, the company is filling for accelerated approval [16]. Identifier NCT02301156. Another clinical study known as UNITY-CLL evaluated the efficacy and safety of the combination of ublituximab and P13K inhibitor. Identifier NCT02612311. For detail information see www.clinicaltrials.gov.

Coltuximab ravtansine (SAR3419) is a CD19 humanized mAbs conjugated to a semi synthetic maytansinoid compound, an anti-tubulin molecule similar to vincristine, but more potent than vinca alkaloids [17].When used as a monotherapy, it slows the progression of pre B lymphocyte-ALL [17]. When used in combination with a chemotherapy regimen that mimicked the pediatric induction protocols, SAR3419 was effective in prolonging the duration of remission. See MYRALL trial (identifier NCT01440179) for more information [18-19].

Moxetumomab pasudotox-tdfk (CAT 8015) is an anti-CD 33 mAb that is currently being developed for the treatment of pediatric and adult ALL. This drug is a reformulation of BL22, which was an older trial drug with the variable region (F_v) of an anti CD22 that is fused with *Pseudomonas aeruginosa* exotoxin A [17, 20]. In a phase 1 trial for children with relapsed ALL, the drug was well tolerated but with modest benefits; therefore, it is reformulated to contain a F_v fragment with greater affinity for CD22 with an overall activity rate of 70% in children with relapsed ALL [21]. There are several clinical trials ongoing for CLL, B cell non-Hodgkin lymphoma. See identifier NCT00659425, NCT02227108, NCT02227108. Recently, FDA approves moxetumomab pasudodotox-tdfk for advanced hairy cell leukemia in 2108 under the name Lumoxiti® [22].

JNJ-56022473 (CSL 362) is an Fc-engineered mAb targeting IL-3 receptor α chain (CD123) which is highly expressed on acute leukemia cells [23]. The Fc modification increases the affinity for FcγRIIIa (CD16) enhancing ADCC against CD123+ AML blast. The safety and efficacy of this compound are being evaluated in a 2-part phase 2/3 study of decitabine plus JNJ-56022473 vs. decitabine alone in AML patients. [23] For detail information see www.clinicaltrials.gov. Identifier NCT02472145.

Studies on inhibitors of cyclin-dependent kinases (CDKs) have shown that targeting cell cycle regulators is important for treatment of many cancers and leukemia. There are many CDK inhibitors that target subunits such as CDk7, CDk1, CDk2, CDk8, and CDk4/CDK6. Palbociclib (PD0332991) is an oral small molecule inhibitor of CDK4/6 [24-25]. Because of the critical role played by CDK6 in MLL-rearranged AML, ALL, or FLT3-ITD driven AML, targeting this cyclin can affect apoptosis and possibly overcome refractory cancers [26]. Currently, there are more than 25 studies in advanced solid cancers and 5 studies in relapsed ALL, high risk MDS, refractory B-ALL combining palbociclib with dexamethasone, sorafenib, decitabine, and others. See identifier NCT02310243, NCT03472573, NCT03515200. For detail information, see www.clinicaltrials.gov.

Panobinostat, a histone deacetylase inhibitor (HDACis) removes acetyl groups from lysine residues on histone causing a decrease in chromatin and silencing epigenetic regulation [27]. The epigenetic regulation by panobinostat is primarily mediated through the inhibition of class I HDAC enzymes, leading to increased histone acetylation, relaxation of chromatin and alteration of gene expression, such as tumor suppressor genes. A phase 1/2 study known as PANOBEST trial assessed the feasibility of this drug for prolonged prophylactic use after hematopoietic stem cells transplant (HSCT) in AML and myelodysplastic syndrome (MDS). See www.clinicaltrials.gov. Identifier NCT01451268, NCT00946647, and others [27-28].

The JAK/STAT signaling pathway has been identified as a significant mechanism by which leukemic cells can bypass normal growth and proliferation restriction. JAK inhibitors such as ruxolitinib, provide important drugs for the treatment of Philadelphia chromosome (Ph)-like ALL and Cytokine receptor-like factor 2 (CRLF2)-rearranged ALL [29-30]. Trans membrane CRLF2 signals downstream JAK kinases including IL-7, JAK1 and JAK2 causing mutation and aberrant cell signaling. There are currently 167 clinical studies on JAK inhibitors, 37 of them are related to leukemia. Some drugs use combination of JAK/STAT inhibitor with ibrutinib in CLL, see identifier NTC02912754; with nilotinib in CLL NCT02973711, or in patients that are newly diagnosed with high-risk B-ALL with CRLF2 rearrangements NTC02723994. See other trials on www.clinicaltrials.gov.

NOVEL THERAPIES

Targeting metabolic requirements of the cancer cells, cancer vaccination, adaptive cellular approaches using chimeric antigen receptor T cells (CAR-T), and immune checkpoint blockade are some of the novel therapies being investigated and developed for leukemia treatment.

Aberrant regulation of the sphingolipid metabolism causes progression of cancer malignancy and chemotherapy drug resistant [31-35]. Ceramide, sphingosine, and sphingosine-1-phosphate (S1P) are bioactive sphingolipids that play important role in cell proliferation, apoptosis, autophagy, motility, angiogenesis, and inflammation [31]. Ceramide induces apoptosis, whereas S1P induces cell growth [31]. Sphingosine is catalyzed to SIP by sphingosine kinases (SPHKs). There are two subtypes of SPHK known as SPHK1 and SPHK2 located on chromosome 17 (17q25.2) and 19 (19q13.2), respectively [31]. In CML, SPHK1 and S1P cause enhanced expression of BCR/ABL1 and up regulation of anti-apoptotic MCL1, respectively. In AML, SPHK1 and S1P causes chemotherapy resistant and inhibition of apoptosis [34]. In T-ALL, SPHK1 and SPHK2 inhibit apoptosis and cause autophagy cell death, and in B-ALL, SPHK2 enhances c-MYC expression [33-35]. Highly selective and potent SPHK1 and/or SPHK2 have been used in studies or phase 1/2 clinical trials. For instance, FTY720 known as fingolimod is an analogue of sphingosine that induce cell death in AML –M2, Philadelphia (+) ALL, and BCR-ABL transform myeloid precursor cell lines, respectively. Further investigations are needed to learn the mechanisms and therapeutic efficacy for clinical development [34].

Over the past decades, immunotherapy, defined as the generation of therapeutic response by activating the immune response, has revolutionized treatment of multiple solid and hematologic cancers. The strategy of cancer vaccination is to prime new or enhance pre-existing antigen specific immune responses, which can be useful in cancer such as AML that has low endogenous immunity [36]. Although vaccination results are suboptimal in some studies, the clinical benefits are shown to prolong survival [37]. Vaccination using monocyte derived dendritic cells (DC) are useful for patients' specific immune responses by producing the strongest immune response, but it is very expensive [36-38]. DCs loaded with various antigens are the most commonly used source for DC vaccination in clinical trials [36]. Preliminary results showed that DC vaccination is safe, but it can cause delayed hypersensitivity reaction at the injection site with no serious adverse events. Immune responses were markedly increased by the combination of DC vaccination and azacitidine [39]. There are currently five clinical studies active or recruiting. Some of the vaccinations use *WT1* mRNA-loaded DCs are in phase 1/2. See NCT 01146262, NCT00965224, NCT02405338 and others.

Chimeric antigen receptor T cells (CAR-T) therapy is another novel therapeutic option for relapsed precursor B-cell ALL or AML. Tisagenlecleucel (Kymriah®) is the first CAR-T approved by the FDA and the first gene therapy approved in the US [40]. CAR-T involves modified T cells that express engineered chimeric antigen receptors (CAR) targeting CD19 positive B-cells. After patients' T cells were harvesting via leukophoresis, lymphocytes are engineered ex vivo to enforce immune response targeting leukemic cells [40]. To date, the most prominent target antigen for CAR-T cell therapy is CD19, due to its restrictive expression pattern and good safety profile [36]. There are more than 80 clinical trials in phase 1 or 2 involving use of anti-CD19 CAR-T therapy at www.clinicaltrials.gov. Despite the promising early results and expanding number of anti-CD19 CAR-T trials, this novel drug format is still not completely understood. As "living drugs," the effect of CAR-T cells depends on different conditioning chemotherapy regimens, manufacturing protocols, and co-stimulatory domains. The potential of inducing severe systemic and neurological adverse events also needs to be considered [36]. Besides CD19, other potential mAb using CDs are CD33, CD123, NKG2D-ligand, and anti-LeY CAR-T cells. Dual targeting CD33 and CD123 were superior to monotherapy approach for specific cytotoxicity and to prevent antigen escape mechanisms [41-41]. See identifier NCT01864902, NTC02203825 and others. Figure 1 depicts how CAR-T works.

Immune checkpoint blockade has revolutionized the treatment of solid cancers and Hodgkin's lymphoma, in particular PD-1 and CTL4 blockade. Programmed cell death receptor (PD-1) on activated T-cells with its ligand (PD-L1) maintains immunologic tolerance through suppression of T cell killing of cancer cells. By blocking PD-1/PD-L1, drugs such as nivolumab or pembrolizumab that have been approved by the FDA to treat lung cancer may also have benefit for leukemia by causing T cells to kill leukemic cells. The PD-1/P-L1 pathway plays an important role in immune escape in CML, CLL and MDS. PD-L1 is expressed at higher levels on leukemic blasts in high risk MDS and causes more resistant disease [43].

CTL4 is another checkpoint that is expressed on the cancer cell surface and the cytoplasm of most patients with AML, CML and CLL [44-45]. Patients with AML with the CTLA-4CT 60AA genotype have worse outcomes and high rates of relapse after induction therapy [44]. Clinical trials using checkpoint blockade are currently limited to early phase clinical trials of 1 or 1/2 [43]. Currently, there are more than 25 clinical trials using CTLA-4, or PD-1 or PD-L1 inhibitors in phase 1 or 1/2 using nivolumab, iplimumab, pembrolizumab, atezolimab, or darvalumab in combination with decitabine, lenalidomide, fludarabine and others for AML, CLL, MDS, or relapse AML [43]. For detail information, see clinical trials www.clinicsltrials.gov.

REPURPOSING DRUGS

Repurposing is a strategy in drug discovery and deployment where drugs that have been approved for treatment of an original condition, are sometimes also useful to treat other conditions [46-47]. Since the development of novel drugs takes between 13 to 15 years from bench top to bedside and the estimated cost is between 2 to 3 billion US dollars, repurposing drugs is a valuable opportunity since the toxicity profiles of the drugs is already known and the cost of the drug is reasonable [48-49]. Repurposing/repositioning is often associated with the discovery of a new mechanism of action and elucidation of a novel molecular target [50].

Repurposing can be using drugs from one cancer for another type of cancer. For example, hydroxyurea is a drug used to decrease the level of white blood cells in AML, but it does not improve survival compared to best supportive therapy [51]. Preclinical data showed hydroxyurea in combination with valproic acid (VA), anti-epileptic agent, has promising results [52].

Non-chemotherapy repurposing of drugs that have been studied or are in clinical trials include metformin, statins, VA and others. Metformin (Glucophage®) an active biguanide extracted from the French Lilac (*Galega officinalis*) has been prescribed asfirst-line treatment of type 2 diabetes [53]. In 2001, metformin appeared on the "cancer scene" when it was found that it stimulated the AMP-activated serine threonine protein kinase (AMPK), a sensor of the energetic cellular status that plays an important role in tumor suppressor pathway [54-55]. It was shown that metformin was associated with a lower risk of cancer in diabetic patients taking metformin [56]. Metformin inhibits oxidative respiration by acting on the complex I of the mitochondrial respiratory chain leading to a drop in ATP synthesis, tilting the AMP/ATP balance toward AMP, which stimulates AMPL [55, 57-58]. The AMPK pathway plays an important role in inhibition of constitutive mTOR and prevents initiation of genes that crucial for cancer proliferation such as c-myc, cyclin D1, BCl-xL [59]. Metformin shows additive effects with anthracyclines in T-ALL and ALL [60-61]. There are more than 300 registered clinical trials on metformin usage on cancer to determine the appropriate dose and its effects. Trials study a nano carrier formulation of metformin or study the effect of metformin derivatives are ongoing [55, 62-64].

Statins, HMG-CoA reductase inhibitors, which have been used for hyperlipidemia, are being explored as anti-leukemic in AML. As monotherapy, statins have not been showing convincing results, but in combination with idarubicin and cytarabine, they show promising results [49]. In experimental study, statins were shown to have immunomodulatory properties by increasing tumor infiltration affecting CD8-T cells and M2-like tumor associated macrophages. This makes statins novel therapy worth further development in combination with anti-leukemic drugs [65].

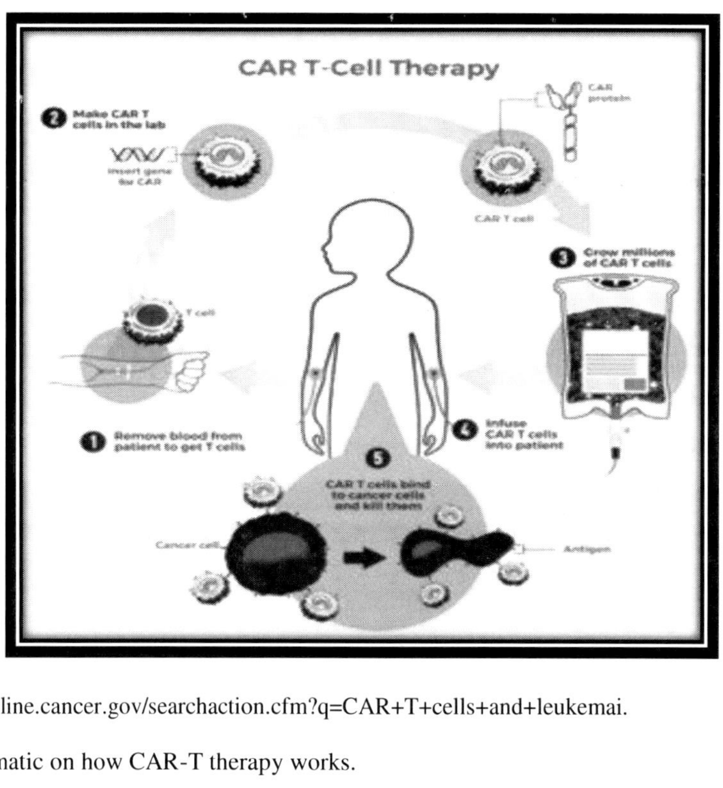

https://visualsonline.cancer.gov/searchaction.cfm?q=CAR+T+cells+and+leukemai.

Figure 1. Schematic on how CAR-T therapy works.

The benzimidazole family of anthelminthic drugs has been evaluated for anti-leukemic effects in cancer cells lines. The drugs are proposed to work by inhibiting amino peptidase activity and glutamate catabolism, reducing glucose uptake, increasing intracellular calcium, and inhibiting microtubule formation [66]. The drugs also have a synergistic effect with vincristine in animal models [67]. No clinical trial has yet been initiated using these anthelmintic agents [49].

Actinomycin D has been approved for use in rare cancers such as Wilms tumor, rhabdomyosarcome, Ewing's sarcoma, testicular and ovarian cancers [68]. This antibiotic works by interacting with DNA and blocking RNA synthesis by inhibiting RNA polymerase I, II and III even at low dose [69]. Recently, actinomycin D at a low dose was reported to treat AML with NPMI mutation; therefore, at a low dose actinomycin D could be a drug useful to investigate in AML. About one third of AML patients carry NPMI mutation [49, 70-71].

Valeric acid or valproic acid (VA) (Depakote®, Deprakine®) is derived from the valerian plant *Veleriana officinalis* that has been used for long term treatment of epilepsy and as a mood stabilizing drug for bipolar disorder [67]. VA was rediscovered to have anticancer activity as histone deacetylase (HDACs) inhibitor and can induce differentiation and apoptosis of AML cells from patients [72-73]. HDACs are often co-expressed in cancer and AML cells [74]. VA is currently involved in many different anticancer clinical trials [67]. In addition, VA often enhances or synergizes with many drugs [75]. Recently, VA was combined with standard induction therapy in elderly AML patients and increased the 5-year-relapse-free survival [49, 76].

CONCLUSION

Incidence of relapsed and refractory in leukemia is common; therefore, the development of low-toxic compounds derived from plants, or repurposing drugs that have been successful used for treatment of other diseases, may be an attractive option to investigate. Repurposing has the potential to rapidly bring old drugs for use in new diseases and could serve to identify compounds that maybe chemically modified to target the cancer cells, but with reduced toxicity. "Naked" monoclonal antibodies (mAb) with no addition of other compounds have been used successfully in leukemia treatment. Recent studies showed addition of synthetic compounds or exotoxins from bacteria has increase cytotoxicity of the mAbs. There are several clinical trials ongoing for this conjugated mAbs. Since the success of the first gene therapy, Kymriah ®, a chimeric antigen receptor T cells (CAR-T), several other CAR-T are in the development or are in clinical trials.

REFERENCES

[1] *Newly Approved Drugs for AML; how to use them in practice*. Feb 2, 2018.

[2] Watts J, Nimer S. Recent advances in the understanding and treatment of acute myeloid leukemia. *F1000 Research* 2018; 7(F1000 Faculty Rev):1196.

[3] Evangelisti C, Charini F, McCubrey JA, et al. Therapeutic targeting of mTOR in T-cell acute lymphoblastic leukemia: an update. *Int J of Mol Sci* 2018.

[4] Steelman LS, Martelli AM, Cocco L,et al. The therapeutic potential of mTOR inhibitors in breast cancer. *Br. J. Clin. Pharmacol.* 2016, 82, 1189–1212.

[5] Martelli AM, Chiarini F, Evangelisti C, et al. Two hits are better than one: Targeting both phosphatidylinositol 3-kinase and mammalian target of rapamycin as a therapeutic strategy for acute leukemia treatment. *Oncotarget* 2012, 3, 371–394.

[6] Lee JS, Vo TT, Fruman, DA. Targeting mTOR for the treatment of B cell malignancies. *Br. J. Clin. Pharmacol.* 2016, 82, 1213–1228.

[7] Batista A, Barata JT, Raderschall E, et al. Targeting of active mTOR inhibits primary leukemia T cells and synergizes with cytotoxic drugs and signaling inhibitors. *Exp. Hematol.* 2011, 39, 457.e3–472.e3.

[8] Zhang YP, Huang YT, Huang TS, et al. The mammalian target of rapamycin and DNA methyltransferase 1 axis mediates vascular endothelial dysfunction in response to disturbed flow. *Sci. Rep.* 2017, 7, 14996.

[9] Teachey DT, Sheen C, Hall J, et al. mTOR inhibitors are synergistic with methotrexate: An effective combination to treat acute lymphoblastic leukemia. *Blood* 2008, 112, 2020–2023.

[10] Wu KN, Zhao YM, He Y, et al. Rapamycin interacts synergistically with idarubicin to induce T-leukemia cell apoptosis in vitro and in a mesenchymal stem cell simulated drug-resistant microenvironment via Akt/mammalian target of rapamycin and extracellular signal-related kinase signaling pathways. *Leuk. Lymphoma* 2014, 55, 668–676.

[11] Zhang Y, Hua C, Cheng H, et al. Distinct sensitivity of CD8+ CD4− and CD8+ CD4+ leukemic cell subpopulations to cyclophosphamide and rapamycin in Notch1-induced T-ALL mouse model. *Leuk. Res.* 2013, 37, 1592–1601.

[12] Tosello V, Saccomani V, Yu J, et al. Calcineurin complex isolated from T-cell acute lymphoblastic leukemia (T-ALL) cells identifies new signaling pathways including mTOR/AKT/S6K whose inhibition synergize with calcineurin inhibition to promote T-ALL cell death. *Oncotarget* 2016, 7, 45715–45729.

[13] Chiarini F, Grimaldi C, Ricci F, et al. Activity of the novel dual phosphatidylinositol 3-kinase/mammalian target of rapamycin inhibitor NVP-BEZ235 against T-cell acute lymphoblastic leukemia. *Cancer Res.* 2010, 70, 8097–8107.

[14] Yun S, Vincelette ND, Knorr KL, et al. 4EBP1/c-MYC/PUMA and NF-κB/EGR1/BIM pathways underlie cytotoxicity of mTOR dual inhibitors in malignant lymphoid cells. *Blood* 2016, 127, 2711–2722.

[15] Sharman JP, Farber CM, Mahadevan D, et al. Ublituximab (TG-1101), a novel glycoengineered anti-CD20 antibody, in combination with ibrutinib is safe and highly active in patients with relapsed and/or refractory chronic lymphocytic leukaemia: results of a phase 2 trial. *Br J Haematol* 2017; 176:412–20.10.1111/bjh.14447.

[16] Kaplon H, Reichert JM. Antibodies to watch in 2018. *MAbs* 2018;10(2): 183-203.

[17] Terwilliger T, Abdul-Hay M. Acute lymphoblastic leukemia: a comprehensive review and 2017 update. *Blood Cancer J* 2017;7, e577.

[18] Jabbour EJ, Faderl S, Kantarjian HM. Adult acute lymphoblastic leukemia. *Mayo Clin Proc* 2005; 80: 1517-1527.

[19] Treneny M, Verhoef G, Dyer M, et al. A phase II multicenter study of the anti-CD19 antibody drug conjugate coltuximab ravtansine (SAR3419 in patients with relapsed of refractory diffuse B-cell lymphoma previously treated with rituximab-based immunotherapy. *Haematologica* 2018; 103 (18):1351-1358.

[20] Kreitman RJ, Pastan I. Antibody fusion proteins: anti CD22 recombinant Immunotoxin Moxetumomab Pasudotox. *Clin Cancer Res* 2011;17:6398-6405.

[21] Wayne AS, Bhojwani D, Silverman LB, et al. A novel anti CD22 immunotoxin, Moxetumomab Pasudotox: phase 1 study in pediatric ALL. *Blood* 2011;118:248.

[22] https://www.businesswire.com./FDA-Approves-LUMOXITI.

[23] Reichert JM. Antibodies to watch in 2017. *Mab* 2017;9(2):167-181. doi: 10.1080/19420862.2016.1269580.

[24] Fry DW, Harvey PJ, Keller PR, et al. inhibition of cyclin-dependent kinase 4/6 by PD03332991 and associated antitumor activity in human tumor xenografts. *Mol Cancer Ther* 2004;3:1427-1438.

[25] Aleem E, Arceci RJ. Targeting cell cycle regulators in hematologic malignancies. *Front. Cell Dev Biol* 2015; 3;16. Doi:10.3389/fcell.2015.00016.

[26] Bose P, Simmons GL, Grant S. Cyclin-dependent kinase inhibitor therapy for hematologic malignancies. *Expert Opin. Investig. Drugs*.2013;22:723-738.

[27] Bug G, Burchert A, Wagner EM, et al. Phase I/II study of the deacetylase inhibitor panobinostat after allogenic stem cell transplantation in patients with high risk of MDS or AML (PANOBEST trial). *Leukemia* 2017; 31(11):2523-2525.

[28] Garcia-Manero G, Sekeres MA, Egyed M, et al. A phase 1b/2b multicenter study of oral panobinostat plus azacitidine in adults with MDS, CMML or AML with less than 30% blasts. *Leukemia* 2017; 31(12):2799-2806.

[29] Jain P, Keating M, Renner S, et al. Ruxolitinib for symptoms control in patient with CLL: a single phase 2 trial. *Lancet Hematol* 2017; 4(2):PE67-PE74.

[30] Konoplev S, Lu X, Konopleva M, et al. CRLF-2 Positive B cell ALL institution experience. *Am J Clin Pathol* 2017;147(4): 357-363.

[31] Evangelisti C, Buontempo F, Lonetti A, et al. Therapeutic potential of targeting sphingosine kinases and sphingosine 1-phosphate in hematological malignancies. *Leukemia* 2016;30:2142-2151.

[32] Cuvillier O, Levada T. Sphingosine 1-phosphate antagonizes apoptosis of human leukemia cells by inhibiting release of cytochrome c and Smac/DIABLO from mitochondria. *Blood* 2001;98:2828-2836.

[33] Wallington-Beddoe CT, Powell JA, Tong D, et al. Sphingosine kinase 2 promotes acute lymphoblastic leukemia by enhancing MYC expression. *Cancer Res* 2014;74:2803-2815.

[34] Evangelisti C, Teti G, Chiarini F, et al. Assessment of the effect of sphingosine kinase inhibitors on apoptosis, unfolded protein response and autophagy of T-cell acute lymphoblastic leukemic cells indications for novel therapeutics. *Oncotarget* 2014;5:7886-7901.

[35] Kitatani K, Taniguchi M, Okazaki T. Role of sphingolipids and metabolizing enzymes in hematological malignancies. *Mol Cells* 2015; 38(6):482-495.

[36] Lichtenegger FS, Krupka C, Haubner S, et al. Recent developments in immunotherapy of AML. *J of Hematology & Oncol* 2017;10:143.

[37] Yang Y. Cancer immunotherapy: harnessing the immune system to battle cancer. *J Clin Invest* 2015;125(90: 3335-3337.

[38] Sabado RL, Balan S, Bhardwaj N. Dendritic cell-based immunotherapy. *Cell Res* 2017;27:74-95.

[39] Lichtenegger FS, Deiser K, Rothe M, et al. Induction of antigen-specific T cell responses through dendritic cell vaccination in AML: resultds of a phase I/II trial and ex vivo enhancement by checkpoint blockade. *Blood* 2016; 128(22):764.

[40] Maude SL. Future directions in chimeric antigen receot T cell therapy. *Curr Opin Pediatr* 2017; 29 (1):27-33.

[41] Zah E. Lin MY, Silva-Benedict A, et al. T cells expressing CD19/CD20 bispecific chimeric antigen receptors prevent antigen escape by malignant B cells. *Cancer Immunol Res* 2016; 4:498-508.

[42] Arndt C, Feldmann A, Koristka S, et al. Improved killing of AML blasts by dual-targeting CD123 and CD33 via UniTARG a novel antibody-based modular T cell retargeting system. *Blood* 2015;126:2565.

[43] Pianko MJ, Liu Y, Bagchi S, Lesokhin AM. Immune checkpoint blockade for hematologic malignancies: a review. *Stem Cell Investig* 2017; 4: 32 doi:10,21037/sci.2017.03.04.

[44] Perez-Garcia A, Brunet S, Berlangga JJ, et al. CTLA-4 genotype and relapse incidence in patients with acute myeloid leukemia in first complete remission after induction chemotherapy. *Leukemia* 2009;23:486-491.

[45] Ciszak L, Frydecka I, Wolowiec D, et al. CTLA-4 affects expression of key cell cycle regulators of G0/G1 phase in neoplastic lymphocytes from patients with chronic lymphocytic leukemia. *Clin Exp Med* 2016;16:317-332.

[46] Sukhai MA, Spagnuolo PA, Weir S, et al. New sources of drugs for hematologic malignancies. *Blood* 2011;117:6747-6755.

[47] Gupta SC, Sung B, Prasad S, et al. Cancer drug discovery by repurposing: teaching new tricks to old dogs. *Trends Pharmacol Sci* 2013;34:508-517.

[48] Nosenga N. Can you teach old drugs new tricks? *Nature* 2016;534-314-316.

[49] Andresen V, Gjertsen BT. Drug repurposing for the treatment of acute myeloid leukemia. *Front Med* 2017;4:211.

[50] Gurova K. New hopes from old drugs: revisiting DNA-binding small molecules as anticancer agents. *Future Oncol* 2009;5 (10):1685-1704.

[51] Burnett AK, Milligan D, Prentice AG, et al. A comparison of low dose cytarabine and hydroxyurea with ot without all trans retinoic acid for acute myeloid leukemia and high risk myelodysplastic syndrome in patients not considered fit for intensive treatmenr. *Cancer* 2007;109:1114-1124.

[52] Leitch C, Osdal T, Andresen V, et al. Hydroxyurea synergizes with valproic acid in wild-type acute myeloid leukemia. *Oncotarget* 2016;7:8105-8118.

[53] Bailey CJ, Turner RC. Metformin. *N Engl J Med* 1996;334:574-579.

[54] zhou G, Myers R, Li Y, et al. Role of AMP-activated protein kinase in mechanism of metformin action *J Clin Invest* 2001;108:1167-1174.

[55] Biondani G, Peyron JF. Metformin, an anti-diabetic drug to target leukemia. *Front. Endocrinol* 2018; 9: 446. Doi: 10.3389/fendo.2018.00446.

[56] Zhang P, Li H, Tan X, et al. Association of metformin use with cancer incidence and mortality: a meta-analysis. *Cancer Epidemiol* 2013;37:207-218.

[57] Owen MR, Doran E, Halestrap AP. Evidence that metformin exerts its anti-diabetic effects through inhibition of complex of the mitochondrial respiratory chain. *Biochem J* 2000; 275:223-228.

[58] El-Mir MY, Noguiera V, Fontaine E, et al. Dimethylbiguanide inhibits cell respiration via an indirect effect targeted on the respiratory chain complex I. *J Biol Chem* 2000;275:223-228.

[59] Green AS, Chapuis N, Maciel TT, et al. The LKB1/AMPK signaling pathway has tumor suppressor activity in acute myeloid leukemia through the repression of mTOR-dependent oncogenic mRNA translation. *Blood* 2010; 116:4262-4273.

[60] Shi WY, Xiao D, Wang L, et al. Therapeutic metformin/AMPK activation blocked lymphoma cell growth via inhibition of mTOR pathway and induction of autophagy. *Cell Death Dis* 2012; 3:e275.

[61] Pan J, Chen C, Jin Y, et al. Differential impact of structurally different anti-diabetic drugs on proliferation and chemosensitivity of acute lymphoblastic leukemia cells. *Cell Cyle* 2012;11:2314-2316.

[62] Higurashi T, Hosono K, takahashi H, et al. Metformin for chemoprevention of metachronous colorectal adenoma or polyps in post-polypectomy patients without diabetes; a multicenter double blind, placebo-controlled, tandomized phase trial. *Lancet Oncol* 2016;17:475-483.

[63] Caraci F, Chisari M, Frasce G, et al. Effects of phenformin on the proliferation of human tumor cell lines. *Life Sci* 2003;74:643-650.

[64] Hundal RS, Inzucchi SE. Metformin: new understanding, new uses. *Drugs* 2003;63:1879-1894.

[65] Mira E, Carmona-Rodríguez L, Tardáguila M, et al. A lovastatin-elicited genetic program inhibits M2 macrophage polarization and enhances T cell infiltration into spontaneous mouse mammary tumors. *Oncotarget* 2013; 4:2288–301.

[66] Spagnuolo PA, Hu J, Hurren R, et al. The antihelmintic flubendazole inhibits microtubule function through a mechanism distinct from Vinca alkaloids and displays preclinical activity in leukemia and myeloma. *Blood* 2010: 115:4824–33.10.1182/blood-2009-09-24305.

[67] Chateauvieux S, Morceau F, Dicato M, Diederich M. Molecular and therapeutic potential and toxicity of valproic acid. *J Biomed Biotechnol* 2010; 2010:479364. 10.1155/2010/479364.

[68] Gaspar N, Hawkins DS, Dirksen U, et al. Ewing sarcoma: current management and future approaches through collaboration. *J Clin Oncol* 2015; 33:3036. 46.10.1200/JCO.2014.59.5256.

[69] Perry RP, Kelley DE. Inhibition of RNA synthesis by actinomycin D: characteristic dose-response of different RNA species. *J Cell Physiol* 1970; 76:127–39.10.1002/jcp.104076020.

[70] Falini B, Brunetti L, Martelli MP. Dactinomycin in NPM1-mutated acute myeloid leukemia. *N Engl J Med* 2015; 373:1180–2.10.1056/NEJMc1509584.

[71] Falini B, Mecucci C, Tiacci E, et al.Cytoplasmic nucleophosmin in acute myelogenous leukemia with a normal karyotype. *N Engl J Med* 2005; 352:254–66.10.1056/NEJMoa041974.

[72] Göttlicher M, Minucci S, Zhu P, et al.Valproic acid defines a novel class of HDAC inhibitors inducing differentiation of transformed cells. *EMBO J* 2001; 20:6969–78.10.1093/emboj/20.24.6969.

[73] Phiel CJ, Zhang F, Huang EY, et al. Histone deacetylase is a direct target of valproic acid, a potent anticonvulsant, mood stabilizer, and teratogen. *J Biol Chem*; 2001: 276:36734–41.10.1074/jbc.M101287200.

[74] Tickenbrock L, Klein HU, Trento C, et al. Increased HDAC1 deposition at hematopoietic promoters in AML and its association with patient survival. *Leuk Res* 2011; 35:620–5.10.1016/j.leukres.2010.11.006.

[75] Stiborova M, Eckschlager T, Poljakova J, et al. The synergistic effects of DNA-targeted chemotherapeutics and histone deacetylase inhibitors as therapeutic

strategies for cancer treatment. *Curr Med Chem* 2012; 19:4218–38.10.2174 /0929867128028842 86.

[76] Tassara M, Dohner K, Brossart P, et al. Valproic acid in combination with all-trans retinoic acid and intensive therapy for acute myeloid leukemia in older patients. *Blood* 2014; 123:4027–36.10.1182/blood-2013-12-546283.

About the Editor

Dr. Lunawati Bennett is a Professor of Pharmaceutical Sciences at Union University College of Pharmacy in Jackson, Tennessee. She has a Ph.D. in Pharmaceutical Sciences and a Pharm.D. degrees in pharmacy. She has taught in pharmacy schools as a pharmacologist for over 10 years teaching drugs used in treating disorders of the endocrine, gastrointestinal, respiratory, cardiovascular, central nervous systems, and drugs for the treatment of blood disorders, pain, cancer, and infectious diseases. She loves teaching her Pharm.D. students to help them becoming competent and caring pharmacists.

She was inducted as a member of Rho Chi Honour Pharmacy Society, and is a practicing licence pharmacist in Tennessee and California. She has published several scientific papers in reputable peer review journals. Her publications includes: role of antioxidants in cardiovascular diseases, diabetes and cancer; drugs for the treatment of Gaucher disease; prostate cancer; certain type of hypercholesterolemia; and naturally occurring polyphenols against metastatic cancer. She has written book chapters on the role of vitamin E and ocular drug delivery. Her recent book published is "*Consumers' Guide to prescription and Over the Counter Medications*". Her research interest includes understanding the role of antioxidants and the use of combinational antioxidants and antineoplastic in cancer treatment.

ABOUT THE CONTRIBUTORS

Ifeoluwa Babatunda PhamD

PhD student Case Western University, Cleveland, Ohio

Emily Brandl PharmD, BCGP

Assistant Professor of Pharmacy Practice, Union University, College of Pharmacy, Jackson, Tennessee

Andrew Castleman PharmD, MS

Assistant Professor of Pharmaceutical sciences, Union University, College of Pharmacy, Jackson, Tennessee

Mitali Gaurav PharmD

Postdoctoral Fellow, Union University, College of Pharmacy, Jackson, Tennessee

Zachery R. Halford, PharmD, BCOP, BCPPS

Associate Professor of Pharmacy Practice, Union University, College of Pharmacy, Jackson, Tennessee

Danya Horchi

Pharmacy Student, Union University, College of Pharmacy, Jackson, Tennessee

Michele Lese PharmD, BCPS

Former Assistant Professor, School of Pharmacy, Palm Beach Atlantic University, West Palm Beach, Florida

Heath McLean

Pharmacy student, Union University, College of Pharmacy, Jackson, Tennessee

Joel S Owen PhD

Vice President Strategic Modeling and Simulation Cognigen Corporation, Buffalo, New York

Adjunct Professor of Pharmaceutical Sciences, Union University, College of Pharmacy, Tennessee

Qingyu S Zhou PhD

Assistant Professor of Pharmaceutical Sciences, University of South Florida, College of Pharmacy, Tampa, Florida

Elizabeth Sykes

Pharmacy student, Union University, College of Pharmacy, Jackson, Tennessee

INDEX

#

A

B

C

D

E

F

G

H

J

K

L

M

N

O

P

Q

R

S

T

U

V

W

X

Y

Z

ζ

Chronic Lymphocytic Leukemia: Diagnosis, Treatment Options and Prognosis

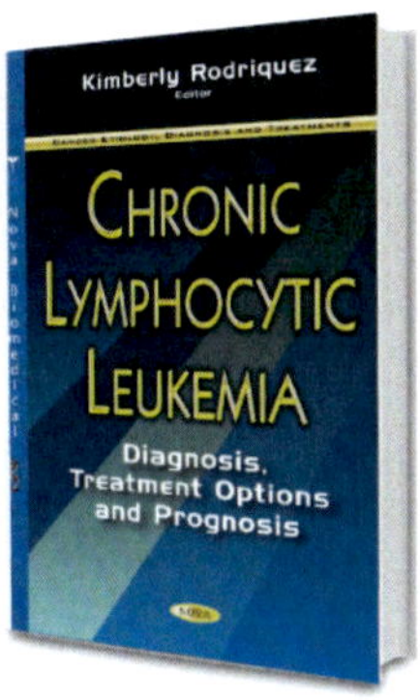

Editor: Kimberly Rodriquez

Series: Cancer Etiology, Diagnosis and Treatments

Book Description: Chronic Lymphocytic Leukemia (CLL) is the most common leukemia in the western world, seen mostly in the elderly age-group and has a very variable clinical outcome. This book reviews the diagnosis, treatment options and prognosis of CLL.

Hardcover ISBN: 978-1-63485-510-5
Retail Price: $160

Acute Myeloid Leukemia: Signs/Symptoms, Classification and Treatment Options

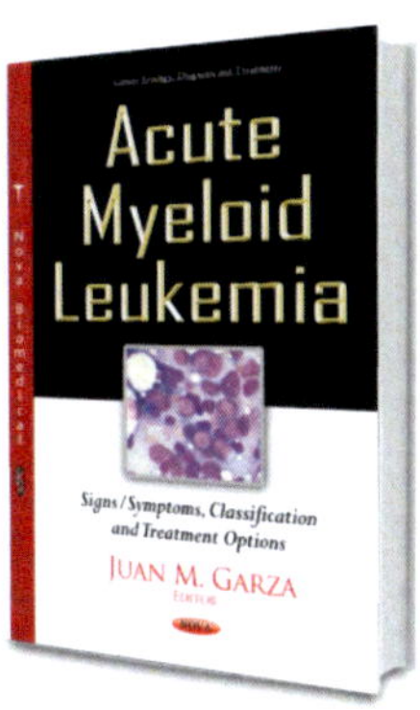

Editor: Juan M. Garza

Series: Cancer Etiology, Diagnosis and Treatments

Book Description: In this book, the clinical presentation of acute myeloid leukemia are presented.

Hardcover ISBN: 978-1-63483-878-8
Retail Price: $130

Chronic Lymphocytic Leukemia: New Research

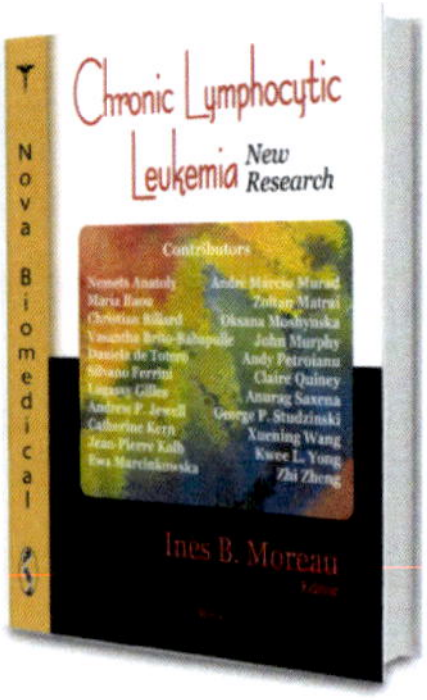

Editors: Inès B. Moreau

Series: Cancer Etiology, Diagnosis and Treatments

Book Description: This new book presents recent and important research on Chronic lymphocytic leukemia (or "chronic lymphoid leukemia"), known for short as CLL, which is a type of leukemia in which too many lymphocytes are produced.

Hardcover ISBN: 978-1-60456-081-7
Retail Price: $170

Experimental Leukemia: History, Biology and Genetics

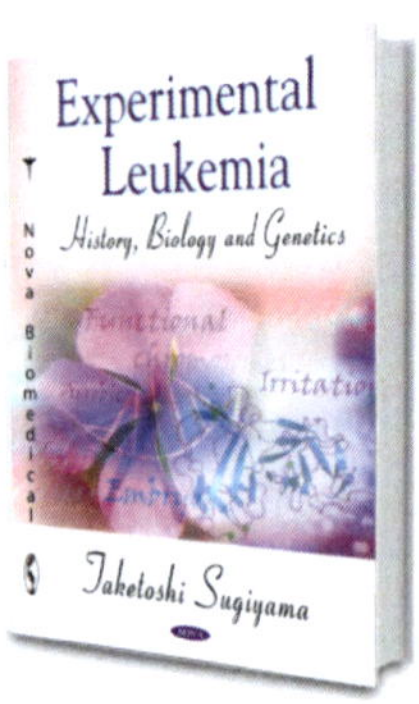

Author: Taketoshi Sugiyama (Kobe University, Kobe, Japan)

Book Description: In this book, the author has arranged the chapters to contrast the pioneer works by Peyton Rous, Jacob Furth, and Ludwik Gross, etc, done more than half a century ago and the recent works by molecular biologists.

Hardcover ISBN: 978-1-60021-497-4
Retail Price: $162